Kinematic MRI of the Joints

Functional Anatomy, Kinesiology, and Clinical Applications

Kinematic MRI of the Joints

Functional Anatomy, Kinesiology, and Clinical Applications

Edited by
Frank G. Shellock, Ph.D.
Christopher M. Powers, Ph.D.

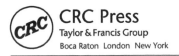

CRC Press
Taylor & Francis Group
Boca Raton London New York

CRC Press is an imprint of the
Taylor & Francis Group, an **informa** business

CRC Press
Taylor & Francis Group
6000 Broken Sound Parkway NW, Suite 300
Boca Raton, FL 33487-2742

First issued in paperback 2019

© 2010 by Taylor & Francis Group, LLC
CRC Press is an imprint of Taylor & Francis Group, an Informa business

No claim to original U.S. Government works

ISBN-13: 978-0-8493-0807-9 (hbk)
ISBN-13: 978-0-367-39746-3 (pbk)

This book contains information obtained from authentic and highly regarded sources. While all reasonable efforts have been made to publish reliable data and information, neither the author[s] nor the publisher can accept any legal responsibility or liability for any errors or omissions that may be made. The publishers wish to make clear that any views or opinions expressed in this book by individual editors, authors or contributors are personal to them and do not necessarily reflect the views/opinions of the publishers. The information or guidance contained in this book is intended for use by medical, scientific or health-care professionals and is provided strictly as a supplement to the medical or other professional's own judgement, their knowledge of the patient's medical history, relevant manufacturer's instructions and the appropriate best practice guidelines. Because of the rapid advances in medical science, any information or advice on dosages, procedures or diagnoses should be independently verified. The reader is strongly urged to consult the relevant national drug formulary and the drug companies' and device or material manufacturers' printed instructions, and their websites, before administering or utilizing any of the drugs, devices or materials mentioned in this book. This book does not indicate whether a particular treatment is appropriate or suitable for a particular individual. Ultimately it is the sole responsibility of the medical professional to make his or her own professional judgements, so as to advise and treat patients appropriately. The authors and publishers have also attempted to trace the copyright holders of all material reproduced in this publication and apologize to copyright holders if permission to publish in this form has not been obtained. If any copyright material has not been acknowledged please write and let us know so we may rectify in any future reprint.

Except as permitted under U.S. Copyright Law, no part of this book may be reprinted, reproduced, transmitted, or utilized in any form by any electronic, mechanical, or other means, now known or hereafter invented, including photocopying, microfilming, and recording, or in any information storage or retrieval system, without written permission from the publishers.

For permission to photocopy or use material electronically from this work, please access www.copyright.com (http://www.copyright.com/) or contact the Copyright Clearance Center, Inc. (CCC), 222 Rosewood Drive, Danvers, MA 01923, 978-750-8400. CCC is a not-for-profit organization that provides licenses and registration for a variety of users. For organizations that have been granted a photocopy license by the CCC, a separate system of payment has been arranged.

Trademark Notice: Product or corporate names may be trademarks or registered trademarks, and are used only for identification and explanation without intent to infringe.

A CIP record for this book is available from the British Library.

Library of Congress Cataloging-in-Publication Data available on application

**Visit the Taylor & Francis Web site at
http://www.taylorandfrancis.com**

**and the CRC Press Web site at
http://www.crcpress.com**

Foreword

An impressive array of new imaging technologies revolutionized diagnostic medicine in the twentieth century. These advances culminated in the harnessing of proton magnetic resonance, and the breakneck speed of discovery and implementation is continuing into the twenty-first century.

This book is the first to comprehensively cover one of the most important of these rapidly advancing disciplines – functional imaging. The last century is known for developing static diagnostic imaging, but in neurologic and orthopedic medicine, functional impairments are the hallmark of disease. With static imaging we often use educated guesses to predict functional impairments, much like the physical examination allowed physicians to guess internal pathology. However, noninvasive visualization of internal pathology has largely replaced the physical examination in diagnosing and staging internal disease. Similarly, kinematic and dynamic imaging now give physicians tools to directly evaluate functional abnormalities.

Drs. Shellock and Powers have brought together an international team of experts to review the mechanics of the most commonly impaired joints. With each joint, they stress the clinical importance of biomechanics in determining the mechanism of injury, the nature and extent of pathology, and proper treatment. An accompanying chapter describes, in detail, magnetic resonance techniques and protocol used to image each joint, including kinematic and dynamic imaging, with and without stress. To my knowledge no other text contains this information under one cover.

The authors have performed a great service by compiling this information. Especially for radiologists, whose training does not traditionally include biomechanics, but also for physical therapists, orthopedic surgeons, osteopaths, sports medicine chiropractors, and sports-oriented physicians of all specialties, this book provides a rapid, thorough course in functional anatomy and pathology of joints. This book is valuable even for radiologists who do not commonly use motion-imaging sequences. Virtually all abnormalities seen with static imaging are caused by abnormal motion, and interpreters untrained in normal and abnormal joint motion may miss many of them. For example, shoulder impingement is caused by abnormal biomechanics, but with proper understanding the diagnosis can often be made on static images. This book is the first to describe joint mechanics in a clinically relevant way and correlate it with kinematic and dynamic magnetic resonance imaging (MRI).

I am certain the twenty-first century will witness great advancement in functional imaging. Two major impediments have hampered joint-motion imaging: the lack of understanding of the biomechanics of normal and abnormal joints and the complexity of magnetic resonance techniques in imaging motion. This book is one source that clearly explains both. With increasing sophistication of joint surgery and the availability of this book to empower dynamic MRI, it is likely that joint-motion imaging will become an increasingly important tool in pre- and post-surgical evaluation of a growing number of patients. This book is invaluable for all radiologists who interpret joint MRI and all clinicians using MRI for assessing their patients.

John V. Crues, III, M.D., F.A.C.R.
Medical Director
Radnet Management, Inc.
Los Angeles, California

Foreword

Kinematic magnetic resonance imaging (KMRI) is a new diagnostic science with great potential. The recently developed ability to rapidly record a sequence of images enables the investigator to document structural displacements and distortions of the soft tissues and articular surfaces as the joint moves. In the past, clinicians have attempted to glean such information by manually palpating the moving tissues or mentally imagining the reactions of the ligaments, tendons, capsule, and muscles based on their knowledge of static anatomy. But both the anatomy and the functional breadth of many joints are too complex for these subjective approaches to resolve the persistent diagnostic dilemmas.

Each of the seven joints reviewed in this volume has unique anatomical complexity. The patellofemoral joint is a gliding contact track between the anterior musculo-retinacular sheath and the anterior articular surface of the knee. Localization of dysfunction in the cervical and lumbar spines is complicated by the fact that there are three joints at each intervertebral level: right and left facet joints and the interbody disc system. Structural differences between the upper and lower portion of the cervical spine add further diagnostic complexity. Ankle joint pathology is obscured by the biplane obliquity of its axis. In addition, interposition of the subtalar joint between the ankle joint and heel denies the examiner a direct grasp of the underside of the ankle joint. Further diagnostic complexity is created by the proximity of long tendons crossing the ankle area as they extend from the shank to the foot. Functional stability of the patella is challenged by the interactions of the fibrous tissue restraints, muscle balance, structural shape of the articular surfaces, and the knee's motion pattern. The diagnostic complexity of the shoulder (glenohumeral) joint lies in its extensive three-dimensional mobility (greatest in the body) and the multiple overlying tissue layers. With every motion the integrity of the near-vertical glenoid labile socket margins is threatened by exposure of the shear forces whenever muscular control is inadequate. Localization of the pathology is obscured by the significant displacement of the soft tissue layers (capsule, rotator cuff, and the deltoid) as the humerus rotates on its scapular base. The temporomandibular joint gains much of its expanded range from the mobility allowed by the fibrous disc which divides the joint into two functional articulations. Distortions of the interactive fibrous tissue structures containing the mandibular condyle are the basis of much of the functional pathology but difficult to identify. The wrist, with two rows of carpal bones as well as intercarpal mobility within the rows, is another area where multiplicity of joints obscures localization of the pathology.

The eleven chapters on KMRI included in this volume identify the current capability of this procedure to differentiate the multiple potential structural causes of dysfunction at the individual joints. With localization of the pathology clinicians can determine an appropriate therapeutic course.

To interpret the KMRI images, however, the analyst must have a comprehensive knowledge of normal static anatomy as a basis from which to identify the changes. As few clinicians are deeply versed in anatomical details, it is customary to seek a reference text in the nearest library. This diversion will not be needed as physical therapists with a strong biokinesiological background have provided an accompanying chapter for each KMRI topic which summarizes the critical reference material on static anatomy. Each chapter also is generously illustrated with very clear line drawings of the key material. This book will impart valuable information to orthopedic surgeons, rehabilitation specialists, and other physicians who are challenged to resolve the diagnostic dilemmas of the musculoskeletal system. Physical therapists and athletic trainers also will find this book a valuable guide for planning their therapeutic programs related to dysfunctional motion.

Jacquelin Perry, M.D., D.Sc. (Hon.)
Medical Consultant
Pathokinesiology Laboratory
Rancho Los Amigas Medical Center
and
Professor Emeritus
University of Southern California
Los Angeles, California

Editors

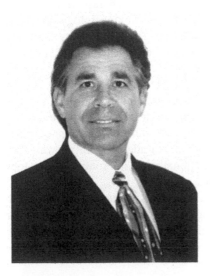

Frank G. Shellock, Ph.D. is a physiologist with more than 15 years of experience conducting laboratory and clinical investigations in the field of magnetic resonance imaging (MRI). He is an Adjunct Clinical Professor of Radiology at the University of Southern California School of Medicine, the President of Shellock R & D Services, and a Special Employee for the Food and Drug Administration. His primary research interests include investigations to develop kinematic MRI techniques for assessment of joint pathology, to identify and implement new clinical MRI applications, to evaluate electromagnetic field-related bio-effects, and to develop instruments and devices used for patient management and interventional MRI procedures.

Dr. Shellock is a member of the Committee for Standards and Accreditation of the Commission on Neuroradiology and MR for the American College of Radiology, the Safety Committee and the Educational Committee for the International Society for Magnetic Resonance Imaging, a former member of the Board of Directors of the Society for Magnetic Resonance Imaging, and a member of the Sub-Committee on MR Safety and Compatibility for the American Society for Testing and Materials. His memberships in professional societies include the American College of Radiology, the International Society for Magnetic Resonance in Medicine, and the Radiological Society of North America. He is a Fellow of the American College of Sports Medicine. Dr. Shellock is the recipient of a National Research Service Award from the National Institutes of Health, National Heart, Lung, and Blood Institute and has received numerous research grants from governmental agencies and private organizations. He is a frequently invited lecturer and visiting professor both in the United States and internationally.

Dr. Shellock has published five textbooks, over 50 book chapters, more than 150 peer-reviewed articles, and 180 scientific abstracts. He has served as a reviewing editor for 14 different medical and scientific journals. As a commitment to the field of MRI safety, Dr. Shellock developed and maintains the popular web site, *www.MRIsafety.com.*

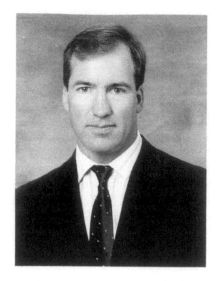

Christopher M. Powers, Ph.D., P.T. is an Assistant Professor in the Department of Biokinesiology and Physical Therapy and Director of the Musculoskeletal Biomechanics Research Laboratory at the University of Southern California. He received a Bachelor's degree in Physical Education from the University of California, Santa Barbara; his Master's degree in Physical Therapy from Columbia University; and a Ph.D. in Biokinesiology from the University of Southern California. Dr. Powers currently teaches courses in biomechanics and the mechanics of human gait. He has been active in kinematic MRI research for the past 8 years, and he has focused on studying the pathomechanics of various orthopedic disorders. He has published over 25 articles and 50 abstracts in the field of orthopedic biomechanics, particularly in the area of patellofemoral joint dysfunction. In addition, Dr. Powers frequently lectures both nationally and internationally on topics related to kinematic MRI, kinesiology, and biomechanics.

Dr. Powers is an active member of the American Physical Therapy Association, the American College of Sports Medicine, the American Society for Testing and Materials, and the Society for Gait and Clinical Movement Analysis. He serves on the editorial board of the *Journal of Orthopaedic and Sports Physical Therapy* and as a reviewer for a number of other scholarly journals.

Acknowledgments

While the authors and editors get all the credit, many other people were responsible for this book. We would like to especially acknowledge our mentors, including the many radiologists, orthopedic surgeons, physiatrists, and other experts — John V. Crues, Jerrold H. Mink, Andrew L. Deutsch, James Fox, Michael Terk, Keith Feder, Richard Ferkel, Bert Mandelbaum, Clarence Shields, Jr., Kevin Stone, Todd Molnar, Joseph Horrigan, Helen Hislop, and Jaquelin Perry — who provided us with guidance, encouragement, support, and most importantly, friendship.

Finally, the excellent illustrations provided by our medical illustrator, Sandra Suycott, are a crucial part of this book.

F.G. Shellock
C.M. Powers

Contributors

Christopher F. Beaulieu, M.D., Ph.D.
Assistant Professor of Radiology
Stanford University Medical Center
Stanford, California

Barbro Danielson, M.D., Ph.D.
Assistant Professor and Senior Radiologist
Department of Radiology
Sahlgrenska University Hospital
Göteborg, Sweden

Marie Dufour, M.D.
Professor of Clinics
Quebec City University Hospital
and
Department of Radiology, Faculty of Medicine
Laval University
Hospital St-François d'Assise
Quebec City, Quebec
Canada

**Wadi M.W. Gedroyc, M.B.B.S.,
M.R.C.P., F.R.C.R.**
Consultant Radiologist and Medical
  Director, MRI
St. Mary's Hospital
London, United Kingdom

Garry E. Gold, M.D.
Assistant Professor of Radiology
Department of Radiology
Stanford University Medical Center
Stanford, California
and
Palo Alto Veterans Administration
  Medical Center
Palo Alto, California

Luc J. Hébert, M.Sc., P.T.
Doctoral Candidate
Department of Rehabilitation, Faculty
  of Medicine
Laval University and
Center for Interdisciplinary Research
  in Rehabilitation and Social Integration
Quebec City, Quebec
Canada

Sally Ho, D.P.T., M.S.
Adjunct Assistant Professor
Department of Biokinesiology
  and Physical Therapy
University of Southern California
Los Angeles, California

Juerg Hodler, M.D., M.B.A.
Professor of Radiology
Head, Department of Radiology
Orthopedic University Hospital Balgrist
University of Zurich
Zurich, Switzerland

Jari O. Karhu, M.D.
Department of Diagnostic Radiology
University of Turku and Turku University
  Hospital
Turku, Finland

Seppo K. Koskinen, M.D., Ph.D.
Radiologist-in-Chief
Department of Radiology
Töölö Hospital and
Helsinki University Central Hospital
Helsinki, Finland

Kornelia Kulig, Ph.D., P.T.
Associate Professor of Clinical
  Physical Therapy
Department of Biokinesiology
  and Physical Therapy
University of Southern California
Los Angeles, California

Susan Mais Requejo, D.P.T.
Lecturer, Department of Physical Therapy
Mount St. Mary's College
Los Angeles, California

Hélène Moffet, Ph.D., P.T.
Associate Professor and FRSQ
  Research Scholar
Department of Rehabilitation, Faculty
  of Medicine
Laval University
and
Center for Interdisciplinary Research
  in Rehabilitation and Social Integration
Quebec City, Quebec
Canada

Christian Moisan, Ph.D.
Head, Interventional MRI Program
Quebec City University Hospital
Adjunct Professor
Department of Radiology
Laval University
Adjunct Professor
Department of Electrical
  and Computer Engineering
Laval University
CHUQ-Hospital St-François d'Assise
Quebec City, Quebec
Canada

Christopher M. Powers, Ph.D., P.T.
Assistant Professor
Director, Musculoskeletal Biomechanics
  Research Laboratory
Department of Biokinesiology
  and Physical Therapy
University of Southern California
Los Angeles, California

John D. Reeder, M.D., F.A.C.R.
Chief, Musculoskeletal Imaging Division
Proscan Imaging
and
Assistant Professor
The Russell H. Morgan Department
  of Radiology and Radiological Science
The Johns Hopkins University School
  of Medicine
Baltimore, Maryland

Gretchen B. Salsich, Ph.D., P.T.
Post-Doctoral Fellow
Musculoskeletal Biomechanics
  Research Laboratory
Department of Biokinesiology
  and Physical Therapy
University of Southern California
Los Angeles, California

Marius R. Schmid, M.D.
Assistant Professor
Department of Radiology
Orthopedic University Hospital Balgrist
Zurich, Switzerland

Nils Schönström, M.D., Ph.D.
Assistant Professor and Senior Surgeon
Department of Orthopedics
Ryhov Hospital
Jönköping, Sweden

Frank G. Shellock, Ph.D., F.A.C.S.M.
Adjunct Clinical Professor of Radiology
University of Southern California
and
President
Shellock R & D Services, Inc.
Los Angeles, California

Elizabeth F. Souza, D.P.T., C.H.T.
Adjunct Clinical Faculty
Department of Biokinesiology
  and Physical Therapy
University of Southern California
Los Angeles, California

Sandra Suycott, M.A.
Medical Illustrator
Monrovia, California

Michael R. Terk, M.D.
Assistant Professor of Clinical Radiology
Division Head, Musculoskeletal Imaging
Keck School of Medicine
University of Southern California
Los Angeles, California

Samuel R. Ward, P.T.
Doctoral Candidate
Musculoskeletal Biomechanics
  Research Laboratory
Department of Biokinesiology
  and Physical Therapy
University of Southern California
Los Angeles, California

Dominik Weishaupt, M.D.
Assistant Professor
Institute of Diagnostic Radiology
University Hospital Zurich
University of Zurich
Zurich, Switzerland

Simon Wildermuth, M.D.
Assistant Professor
Institute of Diagnostic Radiology
University Hospital Zurich
University of Zurich
Zurich, Switzerland

Jan Willén, M.D., Ph.D.
Associate Professor and Senior Spine Surgeon
Department of Orthopaedic Surgery
Sahlgrenska University Hospital
Göteborg, Sweden

Andrew Williams, M.B.B.S., F.R.C.S.
Consultant Orthopaedic Surgeon
Chelsea and Westminster Hospital
London, United Kingdom

Table of Contents

Preface

"Kinematics" is the branch of mechanics dealing with the study of motion. While traditional kinematic analyses (i.e., motion analysis systems that utilize external markers) form the cornerstone to the biomechanical assessment of joint function, interpretation of such data is limited with respect to identifying the internal factors contributing to abnormal joint motion (pathokinematics) and dysfunction. On the other hand, kinematic magnetic resonance imaging (MRI) provides a means by which the intricacies of joint function can be evaluated for both diagnostic and research purposes. The fact that images can be obtained during active motion provides the ability to thoroughly evaluate the interactions of osseous structures and the contribution of muscle action and other soft tissues to joint function.

Kinematic MRI techniques were developed in recognition of the fact that certain pathologic conditions that affect the joints are position-dependent and/or associated with stressed or "loaded" conditions. Information obtained using kinematic MRI procedures often serves to definitively identify and characterize the underlying abnormality or to supplement the information acquired with standard MRI techniques. Combining kinematic MRI with routine MRI views of the joint provides a means of conducting a more thorough examination and can improve the diagnostic yield of the imaging procedure.

The inspiration for this book came from our perceived need for a comprehensive text that would be the definitive resource on this topic. Because the development of most of the kinematic MRI techniques has been the result of the collaborative efforts of radiologists, biomechanists, physical therapists, orthopedic surgeons, and MR physicists, *Kinematic MRI of the Joints* was written by a carefully selected, international panel of leading experts in these various fields.

This book is organized into separate sections for each joint. The first chapter of each section provides information on pertinent functional anatomy and kinesiology, which serves as the foundation for understanding the abnormal conditions that may be assessed using kinematic MRI. Next, each section has one or more chapters devoted specifically to kinematic MRI, which describe the techniques and protocols, as well as a discussion of normal kinematics and pathokinematics seen using this imaging method. Notably, multiple case examples are provided to illustrate the usefulness of kinematic MRI for diagnosis or elucidation of pathologic conditions.

Kinematic MRI of the Joints was written primarily for two audiences: radiologists and clinicians. For the radiologist, this book is designed to be a reference text that guides the technical and practical aspects of performing and interpreting kinematic MRI examinations. For the clinician, this book provides a concise review of normal and abnormal joint function and describes how information obtained from kinematic MRI can be used to better interpret clinical findings and guide appropriate treatment of common orthopedic conditions. Additionally, we feel that orthopedic surgeons will find particular value in this book insofar as the use of MRI is a daily part of their clinical practice. Orthopedic surgeons should become familiar with the spectrum of kinematic MRI applications that exist, which will enable them to improve therapeutic decisions.

The final section of this book describes unique and emerging applications of kinematic MRI (Chapter 17, Kinematic MRI of the Knee: Preliminary Experience Using the Upright, Weight-Bearing Technique and Chapter 18, The Extremity MR System: Kinematic MRI of the Patellofemoral Joint). Finally, we included a Glossary that provides definitions of common terms from the fields of biomechanics and radiology used in this book.

We hope that this book serves to expand the clinical use of kinematic MRI procedures and to stimulate additional research and development that will further contribute to the understanding of normal and pathological joint function.

Frank G. Shellock, Ph.D., F.A.C.S.M.
Christopher M. Powers, Ph.D., P.T.

Dedication

To my loving wife and best friend, Jaana

F. G. Shellock

To my parents and grandparents for their continued support and encouragement during my educational and professional pursuits

C. M. Powers

Part I

Lumbar Spine

1 The Lumbar Spine: Functional Anatomy and Kinesiology

Kornelia Kulig

CONTENTS

I. INTRODUCTION

The lumbar spine provides a stable, yet adaptable musculoskeletal support for the trunk and upper extremities. In addition to the stability requirements, the lumbar spine serves to transfer weight and resist the resulting bending moments of the upper trunk and motion of the upper extremities. Finally, the lumbar spine protects the spinal cord and cauda equina from excessive physiological movements and trauma.

This chapter discusses the lumbar spine with regard to functional anatomy, normal kinesiology, and pathokinesiology. The material in this chapter has been divided into five sections. The functional anatomy section focuses on structures relevant to description of motion and common pathologies. The section on kinesiology analyzes the lumbar spine as a mechanical structure with controlled articulations by levers (vertebrae), pivots (facets and discs), passive restraints (ligaments), and activators (muscles). Section IV presents pathological conditions and their relationship to structure, function, and motion of the lumbar region.

0-8493-0807-0/01/$0.00+$.50
© 2001 by Frank G. Shellock

II. FUNCTIONAL ANATOMY

A. OSSEOUS STRUCTURES AND ARTICULATING SURFACES

There are common aspects of the osseous structures for the five most caudal vertebrae referred to as the lumbar spine (Figure 1.1). The lumbar region serves as a transition between the trunk and pelvis. Structurally, there are three distinct components to each of the lumbar vertebrae: the vertebral body, the pedicles, and the posterior elements (Figure 1.2). Functionally, the lumbar region consists of five functional spinal units (FSU) with L1-L2 being most cranial and L5-S1 most caudal. The FSU is made up of two neighboring vertebrae and the interconnecting soft tissue, devoid of musculature.

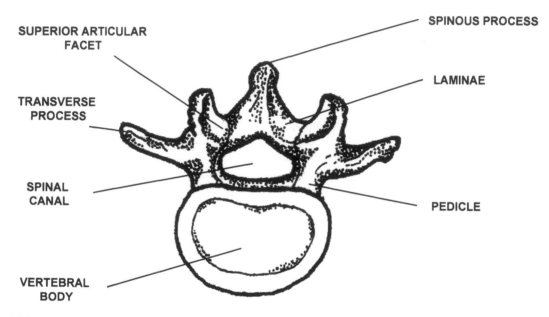

FIGURE 1.1   Typical lumbar vertebra (superior view).

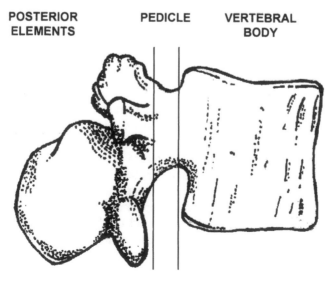

FIGURE 1.2   Typical lumbar vertebra (lateral view). The three functional components of the vertebral body, pedicles, and posterior elements are identified.

The lumbar vertebral body is a box-like structure, oval in the transverse plane, with flat superior and inferior surfaces. The lateral surfaces become slightly concave with age. The posterior surface has visible foramina serving as entry sites for arteries and veins. The main role of the vertebral body is axial load, weight-bearing. The dynamic weight-bearing capabilities of the vertebral body are enhanced by its internal structure of vertical and transverse trabeculae enveloped by a cortical shell.

The lumbar pedicles, two osseous structures projecting posteriorly from the lateral aspect of the vertebral body, are the connectors between the anterior and posterior elements (Figure 1.1). The superior and inferior borders of the pedicle form two neighboring intervertebral foramen. The pedicles are structures well suited to resist tension and bending forces. If fractured due to an excessive extension torque, spondylolisthesis may result.

The posterior elements of a vertebra are the transverse processes, laminae, articular processes, and the spinous process (Figure 1.2). The posterior elements serve as sites of muscle attachment and as structures resisting rotatory and fore-aft forces. The transverse processes project laterally at the level of the inferior vertebral body.

Posterior to each transverse process are superior and inferior articular processes. The medial aspect of the superior articular process has a facet serving as an articular surface with the inferior articular surfaces of the superior vertebrae (zygapophyseal joint). Posterior to the articular processes there is a hemi-lamina, which also serves as a muscle attachment site and protects the neural canal. The right and left hemi-laminas join posteriorly to form a spinous process. The lumbar spinous process is relatively wide, long, and high, providing a long lever for the attaching muscles.

There are four facet surfaces on each lumbar vertebra, two superior (concave medially) and two inferior (convex laterally). Consequently, an FSU has two facet (zygapophyseal) joints. The joint planes transition from the sagittal plane at L1-L2 to almost frontal plane at the L5-S1 FSU (Figure 1.3). Therefore, the L1-L2 FSU has less sagittal motion than L5-S1. In general, the orientation of the lumbar joint surfaces restricts axial rotation at a lumbar FSU.

The role of the facet joint is to direct and restrict motion. Asymmetry of the right and left facet joints is observed in the lumbar spine more frequently than in other regions. This asymmetry may cause aberration of segmental motion. Facet joint surfaces are covered by 2 mm of articular cartilage.

An intervertebral disc is present between each vertebra of the lumbar spine region (Figure 1.4). The disc has a discal joint with both neighboring vertebrae. The primary role of the disc is to distribute weight across the entire vertebral body. The secondary role is to dictate mobility of the FSU (i.e., the higher the disc the more mobile the FSU).

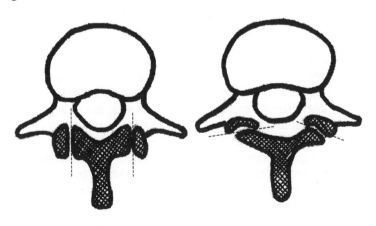

L1 - L2   L5 - S1

FIGURE 1.3 Variability of lumbar facet orientation: L1-L2 and L5-S1.

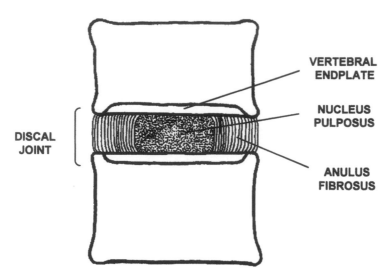

FIGURE 1.4   Frontal view of a lumbar intervertebral disc and neighboring vertebral endplates.

The two distinct components of the disc, the nucleus pulposus and the anulus fibrosus (Figure 1.4), have different roles but can meet these demands only when functioning cooperatively. The nucleus is designed to sustain and transmit pressure with the assistance of the external ring of the anulus. The anulus fibrosus acts like a ligament to restrain movement and to stabilize the FSU. An FSU with a ruptured anulus often presents as being hypermobile (i.e., excessive translatory motion).

B. Ligaments and Joint Capsule

From posterior to anterior there are six ligaments in the lumbar spine, which interconnect the vertebral bodies and are common to the ligaments running from cervical and thoracic regions. The common ligaments (shown in Figure 1.5) are the supraspinous ligament, interspinous ligament, intertransverse ligament (not pictured), ligamentum flavum, apophyseal joint capsular ligaments (not pictured), posterior longitudinal ligament, and anterior longitudinal ligament (Figure 1.5).

In the neutral position, the ligaments are lax. In the sagittal plane, the ligament located anterior to the axis of rotation is taut in extension (anterior longitudinal ligament) and ligaments posterior to the axis of rotation are taut during flexion (the remaining six of the above listed ligaments). During sidebending, the ligaments opposite to the side of sidebending are taut and in rotation all are taut.

The zygapophyseal joint is covered by a joint capsule consisting of transversely oriented collagen fibers at the posterior, superior, and inferior margins of the joint. Anteriorly, the joint capsule is replaced by ligamentum flavum. Posteriorly, the capsule is reinforced by the multifidus muscle. The superior and inferior aspects of the joint capsule are enlarged and contain a small foramen for infiltration of fat into the joint. Intraarticular fat contributes to distribution of articular compression present at end range rotation.

There are additional ligaments unique to the lumbar region: the iliolumbar and false ligaments. The iliolumbar ligaments connect the ipsilateral iliac crest with the transverse processes of L5 and in some cases L4. Its main role is to provide support for L5 and restrict it from anterior translation on the sacrum. The spatial orientation of the iliolumbar ligament, in its five multidirectional parts, provides additional support from excessive flexion, extension, sidebending, and rotation.

The false ligaments (i.e., intertransverse, transforaminal, and mamillo-accessory) are a unique feature of the lumbar spine. However, the false ligaments do not fully meet the criteria of a ligament, that is, a collagenous structure that functions to limit motion between the two bones it connects. The false ligaments either attach to the same bone (mamillo-accessory and transforaminal ligaments)

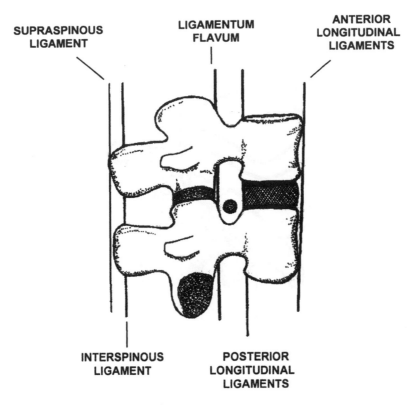

FIGURE 1.5 Ligaments of the lumbar spine.

or appear more membranous than collagenous (intertransverse ligament). The false ligaments play a negligible role in segmental stability.

C. The Vertebral Canal and the Intervertebral Foramen

The consecutive vertebral foramina form the vertebral canal containing the spinal cord (at the L1-L2 level) and the cauda equina (caudally to the terminal end of the spinal cord). Anteriorly, the vertebral canal is formed by the posterior vertebral bodies, discs, and most intimately, by the posterior longitudinal ligament. Posteriorly, the canal is embraced by the ligamentum flavum and the vertebral laminae. Laterally, the vertebral canal is defined by the pedicles, which are intercepted by the intervertebral foramens.

The size of the vertebral canal can be lessened by encroachment of osseous outgrowths, expansion of discal material, buckling of ligamentum flavum, or the presence of developmental anomalies. This narrowing is clinically referred to as spinal stenosis. The pathogenesis of the symptoms related to spinal stenosis will be described later in this chapter.

The lumbar intervertebral foramen is oval shaped and its dimensions have been reported to be 108 mm^2.[1] The size of the intervertebral foramen increases with flexion (24%) and decreases with extension (20%). The intervertebral foramen contains the nerve root with its dural sleeve, radicular vein, radicular artery, and fat. Several structures can decrease the lumen of the intervertebral foramen (i.e., disc, ligamentum flavum, and osseous spurring).

An injury to the intervertebral disc decreases the distance between the vertebral bodies and consequently decreases the size of the intervertebral foramen. Arthrosis of the zygapophyseal joint may result in its enlargement and a decrease of the space defined by the intervertebral foramen. The presence of transforaminal ligaments may contribute to a decrease in size of the intervertebral foramen. These changes may or may not be associated with clinical signs and symptoms.

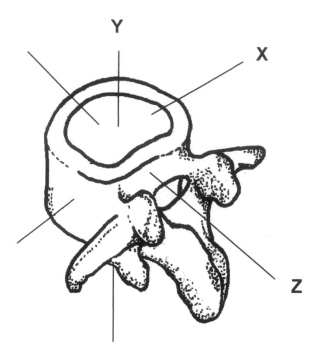

FIGURE 1.6   Orientation of the reference axes.

III. NORMAL JOINT KINESIOLOGY

A. OSTEOKINEMATIC AND ARTHROKINEMATIC MOTIONS

In "neutral" the lumbar spine is positioned in lordosis (a posterior concavity of the lumbar curvature). Movement into lumbar flexion results in relative straightening from the lordotic position. In some cases there is a reversal of the lordotic curve as a whole or its selected segments. During extension of the lumbar spine the lordosis is accentuated. To reach that position, the cranial FSU (e.g., L1-L2) extends and the caudal (e.g., L5-S1) may be required to flex.

Sidebending of the lumbar spine creates a concavity on the side of sidebending. The osseous structure of the lumbar spine produces rotation in association with sidebending. This concomitant rotation varies with the position of the lumbar spine in the sagittal plane, that is, when the spine is flexed the anterior aspect of the vertebral body rotates to the same direction as the sidebending, and to the opposite side when it is extended. Axial rotation is available, but it is quite limited, primarily due to the orientation of the zygapophyseal joints.

By convention, the direction of motion is identified by the position of the anterior aspect of the superior vertebral body. For example, if the description of the position is "L1-L2 is in right rotation," it occurred either by the anterior vertebral body of L1 rotating right or the anterior vertebral body of L2 rotating left. If a motion of a bone at a joint takes place around or along two or more axes, it is referred to as "coupled motion."[2]

Each lumbar FSU has 6 degrees of freedom. The osteokinematic degrees of freedom will be quantified and described in relationship to their axes of rotation. The described motion will be flexion, extension (x-axis), sidebending (z-axis), and rotation (y-axis) (Figure 1.6). Muscles responsible for the movement in each plane and their lever arm will be presented. Additionally, uniplanar and multiplanar motion will be identified.

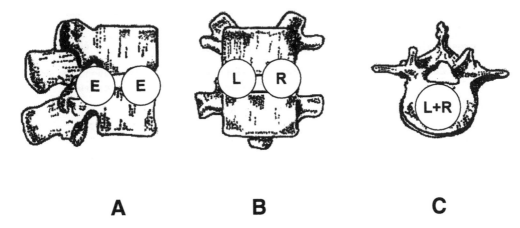

FIGURE 1.7 Approximate locations of the instantaneous axes of rotation in the sagittal (A), frontal (B), and transverse (C) planes at a lumbar functional spinal unit. E, extension; L, left; R, right. (From White, A. A. and Panjabi, M. M., Spinal kinematics, in *The Research Status of Spinal Manipulative Therapy*, NNCDS Monograph, no. 15, U.S. Department of Health, Education and Welfare, Washington, D.C., 1975, p. 93.)

1. Flexion and Extension

Flexion and extension occur in the sagittal plane. These rotatory (osteokinematic) motions are coupled with linear (arthokinematic) motions. The linear motions occur at the discal and facet joints. During flexion, the superior vertebra rotates anteriorly. There is a coupled anterior translation of the superior vertebra on the inferior vertebra of the FSU at the discal joint.[3]

Additionally, due to the presence of the disc, there is a superior and posterior motion of the inferior articular facets in relationship to the superior articular facets. The combination of these motions is referred to as "rocking." Ultimately, the superior facet surfaces glide anteriorly, which results in the anterior translation of the superior vertebra. The shape of the facet joints will dictate the distribution of joint loading. That is, a planar surface will promote even distribution and a joint with a curved articular surface will have more loading anteriorly (see Figure 1.3).

During extension, the superior vertebra rotates posteriorly. Posterior translation of the superior vertebra on the inferior vertebra of the FSU occurs at the discal joint. Conjointly, the superior facet surfaces glide inferiorly and posteriorly along the plane of the facet joints. Extension can be limited by the following: contact of the neighboring spinous processes, inferior articular processes, laminae, and tension of the anterior anulus of the disc.

The axis of rotation for the lumbar FSU is at the level of the intervertebral disc. The axis for flexion is at the posterior aspect of the vertebral body and the axis for extension is at the anterior aspect of the vertebral body (Figure 1.7). For flexion and extension, there is a caudal decrease in the quantity of motion in the sagittal plane (Table 1.1). The quantity of osteokinematic motion at the lumbar spine is the highest in the sagittal plane, followed by sidebending and rotation. The segments with the highest mobility (L4-L5 and L5-S1) are also those with the highest incidence of disc injury.

The arthrokinematic motion of translation is a part of normal spinal mobility and takes place in the three planes. However, if excessive (exceeding 4.5 mm in the sagittal plane), it is considered a measure of clinical instability.[2] Translation for the lumbar spine is typically measured in flexion and extension using x-rays.

2. Sidebending

Sidebending takes place in the frontal plane. This rotatory motion (osteokinematic) is coupled with osteokinematic motion (i.e., rotation) and linear (arthokinematic) motions. The linear motions occur

TABLE 1.1
Representative Values of Segmental Range of Motion in the Lumbar Spine

FSU	Combined Flexion/Extension (degrees)	Lateral Bending (One Side) (degrees)	Axial Rotation (One Side) (degrees)
L1–L2	12	6	2
L2–L3	14	6	2
L3–L4	15	8	2
L4–L5	16	6	2
L5–S1	17	3	1

FSU, functional spinal unit.

Data adapted from White and Panjabi.[2]

at the discal and facet joints. The coupled sidebending and rotation occur as a result of the alignment of the facet joints guiding motion at the FSU. For example, when a motion is initiated with right sidebending and the spine is flexed, right rotation of the superior vertebra will follow. However, when the same right sidebending is initiated with the segment extended, a left rotation will follow.

During sidebending to the right (in extension), the superior vertebra glides right at the discal joint. The right inferior facet of the superior vertebra glides inferiorly while the left glides superiorly along the facet joint surface, thereby causing rotation. Approximation occurs at the zygapophyseal joint, leading to left rotation and separation of the left zygapophyseal joint. These are coupled motions at the lumbar spine.

The axis of rotation for sidebending at the lumbar spine passes from anterior to posterior at the intervertebral disc of an FSU (Figure 1.7). The amount of unilateral sidebending is nearly constant throughout the lumbar spine (5 to 8 degrees), with the exception of the L5-S1 segment, which has the least amount of sidebending (3 degrees). Representative values of segmental range of motion for the lumbar spine are show in Table 1.1.

3. Rotation

Rotation takes place in the transverse plane. Rotation, if initiated in flexion, is coupled with ipsilateral sidebending. If the rotation is taking place to the right, the left facet joint surfaces approximate and consequently the right facet joint surfaces separate. This motion is followed by sidebending if the superior vertebra is rotated to the right. Further sidebending results from superior glide at the left facet joint and inferior glide at the right facet joint.

The axis of rotation for axial rotation at the lumbar spine passes vertically through the center of the vertebral body (Figure 1.7). The amount of unilateral rotation is 2 to 3 degrees, with the least amount of motion at the L5-S1 segment. This pattern of motion reflects the orientation of the facet joints, which are transitioning from a sagittal orientation to an almost frontal orientation.

4. Axial Approximation and Distraction

Axial approximation and distraction for the lumbar spine occur along the vertical axis. Axial approximation (compression) is caused by gravity, external loads, and the forces created by muscle contraction. Consequently, compression is part of all upright positions and most activities. As vertebral bodies approximate, discal height decreases.[4] The vertebral body is able to withstand 3 to 12 kN of compression[5] and its strength is directly related to bone density.[6] Excessive axial loading may cause fracture of the central aspect of the endplate.[7]

The zygapophyseal joints may bear up to 20 to 40% of an applied vertical load.[8,9] The loading on the zygapophyseal joints is dependent on the status of the disc. An FSU with a healthy disc transfers less weight to the zygapophyseal joints, while an FSU with an injured disc would rely more on the zygapophyseal joints for load bearing.

Functionally, axial distraction of the lumbar spine happens much less frequently than axial approximation. However, axial distraction of the lumbar spine is used therapeutically (i.e., "pelvic traction"). Twomey[10] studied the entire cadaveric lumbar spine during sustained axial traction to mimic the clinical procedure and found that traction of 18 lb caused a 7.5 mm lengthening of the entire spine (i.e., 40% of lengthening resulted from flattening of the lumbar lordosis; 60% was due to distraction of the vertebral bodies).

B. Muscles and their Functions

The lumbar muscles protect the spine, interconnect and move the lumbar FSUs, and connect and move the lumbar, thoracic, and pelvic regions. Muscles with direct attachments to the lumbar spine will be discussed first. Then muscles that do not attach to the lumbar spine, but strongly impact on the lumbar spine due to their long lever arms, will be reviewed.

The muscles with direct attachments to the lumbar spine are posterior, lateral, and anterior. The posterior elements of the lumbar spine are covered by the lumbar back muscles, the lateral aspect by the intertransversarii and quadratus lumborum, and the anterior portion is covered by the psoas major muscle (Figure 1.8). Most muscles of the lumbar region are capable of contributing to multidirectional motions. However, each muscle seems to have a dominant lever arm for one type of motion.

The lumbar back muscles include short intersegmental muscles and the polysegmental muscles. The short intersegmental muscles are interspinales and intertransversarii mediales. These muscles are short and small and lie close to the axis of rotation. Therefore, they are not powerful activators. Bogduk[11] states that the value of the intersegmental muscles lies not in the force they can exert, but in the muscle spindles they contain, offering a system of proprioception.

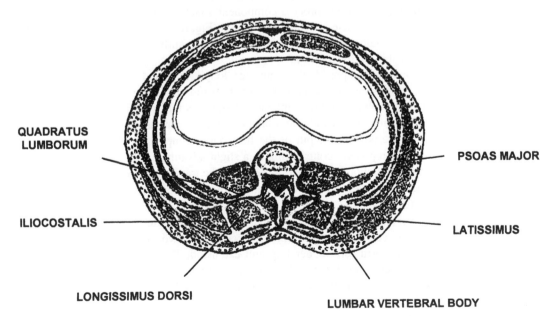

FIGURE 1.8 Transverse view of the muscles of the lumbar spine. (From White, A. A. and Panjabi, M.M., *Clinical Biomechanics of the Spine*, J.B. Lippincott, Philadelphia, 1990. With permission.)

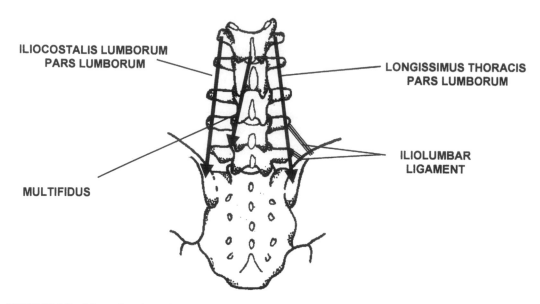

FIGURE 1.9 Line of action of the multifidus and of the lumbar components of the longissimus and iliocostalis. (Adapted from Bogduk, N., *Clinical Anatomy of the Lumbar Spine and Sacrum,* 2nd edition, Churchill Livingstone, New York, 1997, p. 107.)

The polysegmental muscles are the multifidus and lumbar components of the longissimus and iliocostalis (lumbar erector spinae). Multifidus, true to its name, is formed by a large number of independent fascicles and is the most medially located lumbar muscle. There are two distinct components of the multifidus, fibers attaching to the lamina and those attaching to the spinous processes. Both types of fibers attach to the mamillary processes at the posterior aspect of the superior articular process. The laminar component attaches two levels below (i.e., L1 to L3) the iliac crest and sacrum and the spinous process component attaches three levels below (i.e., L1 to L4). The line of action of this muscle is caudal and lateral (Figure 1.9). The vertical component is longer than the horizontal, indicating that multifidus is predominantly an extensor. The horizontal component serves as a stabilizer for rotation.[12]

The lumbar erector spinae, composed of two muscles (longissimus and iliocostalis), lies laterally to the multifidus. The longissimus thoracis pars lumborum runs from the accessory process and transverse process of each lumbar vertebra to the medial aspect of the posterior superior iliac spine. The line of action of this muscle is caudal and lateral, which is similar to that of the multifidus (Figure 1.9). The difference is in the depth of the horizontal component; the longissimus has a longer anterior-posterior component, contributing to a slight advantage as a rotator.

Finally, the iliocostalis lumborum runs from the tip of the transverse process to the iliac crest. Of the three polysegmental muscles, the iliocostalis lumborum has the greatest advantage to produce axial rotation (Figure 1.9).

The intertransversarii and quadratus lumborum are the lateral muscles of the lumbar spine. The intertransversarii medialis connects the mamillary processes of two neighboring vertebrae and, therefore, has a short lever arm for sidebending and extension. This low mechanical advantage coupled with small size categorizes this muscle as an accessory muscle for stabilization. Quadratus lumborum is a rectangularly shaped muscle with its attachments to the iliolumbar ligament posterior iliac crest, the 12th rib, and the transverse processes of L1-L4. This muscle depresses the last rib and if acting unilaterally, it sidebends the lumbar spine.

Anterior to the lumbar spine is the psoas major. It attaches to the transverse processes, the discs, and vertebral margins with the discs of T12 though L5. Its distal attachment is to the lesser trochanter of the femur. The psoas major is able to extend the upper lumbar segments and flex the lower lumbar segments; however, the lever arm for sagittal plane motion is small. Alternately, the psoas is a strong compressor of the lumbar discs.[13]

IV. PATHOKINESIOLOGY: CLINICAL RELEVANCE AND IMPLICATIONS

A. LUMBAR SPONDYLOSIS

Lumbar spondylosis is a degenerative process of activity and age-related changes of the lumbar spine leading to mechanical low back pain. It is thought that the process begins at the intervertebral disc. Subsequently, changes in other structures may follow (deformation of the zygapophyseal joints, osteophytes at the vertebral bodies, ossification of the posterior longitudinal ligament, hypotonic ligamentum flavum). The degenerative process may become symptomatic at any stage.

The symptoms may be placed in one of four categories: back pain, back pain with proximal referral, radicular pain, and myelopathy. Back pain, back pain with proximal referral, and lower extremity radicular pain can be caused by several lumbar structures containing nociceptors, including the disc, nerve root sleeve, facet joints, and ligaments.

In lumbar spondylitic myelopathy, the cauda equina is compromised within the spinal canal. As a result there are degenerative changes of the lumbar spine. Narrowing of the spinal canal, also referred to as spinal stenosis, is another form of spondylosis.

B. STENOSIS

Stenosis is defined as narrowing of the spinal canal. Schonstrom[14] lists seven forms of lumbar stenosis: congenital, developmental, degenerative, metabolic, iatrogenic, post-traumatic, and "miscellaneous." In absolute stenosis, the antero-posterior diameter of the spinal canal is 10 mm or less. Spatially, the spinal stenosis can be central or lateral. Spinal stenosis usually has gradual onset and is seen greatly in persons more than 60 years of age. The main components of a patient's presentation are lower extremity symptoms such as numbness, paresthesia, weakness, and neurogenic claudication. Neurogenic claudication is associated with lower extremity symptoms during walking. Sitting relieves these symptoms. Additionally, walking uphill is easier than on flat surfaces. The management of patients with lumbar stenosis is most often with conservative treatment, but occasionally it requires surgical intervention.

C. SPONDYLOLYTIC INSTABILITY

Spondylolytic instability is most often associated with bilateral spondylolysis. Spondylolysis is associated with a fracture of the pars interarticularis (pedicle). If the vertebra translates forward, the condition will become a spondylolisthesis. A spondylolisthesis can be associated with hypermobility or instability. The symptoms of a patient with instability may include localized low back pain, leg pain, or weakness.

D. FACET SUBLUXATION

Facet subluxation is most commonly of traumatic origin. However, degenerative changes leading to weakening of passive restraints and muscles may also cause subluxation. The patient may present with a painful movement pattern or restriction during an attempt to move the lumbar spine. The management of patients with facet subluxation requires conservative rehabilitation.

V. SUMMARY AND CONCLUSIONS

The lumbar region consists of five FSUs. Its stability depends on the vertebral structure, including the facet joints, and the integrity of the disc, ligaments, and muscles. The lumbar spine exhibits coupling. Sidebending produces axial rotation, and axial rotation produces sidebending. Sidebending produces the same side rotation, and axial rotation produces opposite rotation except for the L4-L5 and L5-S1 FSU where the sidebending is the same.

The common pathologic conditions that affect the lumbar spine are generally of a traumatic or degenerative nature. Pathologies of traumatic origin vary significantly in the extent of injury. Degenerative changes are commonly related to degenerative disc disease, spondylosis, ankylosing spondylitis, stenosis, joint arthrosis, or disc injury.

REFERENCES

1. Panjabi, M. M., Takata, K., and Goel, V. K., Kinematics of lumbar intervertebral foramen, *Spine,* 8, 348, 1983.
2. White, A. A. and Panjabi, M. M., *Clinical Biomechanics of the Spine,* J.B. Lippincott, Philadelphia, 1991.
3. Twomey, L. and Taylor, J., Sagittal movements of the human lumbar vertebral column: a quantitative study of the role of the posterior vertebral elements, *Arch. Phys. Med. Rehab.,* 64, 322, 1983.
4. Adams, M. A. and Dolan, P., Recent advances in lumbar spinal mechanics and their clinical significance, *Clin. Biomech.,* 10, 3, 1995.
5. Hutton, W. C. and Adams, M. A., Can the lumbar spine be crushed in heavy lifting?, *Spine,* 7, 586, 1982.
6. Hansson, T., Roos, B., and Nachemson, A., The bone mineral content and ultimate compressive strength of lumbar vertebrae, *Spine,* 5, 46, 1980.
7. Brown, T., Hansen, R. J., and Yorra, A. J., Some mechanical tests on the lumbosacral spine with particular reference to the intervertebral disc, *J. Bone Joint Surg.,* 39A, 1135, 1957.
8. Nachemson, A., The load on lumbar disc in different positions of the body, *Clin. Orthop.,* 45, 107, 1966.
9. Hakim, N. S. and King, A. I., Static and dynamic facet loads, *Proceedings of the Twentieth Strapp Car Crash Conference,* 1976, p. 607.
10. Twomey, L., Sustained lumbar traction. An experimental study of long spine segments, *Spine,* 10, 147, 1985.
11. Bogduk, N., *Clinical Anatomy of the Lumbar Spine,* 3rd edition, Churchill Livingstone, New York, 1998.
12. Donisch, E. W. and Basmajian, J. V., Electromyography of deep back muscles in man, *Am. J. Anat.,* 133, 25, 1972.
13. Bogduk, N., Pearcy, M., and Hadfield, G., Anatomy and biomechanics of the psoas major, *Clin. Biomech.,* 7, 109, 1992.
14. Schönström, N., Lumbar spinal stenosis, in *Physical Therapy of the Low Back,* 3rd edition, Twomey, L. T. and Taylor, J. R., Eds., Churchill Livingstone, New York, 2000, p. 279.

2 Kinematic MRI of the Lumbar Spine: Assessment in the Axial-Loaded, Supine Position

Jan Willén, Nils Schönström, and Barbro Danielson

CONTENTS

I. INTRODUCTION

The lumbar spine is a highly dynamic structure composed of numerous functional spinal units. It is well documented that changes associated with load and position result in alterations in the space of the spinal canal. For example, narrowing of the canal is seen with axial loading and to a further extent when combined with extension of the lumbar spine.

Since the advent of magnetic resonance imaging (MRI), this noninvasive technique, in most cases, has replaced the use of myelography for preoperative investigation of patients with suspected encroachment of the spinal canal. MRI is superior when analyzing the contents of the canal in more detail but is regularly still performed in a supine relaxed position. This results in unloading of the spine and enlargement of the canal. Therefore, encroachments of the canal may still remain undetected. Notably, a special kinematic MRI technique has recently been developed to examine and characterize the lumbar spine in the axial-loaded, supine position with the intent of obtaining improved diagnostic information to assess this anatomic region.

This chapter presents the functional anatomy of the lumbar spine and the implications for the use of kinematic MRI in the axial-loaded, supine position. The technique used for kinematic MRI of the lumbar spine in the axial-loaded, supine position is described, along with normal findings and those seen in patients with spinal disorders. Finally, the advantages of performing kinematic MRI of the lumbar spine will be presented.

II. BASIC FUNCTIONAL ANATOMY OF THE LUMBAR SPINE: IMPLICATIONS FOR KINEMATIC MRI

The basic function of the spine is to provide a stable base for the locomotor system and at the same time provide a flexible tube containing and protecting the spinal cord and the cauda equina. The linkage system that provides the flexibility is also its weak point, where trauma and degenerative processes can lead to changes impinging on the spinal canal and its neural content. From a clinical point of view, therefore, it is important to focus the description of the basic anatomy of the lumbar spine on one spinal motion segment consisting of two adjacent vertebrae, the intervening disc, and facet joints (i.e., the three joint complex or functional spinal unit).

At the level of the pedicles there is a complete bony ring and very little influence of kinematics. Conversely, at the level of the disc, motion has direct impact on the size and shape of the spinal canal. Furthermore, at each disc level, a pair of spinal nerves exits through the intervertebral foramen and is vulnerable to movements and pathologic changes in the three joint complex.

A. THE SIZE OF THE SPINAL CANAL

The size of the dural sac inside the spinal canal in a healthy individual is sufficient for its neural content, which in the upper lumbar canal consists of the conus medullaris superiorly and the cauda equina inferiorly. It has been shown by Schönström et al.[1] in an *in vitro* study that the transverse area of the spinal canal at the level L3-L4 was reduced by about 40 mm^2 when the spine was moved from flexion to extension. This was a relative reduction of 16%. After a change in axial load from 250 N distraction to 250 N compression, the canal size was reduced by an average of 50 mm^2, corresponding to a relative reduction of 19%. These results were supported by an MRI study on healthy volunteer subjects conducted by Schmid et al.[2] It was reported that the transverse area of the spinal canal was reduced from an average of 268 mm^2 to 224 mm^2 when the spine was brought from an upright flexion to an upright extension position, a reduction of about 44 mm^2. This change was registered at the disc level. No similar change was noted at the pedicle, supporting the statement that no significant positional alterations in the spinal canal takes place at this level. Notably, these changes in canal size are normal and without consequence for a healthy individual. The changes in the size of the spinal canal at the level of the disk can be explained by the bulging of the disc anteriorly and the ligamenta flava posterolaterally.

The space needed by the cauda equina is surprisingly consistent among human subjects. In two *in vitro* studies, the size of the cauda equina at L3-L4 was studied using a pressure recording technique.[3,4] A clamp was applied around the cauda equina in human spine specimens. A thin catheter recorded the pressure among the roots as the clamp was tightened progressively. The transverse area inside the clamp was measured, and at the first sign of a pressure increase, the area was called the critical size. This critical area in the first study was 72 ± 13 mm^2 and in the second study was 77 ± 13 mm^2.

In a clinical study, the transverse area of the dural sac in patients with a central stenosis, confirmed at surgery, was 90 ± 35 mm². On preoperative computed tomography (CT) scans, this corresponded to an anterior-posterior diameter of the dural sac of 9 ± 3 mm.[5] Further clinical experiences have led to the conclusion that the space required for the cauda equina at the L3-L4 level is in the range of 70 to 100 mm². Indirect support for this premise can be seen in the MRI study conducted by Schmid et al.,[2] where none of the asymptomatic volunteers had a transverse area of the dural sac, at any level, below 150 mm².

The changes in dural sac size associated with axial loading of the spine has been studied by several authors using myelography. Using functional myelography in upright flexion and extension, Sortland et al.[6] reported that the diameter of the dural sac was reduced by 6.7 mm in extension for a group of patients with symptoms of spinal stenosis. In a control group the reduction in anterior-posterior diameter of the dural sac was 1.7 mm from flexion to extension.

Penning and Wilmink[7] studied the changes in dural sac size during flexion and extension of the spine using myelography. These authors reported an anterior shift of the dural sac in extension, most likely the result of a thickening of the ligamentum flavum. The anterior-posterior diameter of the dural sac was reduced at disc level in extension, being most pronounced at L3-L4 and L4-L5 levels with average decrease of 2.5 mm at L3-L4 and 3.6 mm at L4-L5. A compensating dilatation of the dural sac was found behind the vertebral body in extension. In a CT study conducted with subjects supine,[8] the same authors found concentric narrowing of the lumbar spinal canal in extension and a widening, with relief of nerve root involvement, in flexion.

B. THE LIGAMENTUM FLAVUM

The ligamentum flavum extends from the midportion of the ventral aspect of the lamina superiorly to the upper edge of the lamina inferiorly. Its function is to protect the spinal canal from behind and permit movement of the three joint complex. The ligamentum flavum is under tension in the neutral position of the spine and is fully relaxed only in full extension.[9] Consequently, the ligamentum flavum has a high content of elastic fibers (60 to 80%).[9] In a study conducted by Schönström et al.,[1] the size of the ligamentum flavum varied between specimens and no conclusion could be drawn concerning its role in contributing to the variability in canal size.

In a separate *in vitro* study, the ligamentum flavum response to tensile stress was studied.[9] The conclusion of this investigation was that an average thinning of 2 mm could be expected under a distraction load of 8 kg. The thinning of the ligamentum flavum was supported by Schmid et al.,[2] who recorded an average of 2.5 mm in an *in vivo* study using MRI on 12 asymptomatic volunteer subjects.

C. THE SEGMENTAL SPINAL NERVES

At each disc level, a pair of spinal nerves leaves the canal. According to Anderson and McNeill,[10] their exit has been divided into three zones in relation to the pedicle. Zone I is in the lateral recess situated between the cranial part of the facet joint and the disc. Zone II is situated below the pedicle. Zone III, the exit zone, is lateral of the pedicle. In the first two zones, changes in size of the available space for the spinal nerves can be recorded as a consequence of movements in the spinal motion segment.

In zone I, the lateral recess, a bulging disc will reduce the space between the disc and the joint. In zone II the caudal facet of the zygapophyseal joint will move upward in extension, reducing the available space for the spinal nerve.

In an MRI study of healthy volunteers performed by Schmid et al.,[2] changes in the size of the foramen (zone II) were observed as a consequence of a change in load and position of the spine. These authors reported a 23% reduction in foraminal size from an upright, neutral position to an upright, extended position. The reduction was 22% from an upright, neutral position to a supine, extended position. If the spine was brought from an upright, neutral to an upright, flexed position the size increased by 19%.

Using MRI, Wildermuth et al.[11] investigated changes in foramen size between different postures and reported that size increases were greater whenever moving from flexion to extension in an upright position compared to a supine position. This indicates that a change in axial load as well as a change in position could have an effect on foraminal size.

D. KINEMATIC MRI OF THE LUMBAR SPINE

Advances in the design of MR systems during the last few years have made it possible to develop specialized open-configured MR systems that permit examinations to be conducted on patients standing upright. These MR systems can be used to evaluate changes in the spinal column and canal during loaded movements. With the well-documented knowledge of the decreasing spinal canal volume in the lumbar spine in an upright, standing posture,[6,12] the demands for development of similar methods for use in MRI examinations have increased.

Harvey[13] described a method for performing kinematic MRI using an open-configured MR system to image the lumbar spine during flexion and extension. With this technique, it was possible to measure the difference in angle between the vertebral bodies from maximal flexion to maximal extension with a precision superior to these measurements made using typical x-ray/myelography techniques. However, subjects had to be well stabilized to avoid motion artifacts during the more than 2 minutes required for image acquisition. The previously described kinematic MRI studies performed by Schmid et al.[2] and Wildermuth et al.[11] also were conducted using a specially designed, vertically opened MR system.

Our early experience of kinematic MRI of the lumbar spine using special positioning techniques has been somewhat limited. The short vertical distance within the available horizontally opened MR system created problems in positioning the surface radiofrequency (RF) coil. The patient had to lie on one side; maintain maximally flexed, neutral, and maximally extended positions; and remain still for the duration of the acquisition time for each posture (Figure 2.1).

III. THE AXIAL-LOADED, SUPINE KINEMATIC MRI TECHNIQUE

A. THE POSITIONING DEVICE

The first attempts to perform functional, axial-loaded examinations of the lumbar spine were undertaken in 1989 at Sahlgren University Hospital, Göteborg, Sweden. By 1992, a specially designed compression device was ready for use. The prototype positioning device was made of stainless steel, and the first studies were done with the CT/myelographic technique. This technique was used until 1994, when the first MR-compatible (i.e., made from materials that would not produce artifacts or distortions of the MR images) device was available. Since that time, all axial-loaded examinations have been performed using this kinematic MRI technique.

The positioning device has, with time, been improved, in cooperation with technicians and designers. It now consists of a plastic compression device and a Neoprene/nylon harness (DynaMed AB, Stockholm, Sweden) (Figure 2.2). The harness is attached to the compression device using nylon straps, which are tightened to provide axial loading of the lumbar spine with the subject in a supine position. The harness is constructed to ensure that the pressure is evenly distributed across the lower part of the chest rather than the shoulders.

It is crucial to ensure that the straps pass posteriorly to the greater trochanter to maintain the lumbar lordosis for an optimal kinematic MRI examination (Figure 2.2). If the lumbar lordosis changes into hypokyphosis, the effect of the axial load will be neutralized. Notably, the load should be approximately 40%, and not exceed 50%, of body weight to avoid injury to the patient. The load is selected according to previous disc pressure measurements at the level L3-L4, with subjects

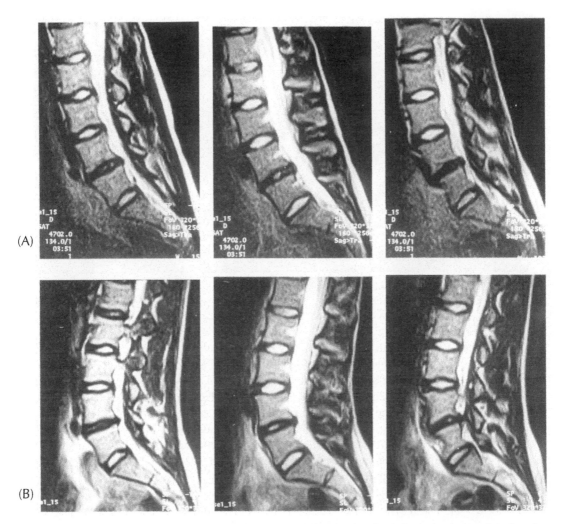

FIGURE 2.1 Examination in a 30-year-old female with low back pain and sciatica in her right leg (i.e., suspected L5 nerve root influence). The examination was performed using an open-configured, 0.2 Tesla MR system. MR images were acquired using 4 mm thick sections and a 0.8 mm intersection gap. (A) Patient in maximal flexion. MR image shows a degenerative L4-L5 disc protruding more in this position than in (B) neutral, and in (C) extension. Right lateral section location (right), central section location (center), and left lateral section location (left) images are shown for A, B, and C. Narrowing of the lateral part of the spinal canal is observed on the *left* and not the *right* side, which was symptomatic for the patient. The remaining levels are without distinction.

standing.[14] The load that is exerted by the device can be regulated by tightening or loosening adjustment knobs at the compression device and the load should be distributed equally on both legs.

The positioning device is compatible with most CT and MR systems and enables examination of patients in a supine position, with straightened legs, thus simulating the axial load on the lumbar spine in an upright position (i.e., the posture associated with most symptoms of sciatica and spinal stenosis). From our experience, it is necessary to maintain the axial load for at least five minutes before the kinematic MRI examination is initiated.

The patients should be asked routinely about any pain in the spine or in the legs during the examination, especially during compression/axial loading. If the patient reports sensations of intractable pain, the load applied by the positioning device may be immediately released.

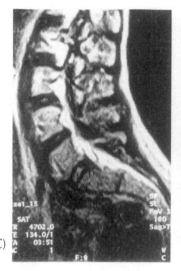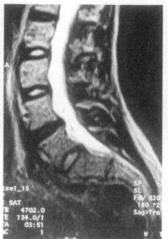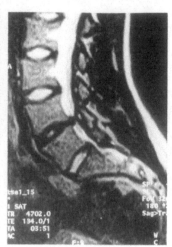

(C)

FIGURE 2.1   (continued).

B. MRI PULSE SEQUENCES

The experience of our group in conducting the axial-loaded, supine kinematic MRI examinations of the lumbar spine was obtained using a 1.0 Tesla MR system and a flat surface RF coil. Subjects were typically examined using sagittal and axial plane, T1- and T2-weighted, spin-echo or fast (or turbo) spin-echo (FSE) pulse sequences. The repetition times (TR) and echo times (TE) were 660 to 900 (TR)/15 to 17 (TE) for the T1-weighted pulse sequences and 2300 to 8350 (TR)/105 to 130 (TE) for the T2-weighted pulse sequences. The section thickness was 4 mm and the field of view (FOV) was 32 cm for the sagittal plane MR images and 25 cm for axial plane MR images. The matrix size was 256 × 256 for sagittal plane MR images and 192 × 256 and 240 × 256 for the axial plane T1- and T2-weighted pulse sequences, respectively. Two excitations (NEX) were used for the T2-weighted MR images, and 3 and 4 NEX for the sagittal and axial plane T1-weighted MR images, respectively.

C. METHOD FOR EXAMINATION

During axial loading or compression in slight extension (or ACE) of the lumbar spine (Figure 2.2A) and the psoas relaxed position (or PRP; Figure 2.2B), the localizer for the axial plane MR image section locations should be parallel to the disc (Figure 2.3) and as evenly distributed as possible. The dural sac cross-sectional area (D-CSA) has been determined using a standard measurement program by our group. In every patient, the image selected should be that in which the dural sac appears to have the smallest area at each actual disc and lateral recess level.

To ensure that the images chosen for measurements are comparable in every position, the radiologist needs to compare nerve roots, other soft tissues, and bony structures such as facet joints and the lamina. Furthermore, it is essential to look for signs of narrowing of the lateral recess and compression or flattening of the nerve roots in any level especially from L3 to S1.

Any deformation of the dural sac should be noted, as well as a suspicion of a disc herniation, narrowing of an intervertebral foramen, ligamentum flavum thickening, or a synovial cyst adjacent to a facet joint. Penning and Wilmink[8] found, in a dynamic CT/myelographic study on patients with suspected spinal stenosis, that the spinal canal area was significantly decreased in lumbar extension in the supine position compared to 45 degrees of lumbar flexion.

In our early kinematic MRI studies on the effect of supine axial compression of the lumbar spine in slight extension (ACE) during CT/myelographic examinations, eight patients with signs

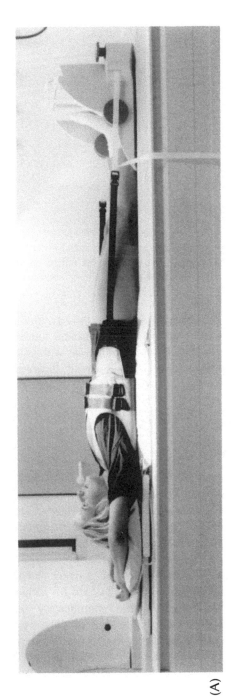

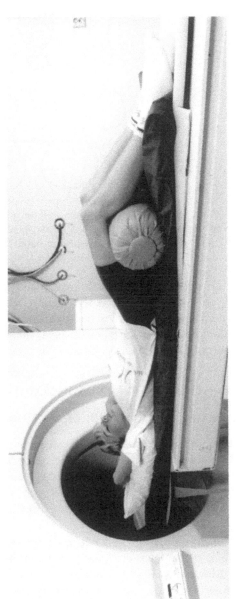

FIGURE 2.2 (A) Patient prepared for a kinematic MRI examination using the ACE (axial compression in slight extension) technique. The patient is placed on a low friction carpet on top of the examination table. The patient harness is connected to a compression device using straps and the axial load is measured by a balance mechanism in the compression device (device made by DynaMed AB, Stockholm, Sweden). (B) Patient in a conventional relaxed supine position on the examination table.

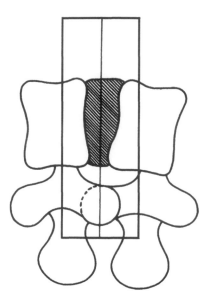

Figure 2.3 A schematic showing the localizer used for selection of transverse section locations for the MR images placed parallel relative to the anatomy of the spine. (From Willén, J. et al., Dynamic effects on the lumbar spinal canal. Axial-loaded CT-myelography and MRI in patients with sciatica and/or neurogenic claudication, *Spine*, 22, 2968, 1997. With permission.)

of sciatica or neurogenic claudication were examined.[15] The decrease of the dural sac cross-sectional area (D-CSA) in 14 disc sites was significantly more pronounced than during supine lumbar extension alone. Thus, on the basis of our experience, we prefer to perform examinations with axial loading to ensure optimal visualization of spinal canal changes. In cases of osteoporosis, however, only examination in lumbar extension should be considered.

IV. NORMAL FINDINGS IN AXIAL-LOADED, KINEMATIC MRI

A. UPRIGHT SEATED, KINEMATIC MRI OF THE LUMBAR SPINE

As previously mentioned, Schmid et al.[2] showed that significant changes in the cross-sectional area of the spinal canal and foramina occur between different body positions. The smallest spinal canal areas were found in the extended position (upright seated or lying supine). They also showed that the ligamentum flavum plays a significant role in changing the D-CSA and that the mean maximum thickness of the structure differs by more than 2 mm between upright flexion and upright extension when the ligament buckles.

There were no differences between the cross-sectional areas in the upright standing and in supine positions, which leads one to conclude that the supine position should be used for patient convenience. However, even the cross-sectional area of the foramina varied significantly and decreased during extension. This was caused by the bulging disc and the thickening of the ligamentum flavum, which decreased the distance between the pedicles of the two vertebrae. Nowicki et al.[16] showed similar changes in an experimental study on human cadaveric materials using CT and MRI examinations.

It should be noted that in the upright seated position, the psoas muscle is relaxed, tending to permit lumbar flexion. However, this is not comparable with the upright standing position, in which the psoas muscle is taut, tending to extend the lumbar spine and increase lordosis. This causes a further decrease in the space within the spinal canal.

B. Comparison between Upright Standing and Axial-Loaded, Supine Kinematic MRI of the Lumbar Spine

In a comparative kinematic MRI study using the vertically opened 0.5 Tesla MR system (Signa SP), the effects of upright standing and axial-loaded, supine positioning on the lumbar spine was assessed in 20 healthy volunteer subjects.[26] The upright standing position was performed in a kneeling position and a spinal compression device (previously described) was used during the procedure. Loading of the lumbar spine was consistently 50% of the subject's body weight.

Changes in the disc and lumbar lordosis were measured consecutively during 30 minutes in each position. Similar effects regarding disc bulges and changes in lumbar lordosis were registered during the two types of loading. However, the lordosis was more pronounced in the upright standing position. This indicates that there may be an option to insert a small pillow beneath the lumbar spine during the supine procedure to get optimal information from the CT and MRI examinations.

C. Axial-Loaded, Supine Kinematic MRI in Asymptomatic Subjects

More than 40 asymptomatic individuals representing different age groups (i.e., 20 to 60 years of age) with no spinal disorders during their lifetimes have been examined using the axial-loaded, supine kinematic MRI technique in PRP and ACE. Progressive degenerative signs in the functional spinal units (FSU) were, as expected, found to be correlated with increasing age. Moreover, the dural sac cross-sectional area (D-CSA) in PRP varied from 250 to 50 mm^2, the latter in the level L5-S1 (Figure 2.4). No radiological signs of stenosis were registered with the exception of one L4-L5 level, where a lateral recess was narrow during ACE. This was seen in a 50-year-old male. However, this narrowing did not provoke any clinical signs of nerve root pressure (Figure 2.5). Radiological findings should, as always, be related to the clinical findings.

Seven of the asymptomatic individuals were selected for examination in PRP and in different degrees of axial loading (ACE, 25 to 50% of their individual body weight). Changes in D-CSA were quantified after 5 to 60 minutes of loading time. A significant decrease in D-CSA was found in five subjects after 5 minutes at a load of 50% of the body weight.[17]

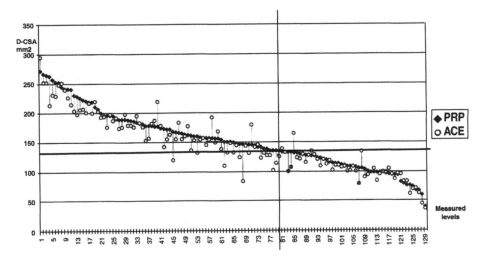

Figure 2.4   The dual sac cross-sectional area (D-CSA) values obtained in psoas relaxed position (PRP) and in axial compression in slight extension (ACE) at each disc level (L3-S1) in asymptomatic individuals (129 disc sites). Note the small amount of significantly decreased D-CSA values below 100 mm^2 at ACE compared to the symptomatic material in Figure 2.6.

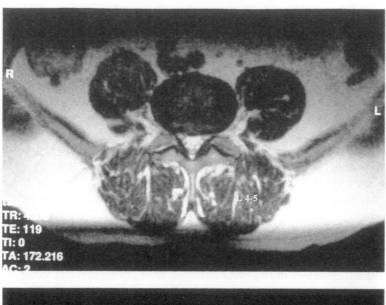

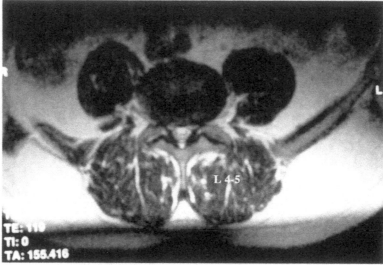

Figure 2.5   Axial-loaded, supine kinematic MRI examination at disc level L4-L5 in a 50-year-old male, showing the most impressive dural sac cross-sectional area (D-CSA) decrease from psoas relaxed position (PRP) (top) to axial compression in extension (ACE) (bottom) among the individuals in the asymptomatic group.

V. AXIAL-LOADED, KINEMATIC MRI IN PATIENTS WITH SPINAL DISORDERS

A. UPRIGHT SEATED, KINEMATIC MRI OF THE LUMBAR SPINE

A quantitative and qualitative assessment of T2-weighted, fast spin-echo MR imaging and myelography, in flexion and extension of the lumbar spine in upright seated and neutral supine positions, was performed by Wildermuth et al.[11] using the 0.5 Tesla MR system (Signa SP). Thirty patients who were referred for lumbar myelography were included in this study. The findings of the two examination procedures correlated well. Only small changes in the sagittal plane diameter of the dural sac and foraminal size between the various testing positions were found.[11] Thus, it was concluded that this particular type of kinematic MRI procedure is equivalent to myelography in most cases and, thus, useful for guiding surgical interventions.

According to Wildermuth et al.,[11] the MRI examination of patients in an upright seated position was difficult because it often caused severe back pain, especially during the flexed and extended positions. Moreover, there were some difficulties in positioning the surface RF coil and in the interpretation of the MR images, especially in patients with degenerative scoliosis. Wildermuth et al.[11] also concluded that the measurement of the cross-sectional area of the spinal canal in axial plane images may be more relevant for the evaluation of the degree and location of spinal canal stenosis than the sagittal diameter alone. This conclusion is in accordance with the findings by Schönström et al.[3-5]

B. Axial-Loaded, Supine Kinematic MRI of the Lumbar Spine

1. Basic Patient Findings

Thirty-four patients with sciatica and/or neurogenic claudication (signs of lumbar spinal stenosis[18]) were analyzed after examination in the traditional supine psoas relaxed position (PRP) and compared with examination using the axial compression, slight extension (ACE), kinematic MRI technique.[15] The dural sac cross-sectional area in disc and lateral recess level (D-CSA) ranged from 300 to 40 mm^2 in PRP. In 40 of the 80 investigated disc sites, there was a significant difference between the measurements in PRP and ACE. Notably, PRP was reduced below 100 mm^2 during ACE (Figure 2.6).

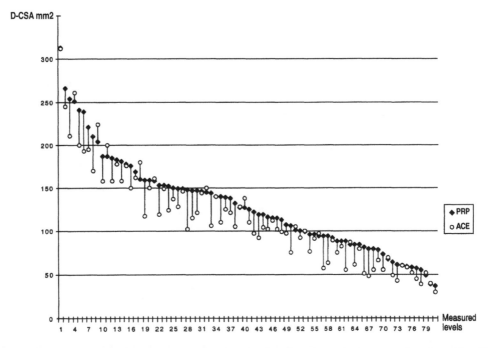

Figure 2.6 Illustration of dural sac cross-sectional area (D-CSA) changes from psoas relaxed position (PRP) to axial compression in slight extension (ACE) in all 80 disc sites in the basic patient material investigated by kinematic MRI. For each disc site, the filled square represents the D-CSA value in PRP and the open circle represents the value in ACE. (From Willén, J. et al., Dynamic effects on the lumbar spinal canal. Axial-loaded CT-myelography and MRI in patients with sciatica and/or neurogenic claudication, *Spine*, 22, 2968, 1997. With permission.)

Twenty-six of the 34 patients had a significant reduction of the D-CSA at one or more sites during ACE. In 11 patients (40 disc sites), there was a statistically significant decrease in D-CSA from PRP to ACE, to levels below the suggested critical values for relative (100 mm^2) or absolute (75 mm^2) central stenosis in one or two sites. Additionally, a narrowing of the lateral recess also was found during ACE in 11 patients (13 disc sites). During this kinematic MRI examination, there was typically a bulging of the disc, thickening of the ligamentum flavum, a changed pattern of the dorsal fat pad, resulting in a deformation of the dural sac and the nerve root(s) at the level of the disc and or lateral recess (Figure 2.7). Narrowing of the lateral recess and the intervertebral foramina and deformation of the nerve roots could be estimated but not measured (Figures 2.8 and 2.9).

The findings in this study suggested that an axial-loaded, supine kinematic MRI examination (ACE) should be performed when the cross-sectional area of the dural sac (D-CSA) in any disc level is below 130 mm^2 in the traditional psoas relaxed position (PRP), or when there is a suspected narrow lateral recess with or without deformation of the anterolateral part of the dural sac or the nerve roots in PRP. Thus, these constitute the so-called "*inclusion criteria*" for the ACE examination.

2. Expanded Patient Findings

When 122 patients were included in the study, a new analysis was performed with an emphasis on the pre-examination clinical diagnosis.[19] The patients were categorized into one of three groups: group 1, classic neurogenic claudication (36 patients); group 2, sciatica showing a clinical picture of rhizopathy (57 patients); and group 3, low back pain with or without referred pain to the lower extremities (29 patients). Existence of a significant reduction of the D-CSA (>15 mm^2) to areas below 75 mm^2 (the borderline value for absolute spinal stenosis)[15] from PRP to ACE or a suspected disc herniation, lateral recess, foraminal stenosis, intraspinal synovial cyst changing to be indisputable from PRP to ACE was regarded as significant information (positive result) of the examination (Figure 2.10).

In 65% of the 36 patients with a history of neurogenic claudication (group 1), positive findings were found, thereby guiding treatment decisions. All of these patients had one to three disc levels with a D-CSA value below 130 mm^2 during PRP.

In the patients with sciatica (group 2), 20 of the 57 patients had a D-CSA value below 130 mm^2 in at least one disc level, or a suspicion of a nerve root compression during PRP. In 50% of these patients, the inclusion criteria for the ACE examination was met. Notably, there was a subsequent positive finding in each of these cases.

However, in the 29 patients with low back pain (group 3), with or without referred pain, there were no positive findings. Thus, these patient studies showed that it is reasonable to recommend a value of 130 mm^2 as a borderline D-CSA value in any disc level in the lumbar spine for a decision to be made to perform a kinematic MRI examination of the lumbar spine using the ACE technique.

VI. ADVANTAGES OF THE USE OF KINEMATIC MRI IN THE EVALUATION OF LUMBAR SPINE DISORDERS

Myelographic examination of the lumbar spine in a standing position, with flexion and extension movements, is a well-established diagnostic procedure for evaluating the patient with suspected narrowing of the spinal canal. It is well documented that a narrowing of the spinal canal is provoked with axial loading and especially in combination with extension of the spine.[6,12]

Since the advent of MRI, this noninvasive technique has replaced myelography in most cases, mainly because of its superior capabilities to analyze the content of the spinal canal in detail. However, to date, most MRI examinations have been performed in a supine psoas relaxed position, which causes unloading of the spine and enlargement of the canal. Thus, certain encroachments of the canal may be undetected.

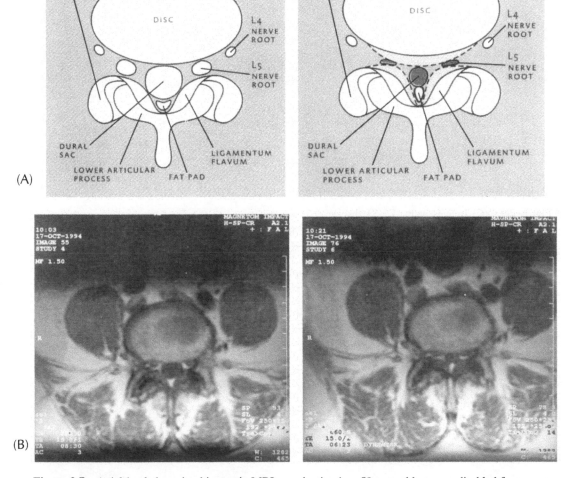

Figure 2.7   Axial-loaded, supine kinematic MRI examination in a 50-year-old woman disabled from neurogenic claudication but without a radiologic diagnosis before the study. Structural changes in and adjacent to the lumbar spinal canal in disc level from psoas relaxed position (PRP) to axial compression in slight extension (ACE) are illustrated by: (A) schematic with explanatory text, right and left; (B) images showing the changes at disc level L4-L5 from PRP to ACE. Note that the dural sac cross-sectional area (D-CSA) is extensively decreased and that the nerve roots are flattened due to the bulging disc, the thickening of the ligamentum flavum, and the changed configuration of the dorsal fat pad at ACE (*note:* PRP, left; ACE, right).

In spite of the on-going development of MR systems, including the so-called vertically opened MR system, substantial problems still remain when attempting to perform examinations in an upright standing or even supine position. Notably, a technique has been developed to assess patients in an upright, seated position described in detail in this textbook (see Chapter 3, Kinematic MRI of the Lumbar Spine: Assessment in the Upright, Seated Position).

Asymptomatic patients are usually able to sit motionless during the examination and it is possible to measure the cross-sectional area of the spinal canal and the foramina with good precision and accuracy.[2] However, examination in a seated position may not be comparable with an upright standing position because the psoas muscle does not affect the lumbar spine in the same way. In other words the lumbar spine tends to flex in the seated position, which enlarges the spinal canal.

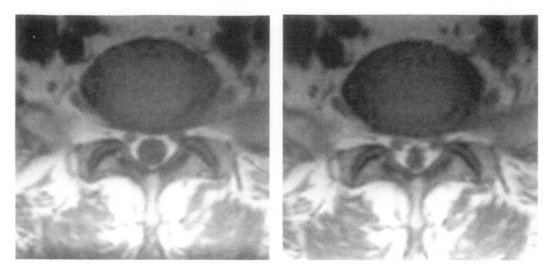

Figure 2.7   (C) Images at the L5-S1 disc level showing changes of the dural configuration and size, but without any sign of nerve root compression (*note:* PRP, left; ACE, right).

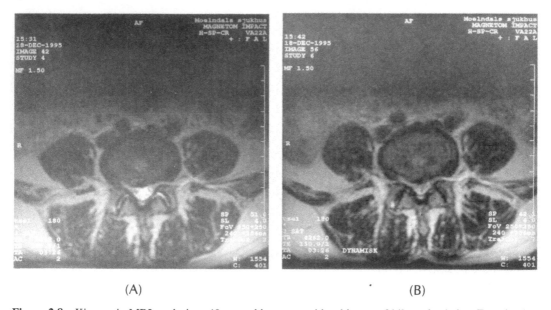

(A)   (B)

Figure 2.8   Kinematic MRI study in a 40-year-old woman with a history of bilateral sciatica. Examination in psoas relaxed position (A) did not show any nerve root compression but in axial loading (B) the dural sac cross-sectional area decreased to 55 mm^2, causing narrowing of the lateral recesses at the L4-L5 level, resulting in pressure on the L5 nerve roots, explaining the patient's pain. (From Willén, J. et al., Dynamic effects on the lumbar spinal canal. Axial-loaded CT-myelography and MRI in patients with sciatica and/or neurogenic claudication, *Spine*, 22, 2968, 1997. With permission.)

In patients with low back pain and sciatica, the overall examination time causes pain, resulting in motion artifacts and difficulties in reproducing the patient position between sequences. Furthermore, examinations in symptomatic individuals have, so far, been performed using only sagittal plane, T2-weighted fast spin echo pulse sequences, not axial plane imaging. The sagittal diameter of the spinal canal can be measured reliably using positional MR imaging.[11] However, according to studies by Schönström et al.,[3-5] the cross-sectional area was more relevant for assessment of the

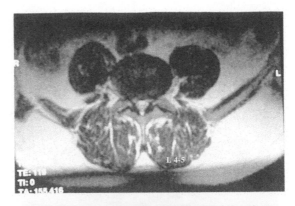

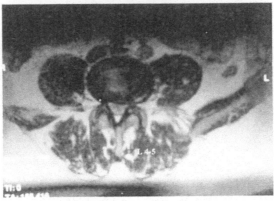

Figure 2.9   Kinematic MRI examination of a woman with L5 neurogenic claudication. There is a decrease in the dural sac cross-sectional area (D-CSA) from psoas relaxed position (PRP) (top) to axial compression in slight extension (ACE) (bottom), with narrowing of the lateral recesses bilaterally at the L4-L5 disc level.

degree of spinal canal stenosis than the sagittal diameter alone. Additionally, differences in foraminal size between flexion and extension were less pronounced in the study on symptomatic patients[11] than in the study on asymptomatic patients.[2]

A drawback in the assessment of the intervertebral foramen was that the sections (5 mm) and intersection gaps (1.5 mm) were relatively thick. However, it is worthwhile noting that there were impressive changes in foraminal size from flexion to extension in some patients, which supports the results by Nowicki et al.,[16] who evaluated human section material using CT and MR in different lumbar spine positions.

As previously mentioned, from our experience, the best results using a kinematic MRI procedure were seen during ACE of the lumbar spine in patients with neurogenic claudication (clinical signs of spinal stenosis). Valuable information from the therapeutic point of view was found in 65% of the 36 patients examined.[19] In the 57 patients with sciatica, only 10 patients showed valuable information at ACE if the inclusion criteria for MR imaging in ACE were not followed. On the contrary, if the inclusion criteria for axial-loaded, supine kinematic MRI were followed, this figure increased to 50% for diagnostic information.

Regarding examination in patients with chronic low back pain with clinical referred pain to the lower extremities, we have not found any reason to continue with an axial-loaded, supine kinematic MRI examination. The message of this study[19] is that it is important to select the correct patients for kinematic examinations to achieve satisfactory results.

Porter and Ward[20] stated in a CT-myelographic study on patients with neurogenic claudication that this disorder is often associated with stenosis of at least two disc sites. This might be multilevel central stenosis or a combination of central, lateral, or foraminal stenosis. Hamanishi et al.,[21] after a CT study

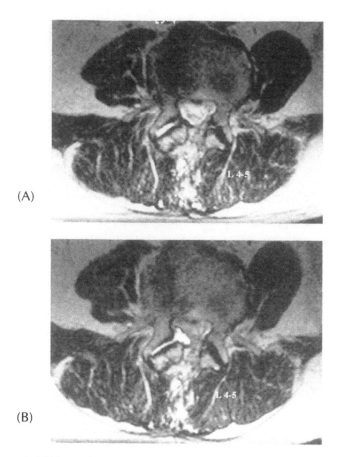

(A)

(B)

Figure 2.10   Kinematic MRI examination performed in an elderly male patient. This patient had a previous surgical procedure for spinal stenosis at the L3-L5 disc levels with a good result. After two years, he experienced a severe L4 rhizopathy at the ventral part of his right thigh. Examination in a relaxed position (A) did not reveal any pathology, but during axial loading (B), a large synovial cyst appeared to bulge from the right facet joint into the spinal canal, explaining the origin of the patient's painful symptoms.

on patients with intermittent claudication considered double lesions with D-CSA values below 100 mm^2 to be a critical factor in the development of this condition. Several experimental studies support the opinion that double level stenosis impairs local nerve blood flow and nerve impulse propagation.[22,23]

In our basic patient study,[15,24] 30% of patients showed a significant decrease of the D-CSA below 100 mm^2 at more than one disc level at ACE. Thus, it is of great importance that all possible stenotic levels are evaluated in every patient. According to our experience it is essential to load the lumbar spine with 40 to 50% of the body weight to get as much as possible out of the examination. This is shown in our study on healthy subjects.[17]

Results of studies on the effects of axial loading on the lumbar spine in asymptomatic, healthy individuals are important to compare with the results achieved in symptomatic patients. In our data on asymptomatic individuals in different age groups, the D-CSA values varied extensively between individuals and disc sites.[17] When comparing the decreases of D-CSA to below 100 mm^2 during ACE, more frequent findings were evident in the symptomatic than in the asymptomatic group (Figures 2.4 and 2.6). Among the asymptomatic individuals very few D-CSA values below 75 mm^2 were found during ACE. No clinical signs of nerve root compression were reported. A prerequisite to perform an MRI examination is a suspected pathologic condition. Of course, an "abnormal" finding of any kind at a radiologic examination has to be correlated to the patient history and the objective findings before making the decision to institute a treatment.[25]

VII. SUMMARY AND CONCLUSIONS

According to present experience, there is a considerable risk of failing to detect an essential narrowing of the spinal canal if only the traditional psoas muscle, relaxed position examination is performed. This is especially true when examining patients with clinical signs of neurogenic claudication. A severe stenosis at one location should not exclude further attempts to investigate the surrounding disc levels carefully, including the evaluation of nerve roots in the lateral recess and in the foramina.

Examination of the lumbar spine in the extended position alone will improve the diagnostic specificity to a certain extent and may be used in elderly people or in patients with clinical signs of osteoporosis. By adding the axial-loaded, supine kinematic MRI examination to the standard investigation, the quality of the preoperative evaluation will be improved. Finally, every MRI examination should begin with a standard investigation to avoid loading on a spine with a malignant disease. The presence of malignancy constitutes a contraindication for the axial-loaded, supine kinematic MRI examination.

To conclude, based on our extensive experience with this procedure, we recommend that the axial-loaded, kinematic MRI examination of the lumbar spine be performed in patients with: (1) neurogenic claudication; (2) sciatica (i.e., if D-CSA in any level is below 130 mm²); (3) suspected disc herniation, narrow lateral recess or foraminal stenosis; and (4) suspected synovial cyst.

REFERENCES

1. Schönström, N. S. R., Lindahl, S., Willén, J. et al., Dynamic changes in the dimensions of the lumbar spinal canal. An experimental study in vitro, *J. Orthop. Res.*, 7, 115, 1989.
2. Schmid, M. R., Stucki, G., Duewell, S. et al., Changes in cross-sectional measurements of the spinal canal and intervertebral foramina as a function of body position: in vivo studies on an open-configuration MR system, *Am. J. Roentgenol.*, 172, 1095, 1999.
3. Schönström, N. S. R., Bolender, N. F., and Spengler, D., Pressure changes within the cauda equina following constriction of the dural sac, *Spine*, 9, 604, 1984.
4. Schönström, N. S. R. and Hansson, T., Pressure changes following constriction of the cauda equina. An experimental study in situ, *Spine*, 13, 385, 1988.
5. Schönström, N. S. R., Bolender, N. F., and Spengler, D. M., The pathomorphology of spinal stenosis as seen on CT-scans of the lumbar spine, *Spine*, 10, 806, 1985.
6. Sortland, O., Magnaes, B., and Hauge, T., Functional myelography with metrizamide in the diagnosis of lumbar spinal stenosis, *Acta Radiol. Suppl.*, 355, 42, 1977.
7. Penning, L. and Wilmink, J. T., Biomechanics of the lumbosacral dural sac. A study of flexion-extension myelography, *Spine*, 6, 398, 1981.
8. Penning, L. and Wilmink, J. T., Posture-dependent bilateral compression of L4 and L5 nerve roots in facet hypertrophy. A dynamic CT-myelographic study, *Spine*, 12, 488, 1987.
9. Schönström, N. S. R. and Hansson, T. H., Thickness of the human ligamentum flavum as a function of load. An in vitro experimental study, *Clin. Biomechanics*, 6, 19, 1991.
10. Anderson, G. B. J. and McNeill, T. W., *Lumbar Spine Syndromes*, Springer Verlag, Vienna, 1989.
11. Wildermuth, S., Zanetti, M., Duewell S. et al., Lumbar spine: quantitative and qualitative assessment of positional (upright flexion and extension) MR imaging and myelography, *Radiology*, 207, 391, 1998.
12. Schumacher, M., Die Belastungsmyelographie, *Fortschr. Röntgenstr.*, 145, 642, 1986
13. Harvey, S. B., Measurement of lumbar spine flexion-extension using low-field open-magnet magnetic resonance scanner, *Invest. Radiol.*, 33, 439, 1998.
14. Nachemson, A. and Elfström, G., Intravital dynamic pressure measurements in lumbar discs. A study on common movements, maneuvers and exercises, *Scand. J. Rehabil. Med. Suppl.*, 1, 1, 1970.
15. Willén, J., Danielson, B., Gaulitz, A. et al., Dynamic effects on the lumbar spinal canal. Axially loaded CT-myelography and MRI in patients with sciatica and/or neurogenic claudication, *Spine*, 22, 2968, 1997.

16. Nowicki, B. H., Haughton, V. M., Schmidt, T. A. et al., Occult lumbar lateral spinal stenosis in neural foramina subjected to physiologic loading, *Am. J. Neuroradiol.,* 17, 1605, 1996.

17. Danielson, B., Axial loading of the lumbar spine in MRI. A study on healthy subjects, *Acta Radiol.,* in press.

18. Amundsen, T., Weber, H., Lilleås, F. et al., Lumbar spinal stenosis. Clinical and radiological features, *Spine,* 20, 1178, 1995.

19. Willén, J. and Danielson, B., The diagnostic effect of axial loading of the lumbar spine during CT and MRI in patients with low back pain, sciatica and neurogenic claudication, *Spine,* in press.

20. Porter, R. and Ward, D., Cauda equina dysfunction. The significance of two-level pathology, *Spine,* 17, 9, 1992.

21. Hamanishi, C., Matukura, N., and Fujita, M., Cross-sectional area of the stenotic lumbar dural tube measured from the transverse views of magnetic resonance imaging, *J. Spinal Disord.,* 7, 388, 1994.

22. Olmarker, K., Spinal nerve root compression. Nutrition and function of the porcine cauda equina compressed in vivo, *Acta Orthop. Scand. Suppl.,* 242, 1, 1991.

23. Takahashi, K., Olmarker, K., Holm, S. et al., Double level cauda equina compression: an experimental study with continuous monitoring of intraneural blood flow in the porcine cauda equina, *J. Orthop. Res.,* 11, 104, 1993.

24. Danielson, B. I., Willén J., Gaulitz, A. et al., Axial loading of the spine during CT and MR in patients with suspected lumbar spinal stenosis, *Acta Radiol.,* 39, 604, 1998.

25. Schönström, N. and Willén, J., Imaging lumbar stenosis, *Radiol. Clin. North Am.,* in press.

26. Lee, S. U., Personal communication.

3 Kinematic MRI of the Lumbar Spine: Assessment in the Upright, Seated Position

Dominik Weishaupt, Simon Wildermuth, Marius R. Schmid, and Juerg Hodler

CONTENTS

I. INTRODUCTION

Magnetic resonance imaging (MRI) has become a standard of reference in the evaluation of patients with low back pain, with or without sciatica.[1,2] Abnormalities of intervertebral disks, including their biochemical status,[3] bone marrow changes in adjacent vertebral endplates,[4,5] facet joint osteoarthritis,[6] as well as the degree of spinal canal and foraminal stenosis caused by various abnormalities can be evaluated using MRI.

So far, MRI of the lumbar spine is performed routinely in supine, neutral position without loading of the lumbosacral spine. The closed, cylindrical configuration of conventional MR systems limits patient position to the horizontal plane. Thus, spinal motion during diagnostic imaging is not possible or only to a very limited degree (e.g., by placing a cushion underneath the lumbar spine to increase lordosis or to provoke rotation).[7]

However, clinical data indicate that a change in body position or certain physical activities may significantly alter symptoms in patients with low back pain. Such effects may relate to axial loading of the spine as it occurs during standing upright, with or without carrying weight, or in the sitting position. Patients with spinal stenosis commonly complain about increasing symptoms during standing upright, walking, and occasionally during sitting or forward lumbar flexion.[8-10]

Previously published biomechanical studies using mostly lumbar cadaveric spine specimens have documented a decrease in spinal canal (or dural sac) cross-sectional area and spinal foraminal dimensions with axial loading, as well as with flexion and extension.[11-16] Using a cadaveric spine model,

0-8493-0807-0/01/$0.00+$.50
© 2001 by Frank G. Shellock

Nowicki et al.[15] reported that flexion and extension, lateral bending, and axial rotation significantly changed the anatomic relationships of the ligamentum flavum and intervertebral disk to the spinal nerve roots in the lumbar spine. The investigators referred to compression of the spinal canal or spinal nerve roots occurring exclusively during axial load and/or spinal motion as "dynamic stenosis."[15]

Based on these data, clinically relevant spinal canal and foraminal stenosis, as well as the degree of nerve root compression, may not be demonstrated on conventional MR systems with the patient in the supine position. In consideration of this, some spinal surgeons still prefer myelography, which allows the ability to obtain so-called "functional images" of the lumbar spine in upright flexion and extension.[17] However, myelography is an invasive test, which is commonly associated with transient side effects such as back pain or headache. Moreover, it is associated with high costs and exposes the patient to ionizing radiation. Therefore, the use of myelography is restricted to selected patients[17] and may be used in preoperative planning in the presence of MR contraindications (i.e., pacemaker, neurostimulators, etc.), severe scoliosis, and/or after surgery with ferromagnetic spinal implants.

Several attempts have been undertaken to overcome the limitations of conventional MR imaging of the spine. For example, Willén et al.[18] have described a portable device allowing for axial-loaded spinal imaging in conventional MR or computed tomography (CT) scanners (see Chapter 2). However, kinematic studies in flexion and extension are still limited by the dimensions of the magnet bore.[19]

Specially designed, open-configuration MR systems permit kinematic MRI examinations to be conducted on the lumbar spine. The double-doughnut, vertically opened MR system designed for interventional MR imaging is especially well suited for kinematic MRI because it has a vertical gap between the magnets, allowing imaging of the patient in an axial-loaded, upright, seated position.[20-22] Recent studies[7,23-28] have shown the feasibility and clinical applications of kinematic MRI of the lumbar spine, as discussed later in this chapter.

This chapter outlines the basic principles and clinical applications of kinematic MRI of the lumbar spine, with an emphasis on imaging in the upright, seated position. The first section provides some background information and addresses the technical prerequisites of kinematic MRI. The introductory section is followed by a discussion of position-dependent changes of the cross-sectional area of the spinal canal and the neuroforamina in normal volunteers. The next section compares kinematic MRI to myelography. In addition, the clinical applications of kinematic MRI of the lumbar spine in patients with low back pain will be discussed. Finally, directions for future research will be presented.

II. TECHNICAL ASPECTS

A. THE MAGNETIC RESONANCE SYSTEM

The most important prerequisite for the performance of a loaded, kinematic MRI examination of the lumbar spine is the availability of a vertically opened MR system that has sufficient space to perform spinal movements. Several different open-configured MR systems have been developed that are used mainly for interventional procedures and intraoperative guidance.[20-22] Open-configuration magnets sacrifice magnetic energy efficiency when compared with closed MR systems. Magnet openings disrupt magnetic flow through the field, resulting in field inhomogeneity. As the static magnetic field increases, this problem becomes more prominent, requiring increasing magnet size, weight, and costs. For this reason open MR systems typically operate at low-field and mid-field strengths up to 0.7 Tesla (although a horizontally open 1.0 T MR system has recently become available from Siemens Medical Systems, Iselin, NJ).

Different types of magnets have been used for open-configured MR systems, including permanent, resistive, and superconducting magnets. Open-configured systems with permanent or resistive magnets have a vertically oriented field between horizontal facing poles. Such designs provide a

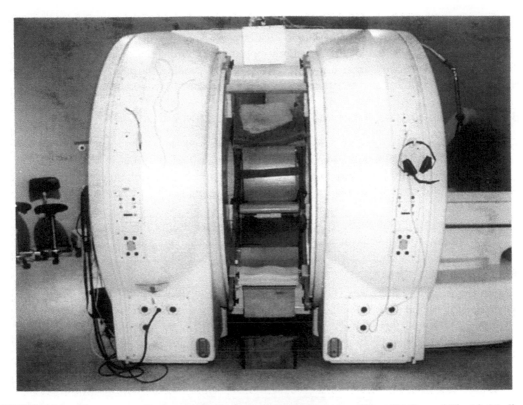

FIGURE 3.1 The superconducting, vertically opened, 0.5 T MR system (Signa SP, General Electric Medical Systems, Milwaukee, WI). Note the chair positioned between this "double-donut" used for kinematic MRI examination of the patient in the upright, seated position.

horizontally oriented gap between the pole faces of approximately 35 cm. This design, using permanent and resistive magnets, is adequate for MR-guided interventional procedures. They have also been employed in kinematic MRI studies of the lumbar spine. Flexion and extension images can be obtained in a lateral decubitus position.[25,26] Obviously, kinematic MRI examinations in upright loaded conditions are not possible using these particular types of MR systems.

The Signa SP (General Electric Medical Systems, Milwaukee, WI) is the first MR system specifically designed for intraoperative MR procedures (Figure 3.1). This MR system has a vertically oriented opening that allows the patient to sit upright and still flex, extend, or rotate the lumbar spine. The static magnetic field strength for this superconducting MR system is 0.5 Tesla, which is higher than that of competing, horizontally open systems with permanent and resistive magnets (typically 0.05 to 0.23 Tesla). Notably, the signal-to-noise ratio of MR systems increases linearly with field strength, providing higher spatial resolution and high temporal resolution.[29] These important aspects of imaging are crucial for MRI examinations of the critical anatomic structures of the lumbar spine.[29]

The superconducting Signa SP magnet is designed with two split coils sharing interconnected cryostats, separated by a 56 cm gap at the center of the magnet. Each of the coaxial split coils produces a 1.5 Tesla magnet field at each isocenter and a 0.5 Tesla magnetic field at the center used for imaging the patient. This design achieves a spherical imaging volume with a 30 cm diameter located coaxially with the two split coils and halfway between them, so that no magnet structure is located in the immediate vicinity of the imaging volume. Due to the diverging field lines at the coil extremities, a split-coil design cannot produce a magnetic field as homogeneous at the position of the patient, as that of a single-coil magnet. Nevertheless, the field homogeneity over the volume of interest is acceptable for MRI examinations.

To prevent collapse of the MR system, strong structural supports are required. There are horizontal supports positioned at the top and the bottom of the magnet, in positions as peripheral as possible. In this configuration, the structural supports are above and below the patient and permit the patient to stand easily in an upright position (i.e., depending on patient height, of course). However, the patient can also be examined in an upright, seated position.

B. Positioning Devices, Techniques, and Radiofrequency Coils

The patient table of the Signa SP MR system can be removed, and a chair can be installed in the gap between the two split coils. Since the two supports at the top and at the bottom of the MR system are sufficiently far from the isocenter of the magnet, it is possible to comfortably perform kinematic MRI of the lumbar spine in seated patients weighing up to 100 kg with a body height of up to 1.9 m.[20]

A chair used for the kinematic MRI procedure can be made from either wood, polyvinyl chloride (PVC), or other nonmagnetic materials (Figure 3.2). Such chairs may be brought into stable, incremented positions using special support mechanisms fastened to the inner surfaces of the two magnets of the MR system.

The chair used for kinematic MRI must be adjustable in height to properly position the lumbar spine of the patient at the isocenter of the MR system (i.e., adjustable based on the size of the patient). The vertical back support of the chair should also be adjustable to accommodate different types of patients and to enable different degrees of spinal extension. A noncompressible cushion is commonly placed posterior to the back for extension studies (Figure 3.3).

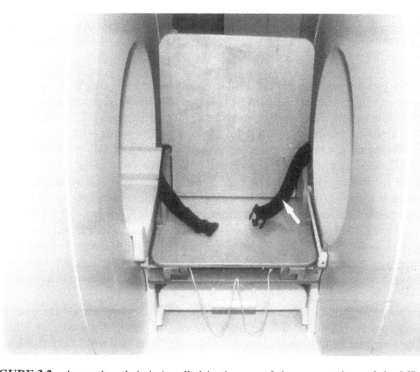

FIGURE 3.2 A wooden chair is installed in the gap of the magnet rings of the MR system to perform kinematic MRI examinations of the lumbar spine of the patient in the upright, seated position. The patient sits on the chair and the pelvis is fixed with a belt (white arrow). (From Wildermuth, S. et al., *Radiology,* 207, 391–398, 1998. With permission.)

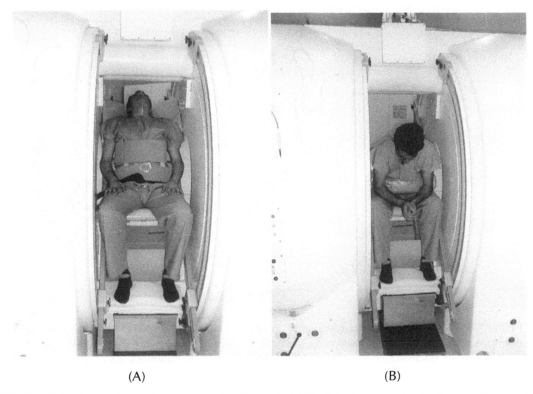

(A)　　　　　　　　　　　　　　　　　(B)

FIGURE 3.3　Positioning techniques used for kinematic MRI of the lumbar spine in the upright, seated position. (A) Subject in the upright, seated extended position. (B) Subject in the upright, seated flexed position. Note the subject is bending over a cushion placed on top of the thighs.

For kinematic MRI in seated, flexed positions, a noncompressible cushion is placed on the patient's legs, over which the body is bent. For this purpose, a commercially available neck pillow is used. This technique is relatively comfortable for the patient. Additionally, it not only leads to consistent increments of flexion positions, but also decreases motion artifacts during the kinematic MRI examination. Based on discussions with spine surgeons interested in biomechanical studies, our group decided to equip the chair with a belt that fixes the pelvis to the chair. This is especially important for kinematic MRI examinations performed during spine extension, because it prevents the patient from slipping anteriorly (Figure 3.3).

Standard radiofrequency (RF) coils typically used for conventional MR systems cannot be used easily for kinematic MRI studies in the Signa SP MR system because their design is too rigid. In addition, these RF coils do not follow the anatomic shape and changes that occur during spinal movements.

For interventional MR procedures, flexible rectangular wrap-around surface coils have been specifically developed (Figure 3.4). Fortunately, these RF coils also can be used for kinematic MRI studies of the lumbar spine. The coil has the form of a butterfly with two connected loops or wings and operates in the transmit and receive mode. The flexible design of the coil allows it to follow the anatomic contours of the patient's back during flexion or extension motion of the lumbar spine. Thus, uniform signal intensity is achieved in the region of interest during the kinematic MRI examination. Kinematic MRI of the lumbar spine also may be performed using a transmit and receive RF coil that is built into the vertical back support of the chair (i.e., installed in the gap between the magnet rings).[20] This design also permits imaging of the lumbar spine in the upright, seated position in different increments of extension and flexion.

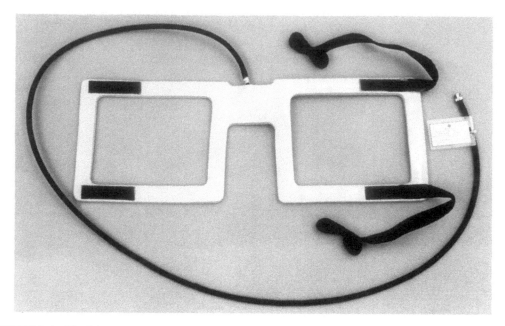

FIGURE 3.4   Flexible transmit and receive RF surface coil used with the Signa SP MR system. The two flexible wings of the coil are placed on the two opposite sides of the body to facilitate MRI of the lumbar spine during the kinematic examination. (From Wildermuth, S. et al., *Radiology,* 207, 391–398, 1998. With permission.)

C. IMAGING PARAMETERS AND PROTOCOL

The protocol for kinematic MRI of the lumbar spine includes image acquisition in the upright, seated, neutral, flexed, and extended positions (Figure 3.3). Alternatively, kinematic MRI may be limited to the seated flexion and extension because the neutral position does not add relevant information in many situations.[27]

The imaging sequences required to obtain sufficient image quality for the diagnostic assessment of the lumbar spine are relatively long (e.g., 5 minutes). This relates to the fact that small structures, such as the facet joints of the lumbar spine, must be imaged with reasonable resolution. Such examination times typically do not allow for acquisition of more than 3 to 6 pulse sequences in patients suffering from pain.

When both sagittal and axial images are needed (which is commonly required for thorough MR imaging of the lumbar spine), the number of available spinal positions is limited. To our knowledge, kinematic MRI examinations with multiple images obtained in many different positions have not been performed in the lumbar spine. However, such kinematic MRI examinations have been performed on other joints using incremental, passive-movement and active-movement, kinematic MRI techniques.[30]

It should be realized that, even with an examination limited to few positions of the spine, patients may report increased symptoms in the upright, seated position and, therefore, may not be willing or able to permit imaging at maximal ranges of motion. Even without maximum extension or flexion spinal movements, there may be increasing pain during the kinematic MRI examination and motion artifacts are not uncommon during acquisition of MR images in the upright, seated position.

The use of the following protocol for the kinematic MRI examination of the lumbar spine in the upright, seated position is recommended:

1. A standard, fast gradient echo pulse sequence is used to acquire images to verify the correct position of the RF surface coil. MR images are obtained in both the sagittal and axial planes.
2. A sagittal plane, T2-weighted, fast spin-echo pulse sequence with an echo train length of 12 has proved to represent a reasonable compromise between image quality, image contrast, imaging time, and motion artifacts. The repetition time (TR) used at our institution is typically 3000 to 4000 msec; the echo time (TE) is 90 to 100 msec; the field-of-view (FOV) is 20 to 22 cm; the section thickness is 4 to 5 mm with an intersection gap of 0.5 mm. Four excitations (NEX) are used with a matrix size of 256×192. On the sagittal plane images obtained with these parameters, the entire lumbar spine, including the conus medullaris, can be evaluated.
3. In addition, "angled" (i.e., relative to the spinal anatomy) axial plane, T2-weighted fast-spin echo images are acquired at all abnormal intervertebral levels. For this pulse sequence a FOV of 20 cm, a section thickness of 4 mm with an intersection gap of 0.5 mm, and a matrix size of 256×192 are used.

T1-weighted images are not routinely used for the kinematic MRI examination because any potential additional information is offset by the increased examination time. The MR image acquisition time for the aforementioned pulse sequences is approximately 5 minutes. In our experience, most patients are able to comply with this imaging protocol when asked to assume extended and flexed body positions.

The evaluation of the kinematic MRI study commonly requires transferring the images to a workstation to allow precise, quantitative measurements to be obtained, because qualitative morphological parameters commonly do not change in an impressive manner. Additionally, qualitative techniques are not precise enough for formal evaluations required in a research setting.

Commonly used quantitative parameters for characterization of the spine include the measurement of the cross-sectional area of the dural sac, which is measured on a transverse angled section through the central part of the disk. Sagittal and transverse diameters of the dural sac have also been evaluated on angled axial images, as well as diameters of the lateral recess and the foramen. Our group prefers to measure foraminal size on sagittal images, which best represent this anatomic structure.[27]

Qualitative evaluations have been applied to disk abnormalities,[28] degree of nerve root compromise,[28] facet joint osteoarthritis,[28,31] and foraminal size.[23,28] For assessment of foraminal size, our group uses a four point scoring system. A score of 1 is defined as normal (normal dorsolateral border of the disk and normal form of the intervertebral epidural fat [oval or inverted pear shape]); a score of 2 is defined as slight foraminal stenosis (slight foraminal stenosis and deformity of the epidural fat); and a score of 3 is defined as marked foraminal stenosis (epidural fat only partially surrounding the nerve root). Finally, a score of 4 is defined as advanced stenosis with complete obliteration of the foraminal epidural fat. This scoring system has been shown to provide good interobserver agreement.[23]

III. KINEMATIC MRI FINDINGS IN NORMAL SUBJECTS

To properly analyze kinematic MRI examinations obtained in patients with low back pain, exact knowledge of physiological changes of the spinal canal and foraminal size in healthy subjects is important. Different methods, usually based on cadaveric models, have been used to assess physiological findings. Most of these studies were performed using either CT and/or MR imaging.[11-16] Other work was based on assessments using either conventional radiographs or myelograms.[32] Furthermore, some investigations were simply limited to biomechanical methods without radiological correlation.[33,34]

Understandably, the results from such cadaveric studies may not easily be applied to living subjects. For example, muscles and other surrounding soft tissue structures are dissected in cadaveric studies and axial loading is either absent or simulated by a compression device. This may result in an overestimation of position-dependent changes of the neuroforamina and spinal canal.

Quint et al.[33] evaluated the effect of either present or absent intersegmental agonist and antagonist muscles using a cadaveric model. Notably, the investigators reported a decreased range of motion in the cadaveric spine with muscle simulation compared with an identical model without muscle simulation.

To date, there has been limited experience with the *in vivo* use of kinematic MRI of the lumbar spine in healthy volunteers.[7,19,24,26,27] Kinematic MRI examinations of healthy subjects have been performed using conventional[7,19] or open-configured MR systems.[24,26,27] For example, Fennell et al.[19] reported migration of the nucleus pulposus within the intervertebral disc during flexion and extension of the lumbar spine.

The variability of range of motion in healthy volunteers with regard to flexion and extension movements has been demonstrated by Harvey et al.[26] Using an open-configured, low-field-strength MR system with horizontal access, these investigators found a large variability in the motion of the lumbar spine, as measured on sagittal plane MR images. Furthermore, there was a significant correlation between age and the range of motion in flexion and extension of the spine, indicating a progressive reduction in spinal motion with advancing age.

Schmid et al.[27] evaluated the physiologic changes of the cross-sectional area of the spinal canal and neural foramina *in vivo*. A group of young healthy volunteers (n = 12, age range 19 to 33 years) was included in the investigation. All examinations were performed on a superconducting Signa SP MR system using the flexible transmit-receive surface coil as described above. T2-weighted, fast spin-echo sequences were acquired in the sagittal and angled axial planes. The angled axial T2-weighted sequence was restricted to the L4-L5 level. Both sequences were repeated in different positions, as follows: upright, seated neutral; upright, seated flexed; upright, seated extended; and supine extended.

The cross-sectional area of the spinal canal was measured on the angled axial images at the level of the disk using an electronic caliper. A second measurement was obtained at the level of the L4 pedicle. At this level, the diameter of the spinal canal is exclusively determined by bony landmarks and is not influenced by body position. Therefore, such measurements were used as an internal control. The cross-sectional area of the neural foramina was measured on the sagittal plane images.

In this study,[27] the cross-sectional area of the spinal canal decreased 16.4% from the upright, seated flexed position to the upright, seated extended positon (268 to 224 mm², $p < 0.0001$).[27] In addition, statistically significant differences were found comparing the upright, seated neutral, extended position to the supine, extended position. A major factor contributing to the decrease of the cross-sectional area of the spinal canal in the upright, seated extended position was an increase in thickness of the ligamentum flavum (Figure 3.5). The mean thickness of the ligamentum flavum increased from 1.8 mm in the upright, seated flexed position to 4.3 mm in the upright, seated extended position ($p < 0.001$). Ligamentum flavum thickness values for both of the other positions were between these two values (upright, seated neutral position, 2.3 mm; supine extended position, 3.3 mm).

The ligamentum flavum is a segmentally organized structure that connects the vertebral laminae. Fibers that are oriented almost perpendicularly attach to the lower anterior surface of the lamina and the posterior surface of the lamina below.[35] The ligamentum flavum blends with the capsule of the facet joints. Dorsally, the ligamenta flava connect to the ligamenta interspinalia.[36]

The results of the aforementioned study of Schmid et al.[27] suggested that the ligamenta flava reduces the cross-sectional area of the spinal canal during upright or supine extension. The ligamentum flavum buckles during extension, presumably as a result of a decrease in the vertical distance between the adjacent laminae.

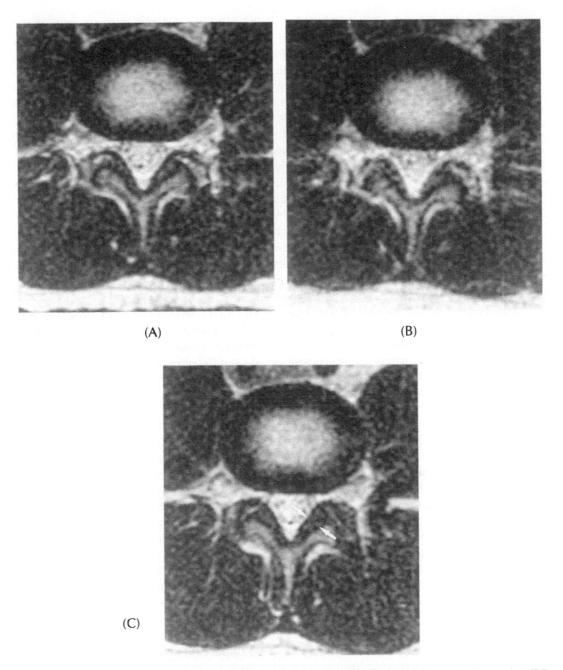

(A)   (B)

(C)

FIGURE 3.5 Angled, axial plane, T2-weighted fast spin-echo (TR/TE, 3000/102 msec) kinematic MRI examination at the L4-L5 disk level of a 26-year-old male volunteer demonstrates the influence of different body positions on the ligamentum flavum: (A) upright, seated, neutral position; (B) upright, seated, flexed position; (C) upright, seated, extended position. The ligamentum flavum (arrows) is thicker in the upright, seated extended position (C) than in (A) and (B) (mainly on the left side).

Position-dependent changes of the ligamenta flava also have been demonstrated by Chung et al.[7] This group reported results of examinations of asymptomatic volunteers studied in various spinal positions in a conventional MR system. Such findings correlated with the results of a cadaveric study using cryomicrotomy on spines. Tajima and Kawano[37] reported an increased thickness of the human lumbar spine ligamentum flavum during extension.

In a different cadaveric study conducted by Revel et al.[11] the decrease in cross-sectional area of the spinal canal of the lumbar spine caused by folding of the ligamentum flavum was confirmed. In addition, these investigators observed narrowing of the cross-sectional area of the spinal canal by posterior bulging of the intervertebral disk in the extended position.

The position dependence of disk morphology and its contribution to narrowing of the spinal canal also was demonstrated by two other studies using cadaveric spines.[14,16] Although Schmid et al.[27] found no statistically significant reduction of the anteroposterior diameter of the spinal canal in the extended spine position *in vivo*, the contribution of the intervertebral disk to narrowing of the cross-sectional area of the spinal canal appears to be relevant.

Taking into consideration the large proportion of the spinal canal border formed by the disk, even minor disk bulging during extension may decrease the cross-sectional area of the spinal canal and dural sac substantially. Using CT, Schönström et al.[12] found a significant decrease of the cross-sectional area of the spinal canal in extension (16% reduction compared with flexion of the lumbar spine) mainly due to disk bulging in cadaveric lumbar spines. These investigators believed that the ligamentum flavum did not significantly influence the dimension of the spinal canal. However, based on the evidence of the various studies presented above, the reduction of the cross-sectional area of the spinal canal in supine and upright, seated extended positions is a result of both folding of the ligamentum flavum and posterior bulging of the disk.

The diameter of the spinal canal is influenced not only by flexion and extension movements of the spine, but also by axial loading. Schmid et al.[27] measured the cross-sectional area of the spinal canal in both the supine and upright, seated extended positions. They found a slightly smaller cross-sectional area in the upright, seated position. These differences were not statistically significant, but may still indicate that imaging under axial loading may demonstrate additional findings, at least in selected cases.

Willén et al.[18] demonstrated a statistically significant reduction in the cross-sectional area of the dural sac during axial loading in the supine position compared with standard unloaded conditions. This study group consisted of patients with low back pain. Thus, it is possible that axial loading leads to more pronounced morphological changes in symptomatic patients.

The size of the neural foramina also appears to be position dependent. Several cadavaric studies reported that the size of the lumbar neural foramen increases during flexion and decreases during extension positions of the spine.[13,15,16] In the study performed by Schmid et al.,[27] positional changes of the foraminal size in asymptomatic volunteers were evaluated using kinematic MRI. In this study, position-dependent changes in the size of 54 neural foramina were assessed in 20 volunteers.

The lumbar vertebral foramina that were examined were located as follows: L1-L2 (n = 3), L2-L3 (n = 11), L3-L4 (n = 16), L4-L5 (n = 18), and L5-S1 (n = 6). The cross-sectional area of the neural foramen was measured on sagittal plane images using an electronic caliper. With the exception of the L1-L2 segment, in which only a few foramina were available for comparison, statistically significant differences were found between most body positions for most neural foramina. The limited number of available L1-L2 neuroforamina was caused by the fact that, in most volunteers, these foramina were outside or at the edge of the field-of-view determined by the RF surface coil. The mean cross-sectional area for all evaluated neural foramina combined decreased by 35.6% from the upright, seated flexed position (167 mm^2) to the upright, seated extended position (108 mm^2, $p < 0.0001$) (Figure 3.6). The cross-sectional area of the neural foramina in supine, extended position (109 mm^2) was almost identical to the upright, seated extended position. The upright, seated neutral position had a mean value of 140 mm^2.

Several factors may contribute to the position dependence of neural foramina. In the extended position, the intervertebral disk bulges slightly[11,19] and leads to a compression of the anterior border of the neural foramen. In addition, the height of the foramen decreases because of the compression of the posterior part of the intervertebral disk and decreasing distance between the adjacent pedicles. Last, the ligamentum flavum may bulge posteriorly and narrow the opening of the neural foramen.[11]

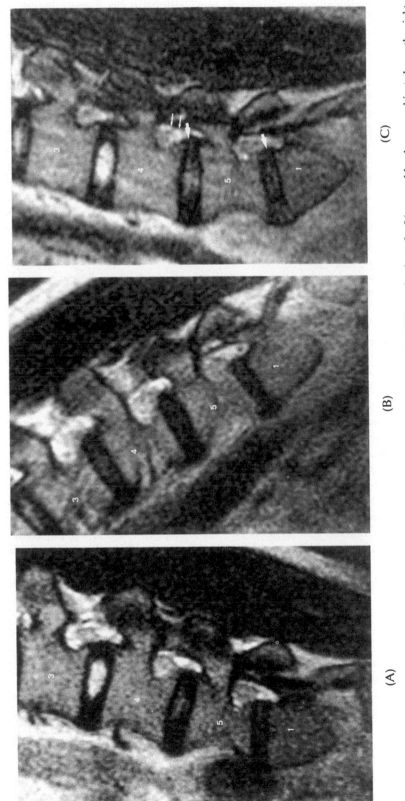

(A)

(B)

(C)

FIGURE 3.6 Sagittal plane, T2-weighted, fast spin-echo (TR/TE, 3000/100 msec) kinematic MRI examination of a 21-year-old volunteer subject shows the right L4-L5 and L5-S1 foramen in different body positions. (A) The upright, seated, neutral position; (B) the upright, seated flexed position; (C) the upright, seated, extended position. There is an increase of foraminal cross-sectional areas of both neuroforamina shown in (B) and (C) compared with that seen in (A). There is a decrease in cross-sectional area of both foramina caused by slightly bulged disks (arrows) and thickening of the ligamenta flava (thin arrows). Numbers indicate the lumbar and sacral vertebrae.

Owing to the multiplanar imaging capabilities of kinematic MRI, the dimensions of the spinal canal may be assessed in the sagittal as well as in the axial planes. However, the relevance of measuring the anteroposterior diameter of the spinal canal in the sagittal plane is not uniformly accepted.

Gepstein et al.[38] examined 594 cervical and lumbar cadaveric vertebral segments from young adults and found a significant correlation between the cross-sectional area and the anteroposterior diameter of the spinal canal. These findings were confirmed by Schönström et al.,[12] who also found an excellent correlation of both parameters in a CT study.

Conversely, Bolender et al.[39] reported that measurement of the anteroposterior diameter was less reliable using CT compared with findings using myelography. The effectiveness of CT was improved when the cross-sectional area of the spinal canal was measured. These investigators further concluded that assessment of spinal canal stenosis using CT is more reliable when based on the cross-sectional area of the spinal canal rather than the anteroposterior diameter. This conclusion is also supported by the findings of Schmid et al.,[27] who reported that physiologic changes of the spinal canal were better detected by measuring the cross-sectional area in the axial plane than by measuring the antero-posterior diameter in the sagittal plane.

To date, the effects of other lumber spinal movements, including lateral bending or axial rotation, have not been examined using upright MRI *in vivo*. Nowicki et al.[15] compared flexion, extension, lateral bending and rotation of frozen cadaveric lumbar spines in patients with a history of only minor spinal symptoms. Surprisingly, flexion and extension or lateral bending did not induce any foraminal stenosis in the presence of apparently healthy disks, disk protrusion, or disk rotation. However, lateral bending of the spine resulted in stenosis of the neural foramen in 30% of the patients.[15]

Chung et al.[7] investigated the influence of rotation on the lumbar spine in asymptomatic volunteers using a conventional closed 1.5 Tesla MR system. Rotation was obtained by using supports placed under one side of the pelvis, and one leg was crossed over the other. In addition, a stabilization belt was tightened around the shoulder to prevent motion. The results of this study indicated that rotation decreases the sagittal plane diameters and the cross-sectional area of the spinal canal.[7] However, foraminal size, as measured by the suparticular diameter on transaxial images, was not influenced by rotation.

In summary, kinematic MRI of the lumbar spine in asymptomatic volunteers allows *in vivo* imaging of position-dependent changes of neural and bony structures of the lumbar spine. Image quality provided by open-configured MR systems is good enough to evaluate the physiologic changes of the spinal canal, dural sac, and neural foramina in various body positions, even under axial loading conditions.

The results of such studies correlate to some of the prior investigations using standard MR systems as well as cadaveric investigations. In asymptomatic volunteers, the upright, seated flexed position of the spine results in an increase in the cross-sectional area of the spinal canal and of the neural foramina.

Conversely, the upright, seated extended position of the lumbar spine results in a decrease in the cross-sectional area of the spinal canal because of an increase in diameter of the ligamentum flavum and additional posterior bulging of the intervertebral disk. The size of the neural foramen decreases in the extended position as a result of decreased interpedicular distance, posterior bulging of the disk, and anterior bulging of the ligamenta flava.

IV. KINEMATIC MRI FINDINGS IN COMPARISON WITH MYELOGRAPHY

Spinal stenosis, acquired or congenital, may involve the central spinal canal, the neural foramen, or the lateral recess.[40,41] In the lumbar spine, spinal stenosis is typically acquired and caused by spondylosis, disk protrusions or extrusions, ligamentous degeneration, spondylolisthesis, or a combination of these disorders. Accurate determination of pathology and exact diagnosis in terms of location, nature, and extent of spinal stenosis is important in preoperative planning for decompressive surgery of the lumbar spine.[42,43]

Both CT and MR imaging show the reduced diameter of the dural sac in spinal stenosis, and the impingement of neural structures secondary to bony and soft tissue changes in the supine position. Nevertheless, some surgeons still prefer to use myelography or CT myelography, especially in the presence of surgical implants, severe scoliosis, or when an important positional component is considered to be present.[17]

Following intrathecal injection of contrast medium, myelography provides excellent depiction of intrathecal structures, especially in combination with CT (CT myelography). Myelography still is preferred by many spinal surgeons for preoperative assessment, because it can easily be compared with intraoperative fluoroscopic and anatomical findings on MR images. In addition, myelography may better identify changes relevant for surgical planning when upright images are obtained (especially in the upright flexion and extension positions).[43,44]

The rationale for the use of myelography with the patient in an upright position is to provoke narrowing of the spinal canal. However, myelography is an invasive procedure and exposes the patient to ionizing radiation. Moreover, myelography may cause significant patient discomfort during and after the examination.[45,46]

The use of the vertically opened Signa SP MR system for assessment of the spine potentially replaces the diagnostic information gained by functional myelography. Recently, Wildermuth et al.[23] performed a study that compared findings of kinematic MRI and myelography of the lumbar spine. In this prospective study design, 30 patients (13 men and 17 women; age range: 27–84 years, mean 58 years) were included. All patients were referred for functional lumbar myelography. Indications for lumbar myelography were preoperative planning in 19 patients (spondylolysis with spondylolisthesis [n = 5], instability [n = 3], and segmental stenosis [n = 11]), persistent symptoms without diagnosis in 4 patients, and difficult postoperative situations in 7 patients (persistent symptoms without diagnosis [n = 4] and recurrent symptoms of segmental stenosis [n = 3]).

Lumbar myelography was performed in a standardized fashion and included radiographs in the lateral decubitus (lateral radiograph), prone (posteroanterior radiograph), and left and right posteroanterior oblique projections. Upright anteroposterior and lateral images were obtained in positions of flexion and extension. Subsequently, all 30 patients underwent kinematic MRI of the lumbar spine using the Signa SP, vertically opened MR system. The imaging protocol for kinematic MRI included a sagittal plane, T2-weighted, fast spin-echo sequence with the patient in the upright, seated neutral position; the upright, seated extended position; and the upright, seated flexed position.

The sagittal diameter of the lumbar dural sac was analyzed on both myelography and kinematic MR images for all five intervertebral levels. Measurement of the sagittal diameter of the dural sac on myelographic images is considered to be a reliable parameter for the diagnostic work-up of central spinal stenosis.[39] On lateral myelographic images the sagittal diameter of the dural sac was measured between the anterior and posterior borders of the dural sac, parallel to the endplate. To compensate for projectional effects, measurements on the myelograms were corrected by a factor of 0.87 and 0.83, respectively, for the upright and lateral supine images (based on the known film-focus distance of 150 and 115 cm, respectively, and assuming a 20 cm distance between the spinal canal and the film in an average patient).

On MR images, measurements of the dural sac were obtained on the image that was closest to the midline. The measurements were obtained on hard copies, using the ruler printed on the film. Although mean measurements obtained from MR images were slightly smaller than those obtained from the myelograms, linear correlation analysis showed a good correlation between the sagittal diameters of the dural sac measured on myelography and those measured on MR imaging for all different body positions (Figure 3.7).

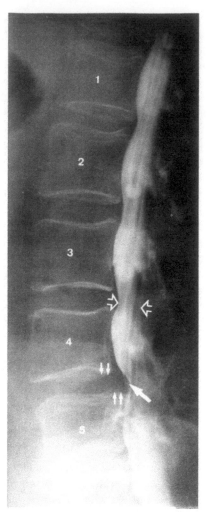

(A)

FIGURE 3.7   Correlation of myelography and MR imaging using the vertically opened configuration MR system. (A) Myelogram and (B) sagittal plane, T2-weighted, fast spin-echo MR image (TR/TE, 3000/85 msec) obtained in the upright, seated extended position. Degeneration of the L4-L5 disk level with anterolisthesis (short arrows) and disk protrusion (arrow) is seen on myelogram (A), as well as on the MR image (B). The sagittal diameter (short arrows) of the dural sac at the levels of the intervertebral disks, parallel to the intervertebral space, can be measured on MR images similarly to myelographic images (open arrows). Numbers indicate the lumbar and sacral vertebrae.

In the study by Wildermuth et al.,[23] patient acceptance of both the myelography and kinematic MRI procedures was assessed. After completion of both examinations, the patients were asked about their preferences with regard to myelography and kinematic MRI. Seventy-six percent of the patients reported relevant pain and 64% felt anxiety during myelography. Kinematic MRI was less painful. When asked whether they preferred lumbar myelography or kinematic MRI for any future evaluation, 64% of the patients favored kinematic MRI, and only 16% preferred lumbar spine myelography. These results demonstrated that kinematic MRI has better patient acceptance than myelography.

Based on these data, we conclude that myelography and kinematic MRI are comparable for quantitative assessment of sagittal dural sac diameters. The higher patient acceptance of kinematic MRI in combination with the better soft tissue contrast and the multiplanar imaging capabilities favors the use of kinematic MRI for assessment of the lumbar spine.

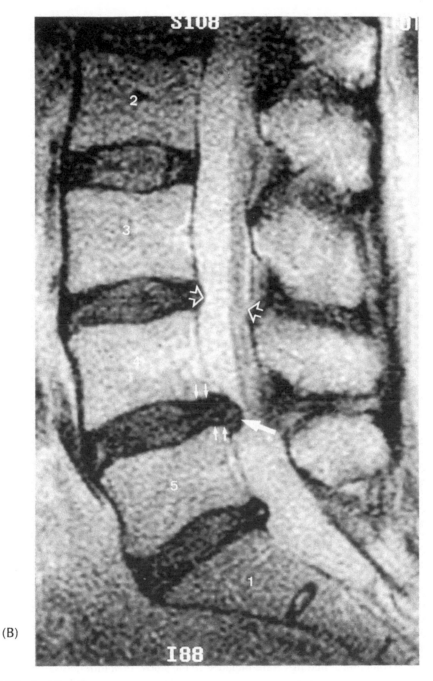

(B)

FIGURE 3.7   (continued).

V. CLINICAL APPLICATIONS

Low back pain is the second most common reason for patients to seek medical attention.[47] The lifetime prevalence of low back pain may be as high as 84%,[48] and low back pain is the leading cause of disability during the working lives of both men and women.

Although 90% of those patients who suffer from low back pain will recover within about 6 weeks irrespective of the type of treatment,[49] the cost of medical care for patients with low back pain is extremely high. It has been estimated that over 25 billion dollars are spent per year in the U.S. in direct medical costs related to low back pain.[50]

MR imaging has been used extensively in the identification of abnormal conditions of the lumbar spine and has become the gold standard in evaluation of spinal pathology.[2] However, in studying patients with low back pain, there is often a discrepancy between symptoms reported by the patient and findings as documented by MR imaging.

Previous studies have documented a high rate of abnormal imaging findings in the lumbar spine of asymptomatic volunteers.[47,51-54] Boden et al.[51] studied 67 asymptomatic individuals with an age range from 20 to 80 years using MR imaging. This group found at least one herniated disk in 20% of the volunteers below 60 years and in 36% of those older than 60 years.

Using MRI, Jensen et al.[47] reported on a study of 98 asymptomatic individuals (20 to 80 years old) all studied by MR. Of the 98 asymptomatic individuals evaluated, 27% had a protrusion and 1% had an extrusion. Boos et al.[52] found a substantially higher frequency (76%) of disc herniations than previously reported in asymptomatic subjects. The authors of the latter study also showed that by matching asymptomatic volunteers to patients with symptomatic disk herniation, the only substantial morphological difference between symptomatic patients and asymptomatic controls was the presence of neural compromise. Another study[54] confirmed the high prevalence of morphological disk abnormalities in asymptomatic individuals 20 to 50 years of age. Such abnormalities included disk bulging, disk protrusion, and anular tears, revealed as high signal intensity zones (HIZ). Conversely, disk extrusion, disk sequestration, and nerve root compression were found to be infrequent in asymptomatic individuals, suggesting that such findings in symptomatic patients may be clinically relevant.

The other end of the spectrum regarding the discrepancy between findings on diagnostic imaging and the clinical symptoms of low back pain is illustrated by the fact that MR imaging may often fail to show compromised neural structures, even in the presence of sciatica.[55] One possible explanation for the negative or indefinite MRI findings is that some of these patients may have nerve root compromise due to bulging of the intervertebral disk or thickening of the ligamentum flavum that resolves in the supine position, that is, the position used for conventional MR imaging of the lumbar spine.

Several biomechanical studies performed on lumbar cadaveric spines have documented a decrease in spinal canal and dural sac dimensions as well as foraminal size with axial loading or motion.[11-16] Moreover, the dynamic process of spinal canal stenosis or foraminal stenosis could theoretically explain why low back pain can be triggered by spinal movements such as forward flexion, extension, and axial loading of the spine, including standing, sitting, or weight bearing.[8,9] These observations suggest that a change in anatomic relationships resulting from axial loading or spinal movements may cause nerve root compression that is not visible on conventional MR imaging of the spine with the patient in a comfortable supine position.

A recent study[28] evaluated whether kinematic MRI of the lumbar spine was able to demonstrate nerve root compromise not visible on conventional MR images obtained with the patient in a supine position. In a prospective study, 30 patients with chronic low back pain or leg pain for more than 6 weeks that was unresponsive to a trial of nonsurgical treatment and surgery was not indicated or not urgent based on clinical findings were included in the study. In addition, disk protrusion and/or extrusion without compression of the neural structures had to be present in at least one intervertebral level as revealed by a conventional MRI examination.

Conventional MR imaging was performed on a 1.0 Tesla MR system using a standard imaging protocol that included sagittal plane, T1- and T2-weighted sequences of the entire lumbar spine, as well as angled axial sequences of at least three intervertebral levels (with inclusion of all degenerated disks). All 30 patients underwent kinematic MRI of the lumbar spine using the vertically opened Signa SP MR system. The patients were imaged in the upright, seated flexed and extended positions. Sagittal plane, T2-weighted MR images of the entire lumbar spine were obtained. In addition, angled axial plane, T2-weighted images were obtained at the same intervertebral levels as during conventional MR imaging.

Both conventional and kinematic MR images were reviewed quantitatively by measuring the cross-sectional area of the dural sac using an electronic caliper and qualitatively by analyzing positional changes with regard to disk abnormality (i.e., normal, disk bulging, disk extrusion, and sequestration), degree of nerve root compromise (i.e., no compromise, nerve root contact, nerve root deviation, nerve root compression), and foraminal size. For assessment of the latter, the scoring system described above[23,31] was used. In addition, the pain intensity was measured using a visual analogue scale with the patients in the upright, flexed and extended positions.

In accordance with cadaveric studies[11-16] and findings in asymptomatic volunteers,[7,24,27] the results of this study showed that the mean cross-sectional area of the dural sac significantly decreased between the supine neutral and the upright, seated extended positions (9.6%; $p < 0.001$) and between the upright, seated flexed and upright, seated extended positions (9.4%; $p < 0.001$) (Figure 3.8). These differences were significant for all subgroups of disk abnormalities, with the exception of the combination of neutral and extended positions in normal disks. No significant differences were found for either normal or abnormal disks between the supine neutral and seated flexion positions.

Based on these results, it was concluded that imaging in the upright, seated flexed position may not be necessary for a kinematic MRI protocol, since this position did not reveal any additional information to imaging the patient supine. However, further studies are needed to determine which sequences are essential in kinematic MRI of the lumbar spine.

The decrease in the cross-sectional area of the dural sac during extension of the spine is caused by several factors, including morphological changes of the intervertebral disk and infolding of the ligamentum flavum.[11,19,27] Although the study of Weishaupt et al.[28] revealed minor morphological changes of the intervertebral disk when comparing disk morphology during the supine position to the upright seated, flexed and extended positions (i.e., a disk with normal appearance in the supine position may become bulged in the upright, seated, extended position), occurrence of a disk extrusion or sequestration which was not visible in the supine position was rare (Figure 3.9).

The kinematic MRI examination frequently demonstrates position-dependent changes in the relationship of the nerve root with the adjacent disk. In the study of Weishaupt et al.,[28] nerve root contact without deviation increased in frequency from the supine position to the upright, seated flexed position (+18.4%), more so than from the supine position to the upright, seated extended position (+7.2%) (Figure 3.10). Moreover, nerve root deviation visible with the patient in the supine position changed to nerve root compression with the patient in the upright, seated extended position in only one of 30 patients (3.3%).

Because neural compromise appears to be more closely related to symptoms of patients with low back pain,[52] kinematic MRI may provide additional information in selected patients with equivocal findings of nerve root compression as seen on supine MR imaging, or in patients with a strong suspicion of dynamic nerve root compromise in the upright, seated extended position (Figure 3.11). Considering that spinal nerves may also be compromised within the neural foramen, the clinical relevance of kinematic MRI as an additional diagnostic tool may be even greater.

As mentioned previously, in a cadaveric study Nowicki et al.[15] demonstrated that foraminal stenosis with subsequent compression of the spinal nerve may be produced by flexion, extension, lateral bending, and axial rotation. The results obtained in the study of Weishaupt et al.[28] further demonstrated the validity of the concept of dynamic foraminal stenosis. This study showed that differences in foraminal size were most frequently observed between the upright, seated flexed and upright, seated extended positions (26.3%). Less frequently, differences between the supine neutral and upright, seated flexed (15.8%) and between the supine neutral and upright, seated extended positions (14.5%) also were present.

In the series reported by Wildermuth et al.,[23] position-dependent foraminal changes occurred less frequently. This difference may be explained by patient selection. Patients in the study of Weishaupt et al.[28] were generally younger in age and possibly more flexible in their lumbar spines.

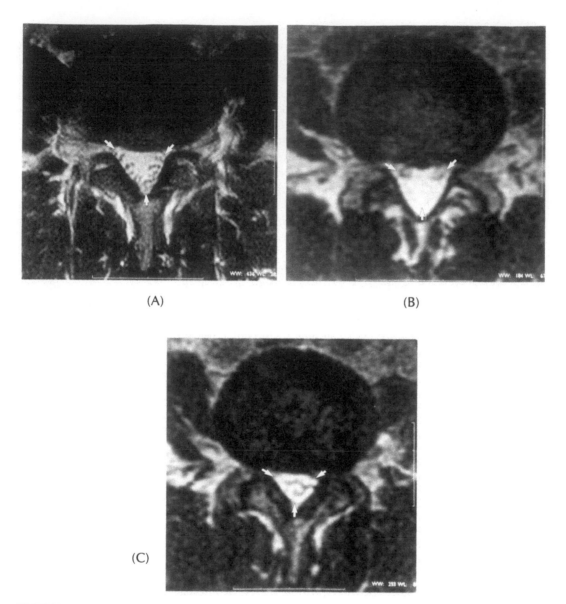

(A)   (B)

(C)

FIGURE 3.8   Angled, axial plane MR images obtained at the L4-L5 intervertebral space in a 49-year-old female patient. (A) MR image (TR/TE, 4000/96 msec) obtained with the patient in a supine position using a conventional 1.0 Tesla MR system, and the corresponding image acquired using a T2-weighted, fast spin-echo kinematic MRI technique (TR/TE, 4200/100 msec) with the patient in upright, (B) seated flexed, and (C) extended positions. The cross-sectional area of the dural sac increased from the supine position (150 mm^2) in (A), to 170 mm^2 in the upright, seated flexed position (B), and decreased to 110 mm^2 in the upright, seated extended position (C). During extension (C) the patient graded the pain intensity as 70% of the maximum pain experienced during his recent lower back problems. In the supine position and during flexion, the patient reported no painful symptoms. Short arrows indicate the dural sac.

An interesting and innovative use of kinematic MRI of the lumbar spine is the possibility to correlate the patient's pain with the positional dependence of morphological changes. In the study of Weishaupt et al.,[28] a visual analogue scale was used. The visual analogue scale is considered to be a valid, reliable, and easily quantified tool for pain assessment.[56] Pain was generally rated higher

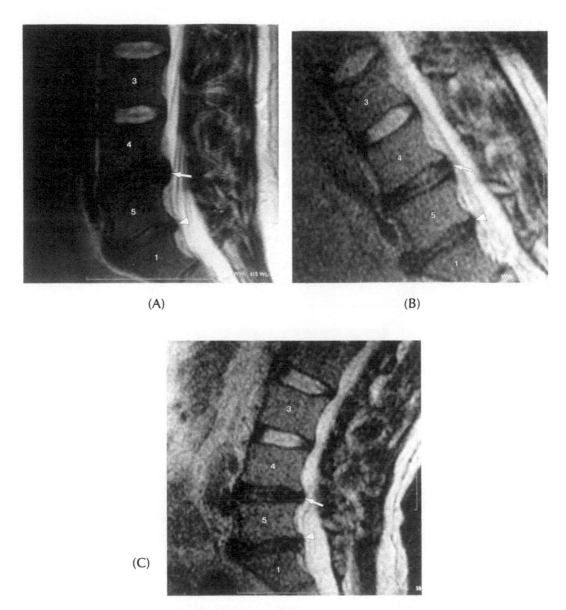

(A)

(B)

(C)

FIGURE 3.9 Positional dependence of the shape of the disk in a 37-year-old male patient with chronic low back pain. (A) Protrusion of the L4-L5 disk (arrow) and L5-S1 disk (arrowhead) on a sagittal plane, T2-weighted, fast spin-echo, conventional MR image (TR/TE, 4500/112 msec). (B) and (C), sagittal plane, T2-weighted, fast spin-echo MR images obtained using the kinematic MRI technique (TR/TE, 4100/95 msec) obtained in the upright, seated flexed (B) and upright, seated extended positions (C). Both the L4-L5 (arrow) and L5-S1 disks (arrowhead) do not reach beyond the posterior vertebral border with the patient in the upright, seated, flexed position and, therefore, were considered to be normal according to the grading system used for assessment. In the upright, seated extended position (C), both disks show protrusion. Numbers indicate lumbar and sacral vertebrae.

in the upright, seated extended position than in the upright, seated flexed position.[28] In certain patients with low back pain, the intensity of painful symptoms, as revealed by score differences, increased when the cross-sectional area of the dural sac decreased, although no statistical significance was seen.[28] However, similar results with statistical significance ($p = 0.046$) were obtained when correlating pain score differences with changes of the foraminal size. These findings also

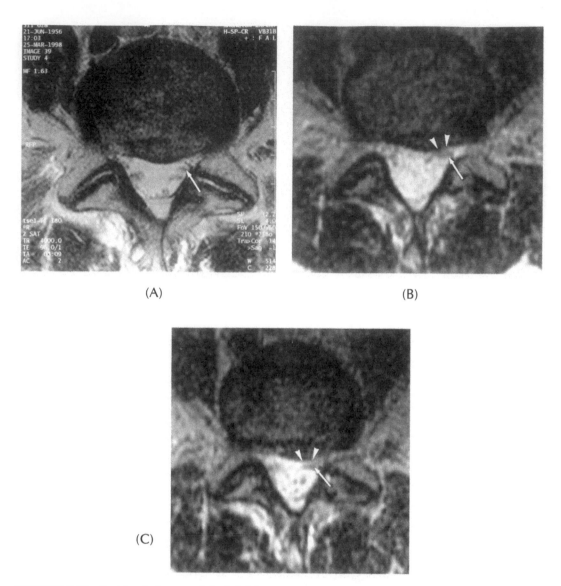

(A)   (B)

(C)

FIGURE 3.10   Positional changes of the left L5 nerve root in a 41-year-old male patient with chronic low back pain. On the conventional, axial plane, T2-weighted, fast spin-echo MR image (TR/TE, 4000/96 msec) (A), there is extrusion of the L4-L5 disk without any contact of the left L5 nerve root (arrow) with the adjacent border of the intervertebral disk. (B) The L5 nerve root contact with the adjacent border of the intervertebral disk (arrowheads) is also present, seen on the kinematic MR image using a T2-weighted, fast spin-echo MR image (TR/TE, 4200/100) obtained with the patient in an upright, seated flexed position. With the patient in an upright, seated extended position (C), the L5 nerve root (arrow) shows deviation by the adjacent intervertebral disk (arrowheads).

support the concept of dynamic foraminal stenosis and contradict previous assumptions that the correlation between foraminal stenosis and symptoms is poor.[57]

Kinematic MRI also may replace functional radiographs of the lumbar spine.[25] Although functional radiographs of the lumbar spine provide the opportunity to measure motion,[58] the diagnostic efficacy of flexion-extension views for diagnosis of segmental instability has been questioned.[59] However, diagnostic criteria for segmental instability are vague even for standard radiographs. A proper definition of instability criteria has yet to be found when using kinematic MRI of the spine.

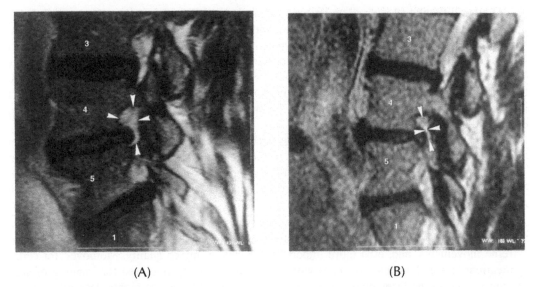

(A)   (B)

FIGURE 3.11   Positional dependence of foraminal size in a 30-year-old male patient. (A) Conventional, sagittal plane, T2-weighted, fast spin-echo MR image (TR/TE, 5000/130 msec). The L4-L5 foramen shows a slight foraminal stenosis with deformity of the epidural fat on the conventional MR image (arrowheads) (A). On the kinematic MR image (TR/TE, 4100/95 msec) obtained with the patient in an upright, seated extended position (B), there is a marked foraminal stenosis at the L4-L5 foramen with epidural fat only partially surrounding the nerve root (arrowheads). On a visual analogue scale, the patient graded his pain as 90% of the maximum pain experienced during his recent problems. The numbers indicate the lumbar and sacral vertebrae.

In summary, kinematic MRI of the lumbar spine opens new diagnostic possibilities to evaluate structural position-dependent changes in patients with chronic low back pain, with and without sciatica, or suspected segmental instability. Based on the current data, conventional MR imaging of the lumbar spine (i.e., in supine position) remains the imaging method of choice in the assessment of degenerative disk disease. In selected patients with equivocal findings on conventional MR imaging, kinematic MRI may be performed in upright (seated) extended and upright (seated) flexed positions in order to demonstrate spinal canal stenosis or neural compromise within the lateral recess or within the neuroforamen.

VI. FUTURE STUDIES AND APPLICATIONS

Vertically opened MR systems are presently available in only a few institutions worldwide (approximately 15). Therefore, kinematic MRI examinations of the lumbar spine with the patient in upright positions will not quickly become a routine imaging tool. Unfortunately, its role will likely remain limited to research.

There remain several questions that have not been investigated with the currently available hardware and software capabilities. These include performance of kinematic MRI procedures with the patient in upright positions with lateral bending (sidewards flexion) and with a rotated spine. Initial results indicate that imaging the spine during rotational movements leads to small but detectable changes in morphology of relevant spinal structures.[7]

Diurnal changes of the intervertebral disks have been previously assessed.[60] However, the kinematic MRI examination may provide additional information, such as the influence of the time of day on height, diameter, and signal intensity of the loaded intervertebral disk.

At the present time, most investigations have concentrated on the demonstration of compression of neural structures.

Another difficult and not well understood subject is instability of the spine. From a radiological point of view, this subject has been evaluated with standard MR images obtained in flexion and extension.[25] Vertebral body translation has typically been used as a parameter for assessing instability. The cutoffs for normal versus abnormal translation are typically about 3 mm.[58] The use of kinematic MRI in suspected instability not only would eliminate the dosage of ionizing radiation but may provide additional insights in the diagnosis of instability. One possible factor related to instability and visible on kinematic MRI may be the sudden separation of the facet joints in flexion due to reduction of capsular strength.

Another potentially promising area of research may focus on positional imaging before and after image-guided injections of nerve roots and facet joints. Although interventions are not the subject of this chapter, one should not forget that the vertically opened MR system and other similar MR systems have been designed for interventions and are also well suited to precisely guide spinal injections such the ones mentioned above.

For other future projects, technical improvements are required. One important subject is improved RF coils allowing for larger fields of view, better adaptation to the body, especially during extreme movements, and, even more importantly, improved image quality. Moreover, for certain applications, faster imaging sequences with better image quality (required for imaging of small structures such as the facet joints, nerve roots, and ligamenta flava) are highly desirable.

With faster MR imaging, the use of a dynamic technique for the kinematic MRI examination, such as that used for peripheral joints,[30] may become feasible for the lumbar spine. The investigation of instability may then go in new directions, again including an interdisciplinary approach. Measurements known from biomechanical studies, such as the determination of the instantaneous centers of rotation during flexion and extension, may be obtained.

The use of faster imaging schemes would have another effect. As mentioned in this chapter, many patients have pain during kinematic MRI and probably do not maintain maximally flexed and extended positions. Thus, position-dependent morphological changes may have been underestimated. The use of faster MR imaging techniques, possibly combined with pain medication, may lead to more impressive results. Although our group is relatively skeptical regarding image processing, more advanced imaging sequences may allow for better representation of morphological findings (for instance, fly-through imaging in various body positions).

VII. SUMMARY AND CONCLUSIONS

MR imaging has several attractive characteristics, including high soft-tissue contrast, spatial resolution, and multiplanar imaging capabilities. Therefore, MR imaging now stands as the preferred imaging modality for a variety of diseases of the lumbar spine, including evaluation of chronic low back pain with and without sciatica. Current MR imaging techniques for the lumbar spine are often performed in a closed magnet with the patient in a supine neutral position. However, it is known that low back pain sometimes worsens under axial load in combination with flexion, extension, or other spinal motion moments.

With the use of the open-configured MR systems, especially those with a vertical gap between their magnet components, it is possible to obtain *in vivo* diagnostic MR images under axial loading conditions and/or in different spinal positions. Using these MR systems it is possible to study physiological as well as pathological changes in the relationships of the intervertebral disk, the spinal canal, and the neural foramina and to assess segmental instability. MR images may be taken in painful positions, and pain may be correlated with morphological changes of the intervertebral disk or other spinal structures.

In accordance with previous studies using cadaveric specimens, kinematic MRI studies obtained in asymptomatic volunteers and symptomatic patients showed an increase of the cross-sectional area of the spinal canal and neural foramen during seated flexion and a decrease of both during seated extension. Kinematic MRI is comparable with myelography for quantitative assessment of the dural sac and, therefore, may replace this examination for this purpose. Although rare, kinematic MRI may demonstrate clinically important neural compromise or foraminal stenosis that are occult on conventional MR imaging in supine position. Therefore, kinematic MRI of the lumbar spine may be performed in selected patients with suspected nerve root compromise, suspected spinal canal stenosis, or suspected stenosis of the neural foramen with equivocal or borderline findings on conventional MR imaging. Additionally, the kinematic MRI examination may be used when a positional component of the symptoms is considered to be present. Thus, kinematic MRI may improve diagnostic performance of conventional MR imaging for evaluating low back pain, and may be of help in elucidating its poorly understood pathogenesis.

REFERENCES

1. Modic, M. T., Masaryk, T. J., Ross, J. S., and Carter, J. R., Imaging of degenerative disk disease, *Radiology,* 168, 177, 1988.
2. Kent, D. L., Haynor, D. R., Longstreth, W. T., and Larson, E. B., The clinical efficacy of magnetic resonance in neuroimaging, *Ann. Int. Med.,* 120, 856, 1994.
3. Boos, N., Dreier, D., Hilfiker, E., Schade, V., Kreis, R., Hora, J., Aebi, M., and Boesch, C., Tissue characterization of symptomatic and asymptomatic disc herniations by quantitative magnetic resonance imaging, *J. Orthop. Res.,* 15, 141, 1997.
4. Pearce, R. H., Thompson, J. B., Berbault, G. M., and Flak B., Magnetic resonance imaging reflects the chemical changes and aging degeneration in human intervertebral disk, *J. Rheumatol.,* 18 (Suppl.), 42, 1991.
5. Modic, M. T., Steinberg, P. M., Ross, J. S., Masaryk, T. J., and Carter J. R., Degenerative disk disease: assessment of changes in vertebral body marrow with MR imaging, *Radiology,* 166, 193, 1988.
6. Weishaupt, D., Zanetti, M., Boos, N., and Hodler, J., MR imaging and CT in osteoarthritis of the lumbar facet joints, *Skeletal Radiol,,* 28, 215, 1999.
7. Chung, S. S., Lee, C. S., Kim, S. H., Chung, M. W., and Ahn, J. M., Effect of low back posture on the morphology of the spinal canal, *Skeletal Radiol.,* 29, 217, 2000.
8. Porter, R. W., Hibbert, C. S., and Wicks, M., The spinal canal in symptomatic disc lesions, *J. Bone Joint Surg.,* 60B, 485, 1978.
9. Kent, D. L., Haynor, D. R., Larson, E. B., and Deyo, R. A., Diagnosis of lumbar spinal stenosis in adults: a metaanalysis of the accuracy of CT, MR, and myelography, *Am. J. Roentgen.,* 158, 1135, 1992.
10. Katz, N., Dalgas, M., Stucki, G., Katz, N. P., Bayley, J., Fossel, A. H., Chang, L. C., and Lipson, S., Degenerative lumbar spinal stenosis. Diagnostic value of the history and physical examination, *Arthritis Rheum.,* 9, 1236, 1995.
11. Revel, M., Mayoux-Benhamou, M. A., Aaron, C., and Amour B., Morphological variations of the lumbar foramina during flexion-extension and disk collapse, *Rev. Rhum. Mal Osteoartic.,* 55, 361, 1998.
12. Schönström, N., Lindahl, S., Willen, J., and Hansson, T., Dynamic changes in the dimensions of the lumbar spinal canal: an experimental study in vitro, *J. Orthop. Res.,* 7, 115, 1989.
13. Mayoux-Benhamou, M. A., Revel, M., Aaron, C., Chomette, G., and Amour, B., A morphometric study of the lumbar foramen. Influence of flexion-extension movements and of isolated disc collapse, *Surg. Radiol. Anat.,* 11, 97, 1989.
14. Nowicki, B. H., Yu, S., Reinartz, J., Pintar, F., Yoganandan, N., and Haughton, V. M., Effect of axial loading on neural foramina and nerve roots in the lumbar spine, *Radiology,* 176, 433, 1990.
15. Nowicki, B. H., Haughton, V. M., Schmidt, T. A., Lim, T. H., An, H. S., Riley, L. H., Yu, L., and Hong, J. W., Occult lumbar lateral spinal stenosis in neural foramina subjected to physiologic loading, *Am. J. Neuroradiol.,* 17, 1605, 1996.
16. Inufusa, A., An, H. S., Lim, T. H., Hasegawa, T., Haughton, V. M., and Nowicki, B. H., Anatomic changes of the spinal canal and intervertebral foramen associated with flexion-extension movement, *Spine,* 21, 2412, 1996.
17. Jeanneret, B. and Forster, T., Anamnesis and myelography in the preoperative assessment of lumbar spinal stenosis: results of a postoperative follow-up study, *Orthopaede,* 22, 217, 1993.

18. Willén, J., Danielson, B., Gaulitz, A., Niklason, T., Schönström, N., and Hansson, T., Dynamic effects on the lumbar spine. Axially loaded CT-myelography and MRI in patients with sciatica and/or neurogenic claudication, *Spine*, 22, 2968, 1997.

19. Fennell, A. J., Jones, A. P., and Hukins, D. W., Migration of the nucleus pulposus of the intervertebral disc during flexion and extension of the lumbar spine, *Spine*, 21, 2753, 1996.

20. Schenck, J. F., Jolesz, F. A., Roemer, P. B. et al., Superconducting open-configuration MR imaging systems for image-guided therapy, *Radiology*, 195, 805, 1995.

21. Jolesz, F. and Silverman, S. G., Interventional magnetic resonance therapy, *Semin. Intervent. Radiol.*, 12, 20, 1995.

22. Lenz, G. and Drobnitzky, M., Interventional MRI with an open low-field system, in *Interventional Magnetic Resonance Imaging*, Debatin, J. F. and Adam, G., Eds., Springer, Berlin, 1998, p. 3.

23. Wildermuth, S., Zanetti, M., Duewell, S., Schmid, M. R., Romanowski, B., Benini, A., Böni, T., and Hodler, J., Lumbar spine: quantitative and qualitative assessment of positional (upright flexion and extension) MR imaging and myelography, *Radiology*, 207, 391, 1998.

24. Zamani, A. A., Moriarty, T., Hsu, L., Winalski, C. S., Schaffer, J. L., Isbister, H., Schenck, J. F., Rohling, K. W., and Jolesz, F., Functional MRI of the lumbar spine in erect position in a superconducting open-configuration MR system: preliminary results, *J. Magn. Reson. Imag.*, 8, 1329, 1998.

25. Funk, C., Beyer, H. M., and Volle, E., Functional MRT of the lumbar spine in an open magnet system — initial results, *RoFo*, 169, 27, 1998.

26. Harvey, S. B., Smith, F. W., and Hukins, D.W., Measurement of lumbar spine flexion-extension using a low-field open-magnet magnetic resonance scanner, *Invest. Radiol.*, 33, 439, 1998.

27. Schmid, M. R., Stucki, G., Duewell, S., Wildermuth, S., Romanowski, B., and Hodler, J., Changes in cross-sectional measurements of the spinal canal and intervertebral foramina as a function of body position: in vivo studies on an open-configuration MR system, *Am. J. Roentgen.*, 172, 1095, 1999.

28. Weishaupt, D., Schmid, M. R., Zanetti, M., Boos, N., Kissling, R., Dvorak, J., and Hodler J., Positional MR imaging of the lumbar spine: does it demonstrate nerve root compromise?, *Radiology*, 215, 247, 2000.

29. Thomas, S. R., Magnets and gradient coils: types and characteristics, in *The Physics of MRI: Medical Physics Monograph no. 21*, Bronskill, M. J. and Sprawls, P., Eds., American Institute of Physics, Woodbory, NY, 1993, p. 97.

30. Shellock, F. G., Kinematic MRI of the joints, *Semin. Musculoskeletal Radiol.*, 1, 143, 1997.

31. Pathria, M., Sartoris, D. J., and Resnick, D., Osteoarthritis of the facet joints: accuracy of oblique radiographic assessment, *Radiology*, 164, 227, 1987.

32. Dai, L. Y., Xu, Y. K., Zhang, W. M., and Zhou, Z. H., The effect of flexion-extension motion of the lumbar spine on the capacity of the spinal canal. An experimental study, *Spine*, 14, 523, 1989.

33. Quint, U., Wilke, H. J., Shirazi-Adl, A., Parnianpour, M., Loer, F., and Claes, L. E., Importance of the intersegmental trunk muscles for the stability of the lumbar spine. A biomechanical study in vitro, *Spine*, 23, 1937, 1998.

34. Panjabi, M. M., Oxland, T. R., Yamamoto, I., and Crisco J. J., Mechanical behavior of the lumbar and lumbosacral spine as shown by three-dimensional load-displacement curves, *J. Bone Joint Surg.*, 76A, 413, 1994.

35. Resnick, D. and Niwayama, G., Anatomy of individual joints, in *Diagnosis of Bone and Joint Disorders*, Resnick, D., Ed., W.B. Saunders, Philadelphia, 1995, p. 672.

36. Zarzur, N. and Kawano, K., Anatomic studies of the human ligamentum flavum, *Anesth. Analg.*, 63, 499, 1984.

37. Tajima, N. and Kawano, K., Cryomicrotomy of the lumbar spine, *Spine*, 11, 376, 1986.

38. Gepstein, R., Folman, Y., Sagiv, P., Ben-David, Y., and Hallel, T., Does the anteroposterior diameter of the spinal canal reflect the size? An anatomical study, *Surg. Radiol. Anat.*, 13, 289, 1991.

39. Bolender, N. F., Schönström, N. S., and Spengler, D. M., Role of computed tomography and myelography in the diagnosis of centralspinal stenosis, *J. Bone Joint Surg.*, 67A, 240, 1985.

40. Lee, C. K., Rauschning, W., and Glenn W., Lateral lumbar spinal canal stenosis: classification, pathologic anatomy and surgical decompression, *Spine*, 13, 313, 1988.

41. Hasegawa, T., An, H. S., Haugthon, V. M., and Nowicki, B. H., Lumbar foraminal stenosis: critical heights of the intervertebral discs and foramina, *J. Bone Joint. Surg.*, 77A, 32, 1995.

42. Hesselink, J. R., Spine imaging: history, achievements, remaining frontiers, *Am. J. Roentgenol.,* 150, 1223, 1988.
43. Bell, G. R. and Ross, J. S., Diagnosis of nerve root compression. Myelography, computed tomography, and MRI, *Orthop. Clin. North Am.,* 23, 405, 1992.
44. Sortland, O., Magnaes, B., and Hauge, T., Functional myelography with metrizamide in the diagnosis of lumbar spinal stenosis, *Acta Radiol.,* 355 (Suppl.), 42, 1977.
45. Badami, J. P., Baker, R. A., Scholz, F. J., and McLaughlin M., Outpatient metrizamide myelography: prospective evaluation of safety and cost effectiveness, *Radiology,* 158, 175, 1986.
46. Peterman, S. B., Postmyelography headache: a review, *Radiology,* 200, 765, 1996.
47. Jensen, M. C., Brant-Zawadzki, M. N., Obuchowski, N., Modic, M. T., Malkasian, D., and Ross, J. S., Magnetic resonance imaging of the lumbar spine in people without low back pain, *N. Engl. J. Med.,* 331, 69, 1994.
48. Cassidy, J. D., Carroll, L., Coté, P., and Senthilselvan, A., The prevalence of graded chronic low back pain severity and its effect on general health: a population based study, *Proceedings of the Annual Meeting of the International Society for the Study of the Lumbar Spine,* Singapore, 1997, p. 9.
49. Waddel, G., A new clinical model for the treatment of low back pain, in *The Lumbar Spine,* Weinstein, J. N. and Wiesel, S. W., Eds, W.B. Saunders, Philadelphia, 1990, p. 38.
50. Freymoyer, J. W. and Cats-Baril, W. L., An overview of the incidence and costs of low back pain, *Orthop. Clin. North Am.,* 22, 263, 1991.
51. Boden, S. D., Davis, D. O., Dina, T. S., Patronas, N. J., and Wiesel, S. W., Abnormal magnetic resonance scans of the lumbar spine in asymptomatic subjects, *J. Bone Joint Surg.* [Am.], 72, 403, 1990.
52. Boos, N., Rieder, R., Schade, V., Spratt, K. F., Semmer, N., and Aebi, M., The diagnostic accuracy of magnetic resonance imaging, work perception, and psychosocial factors in identifying symptomatic disc herniations, *Spine,* 20, 2613, 1995.
53. Stadnik, T. W., Lee, R. R., Coen, H. L., Neirynck, E. C., Buisseret, T. S., and Osteaux, M. J., Annular tears and disk herniation: prevalence and contrast enhancement on MR images in the absence of low back pain and sciatica, *Radiology,* 206, 49, 1998.
54. Weishaupt, D., Zanetti, M., Hodler, J., and Boos, N., MR imaging of the lumbar spine: disk extrusion and sequestration, nerve root compression, endplate abnormalities and osteoarthritis of the facets joints are rare in asymptomatic volunteers, *Radiology,* 209, 661, 1998.
55. Freemont, A. J., Peacock, T. E., Goupille, P., Hoyland, J. A., O'Brien, J., and Jayson, M. I., Nerve ingrowth into diseased intervertebral disc in chronic low back pain, *Lancet,* 350, 178, 1997.
56. Langley, G. B. and Sheppeard, H., The visual analogue scale: its use in pain measurement, *Rheumatol. Int.,* 5, 145, 1985.
57. Devor, M. and Rappaport, Z. H., Relation of foraminal (lateral) stenosis to radicular pain, *Am. J. Neuradiol.,* 17, 1615, 1996.
58. Stokes, I., Reliability of radiographic studies, in *The Lumbar Spine,* Weinstein, J. N. and Wiesel, S. W., Eds., W.B. Saunders, Philadelphia, 1990, p. 337.
59. Penning, L., Wilmik, J. T., and van Woerden, H. H., Inability to prove instability. A critical appraisal of clinical-radiological flexion-extension studies in the lumbar disc degeneration, *Diagn. Imag. Clin. Med.,* 53, 186, 1984.
60. Malko, J. A., Hutton, W. C., and Fajman, W. A., An *in vivo* magnetic resonance imaging study of changes in the volume (and fluid content) of the lumbar intervertebral discs during a simulated diurnal load cycle, *Spine,* 24, 1051, 1999.

Part II

Cervical Spine

4 The Cervical Spine: Functional Anatomy and Kinesiology

Kornelia Kulig

CONTENTS

I. INTRODUCTION

To provide an adaptable musculoskeletal support for the head, the cervical spine is the most mobile region of the spinal column. In addition, the cervical spine functions to transfer weight and resist the resulting bending motions of the head. Finally, the cervical spine protects the spinal cord and vertebral arteries from excessive physiological movement and trauma.

0-8493-0807-0/01/$0.00+$.50
© 2001 by Frank G. Shellock

This chapter discusses the cervical spine with regard to functional anatomy, normal kinesiology, and pathokinesiology. Due to the unique regional characteristics of the head and neck, the material in this chapter has been divided into two sections: the occipito-atlanto-axial region (C0-C1-C2) and the lower cervical region (C2-T1). Each section is further subdivided to allow focus on the functional anatomy, joint kinesiology, and common clinical pathologies related to that region. The functional anatomy subsection focuses on osseous and ligamentous structures relevant to description of motion and common pathologies. The subsection on kinematics analyzes the cervical spine as a mechanical structure with controlled articulations by levers (vertebrae), pivots (facets and discs), passive restraints (ligaments), and activators (muscles). The third subsection presents common pathologies and their relationship to structure, function, and motion of the head and neck.

II. FUNCTIONAL ANATOMY

A. OSSEOUS STRUCTURES AND ARTICULATING SURFACES

1. The Occipito-Atlanto-Axial Region

The occipito-atlanto-axial region (C0-C1-C2) is also referred to as the upper cervical region (Figure 4.1). By convention, two neighboring vertebrae and the interconnecting soft tissue, devoid of musculature, are called a functional spinal unit (FSU).[1] Because of unique functional interactions, the C0-C1-C2 region is also considered a FSU despite its three, and not two, osseous components.[2]

The first cervical vertebra, the atlas, true to the mythological source of its name, functions as a head support. The superior articular surfaces of the atlas are concave, facing medially at both its medial rim and its anterior aspect. The superior atlantal facets mimic human hands that are gracefully holding the head. The flat semicircular vertebral shape and the shape of the facets promote

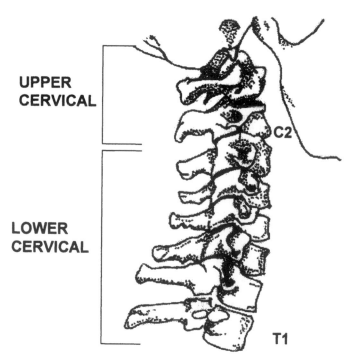

FIGURE 4.1 Functional divisions of the cervical spine: the upper cervical spine and the lower cervical spine. (From Porterfield, J. A. and DeRosa, C., *Mechanical Neck Pain. Perspectives in Functional Anatomy,* W.B. Saunders, Philadelphia, 1995, p. 67. With permission.)

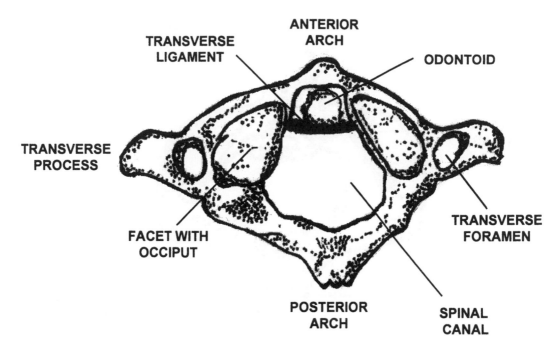

FIGURE 4.2   Superior view of the atlas.

medio-lateral gliding of the atlas between the occiput and the axis, giving it the resemblance of a ball bearing (Figure 4.2).

The relatively large vertebral foramen of the atlas contains the spinal cord and the odontoid process. The odontoid process, a part of the second vertebra in an adult spine, was the body of C1 during early embryonic development. The widely protruding transverse processes serve as attachment sites for suboccipital and cervical muscles, providing a long lever arm for sidebending and axial rotation. The posterior arch of the atlas, with its superior groove, serves as a conduit for the vertebral arteries as they pass from the transverse foramen of the transverse processes to the foramen magnum.

The left and right vertebral arteries share the atlantal groove with the first cervical spinal nerve (suboccipital nerve). The smaller anterior arch, on the dorsal side, serves as an attachment of one of the most vital ligaments in the human body, the transverse ligament (important for spinal cord protection).[3]

The second cervical vertebra, the axis, serves as a pivot for rotation of the occiput and atlas in the transverse plane (Figure 4.3). The former body of the atlas has evolved into the superior extension of the axial vertebral body, and due to its tooth-like shape it has been interchangeably called the dens or odontoid process.

Anteriorly, the dens articulates with the posterior arch of the atlas. Broad variances in the shape of the dens have been observed,[4] including differences in length, anterior or posterior inclination, and presence or absence of posterior groove for the transverse ligament. Slight posterior inclination of the dens may be considered beneficial as it allows for increased extension of the atlas by enabling the atlas to superiorly slide on the odontoid. However, it has been hypothesized that posterior inclination of a short odontoid coupled with weak connective tissue (e.g., with rheumatoid arthritis) may contribute to atlanto-axial instability or subluxation.[5]

The articular surfaces between the atlas and axis promote motion and functionally substitute for the mobility role of intervertebral discs found in other spinal regions. The inferior atlantal facets, when covered with cartilage, are slightly convex and articulate with the superior facets of the axis which are also slightly convex.

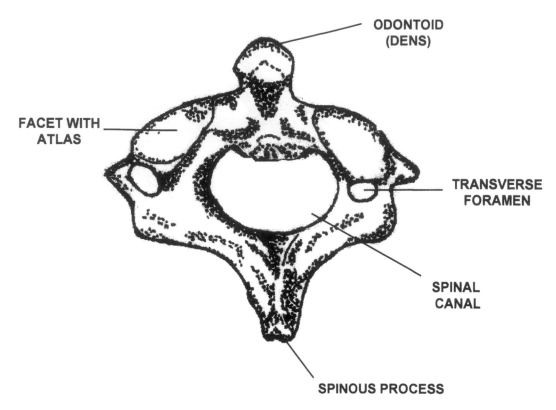

FIGURE 4.3   Superior view of the axis.

The vertical height of the atlanto-axial segment is at its lowest position in neutral rotation. As a result of rotation, the atlantal facets first slide superior and then inferior in relation to the axial facets. Consequently, the vertical height of the atlanto-axial segment first increases and then decreases. This is referred to as a "pistoning effect."[1]

2. The Lower Cervical Region

The lower cervical spine includes the C3-T1 vertebrae (Figure 4.1). However, functionally, the lower cervical region spans the functional spinal units from the C2-C3 to T2-T3 (or T3-T4).[6] Despite strong similarities, there are some unique characteristics of the cervico-thoracic junction. Therefore, this description will focus on the segments from C2 to T1.

A typical lower cervical vertebral body is twice as wide laterally as anterio-posteriorly. The role of the vertebral body is to serve as a load-bearing structure for the weight of the head and forces generated by muscular contractions. The shape of a lower cervical vertebra is well adjusted to its function. In the transverse plane, the lower cervical vertebra forms a triangle with its base (anterior vertebral body and transverse processes) facing anteriorly and apex (spinous process) facing posteriorly (Figure 4.4).

The anterior vertebral body serves as an attachment site for three muscles and the anterior longitudinal ligament. The latero-posterior aspect of the vertebra serves for attachment of multiple muscles and ligaments. The postero-lateral muscles are greater in size and number than the anterior muscles. Consequently, the skeletal and soft tissue structures give the external circumference of the neck a circular appearance.

The superior latero-posterior aspect of the vertebral body has two unique superior projections called uncinate processes (Figure 4.4). These bony projections create a semiconcavity at the superior

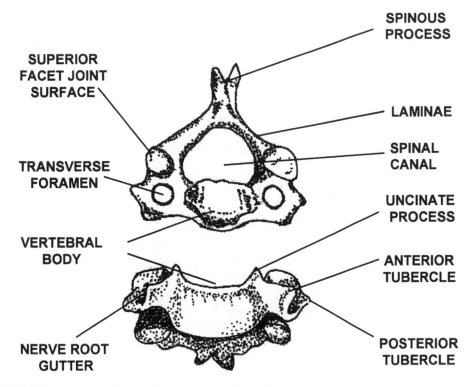

SPINOUS PROCESS

SUPERIOR FACET JOINT SURFACE

LAMINAE

SPINAL CANAL

TRANSVERSE FORAMEN

UNCINATE PROCESS

VERTEBRAL BODY

ANTERIOR TUBERCLE

NERVE ROOT GUTTER

POSTERIOR TUBERCLE

FIGURE 4.4   Typical cervical vertebra: superior and anterior views.

aspect of the cervical vertebral body and contribute to the amount and direction of motion at a cervical FSU.[7] The inferior latero-posterior aspect of the vertebral body has bilateral latero-posterior convexities, which join the uncinate processes of the inferior vertebrae and form the uncovertebral joints (also called the joints of von Luschka). These joints develop in late childhood and are the first to show degenerative changes in adults.[7]

The cervical pedicles, two postero-laterally projecting osseous structures, are the connectors between the anterior and posterior elements. The cervical "transverse processes" projecting latero-ventral are unique due to their gutter-like shape. The gutter contains the nerve root and anterior to it, passing vertically through the transverse foramen, is the vertebral artery. The terminal projections of the "transverse processes" are tubercles serving as attachment sites for several muscles. The anterior tubercle is a terminal projection of a rudimentary rib and the posterior tubercle is the true transverse process.

Spinous processes of the lower cervical spine are bifid (C3-C6) and increase in length from C3 to C7. The bifid shape augments the range of segmental extension by preventing tip-to-tip approximation. The main role of the spinous processes is to provide a distant site of muscle attachment and consequently to create a longer lever arm.

There are four facet surfaces on each cervical vertebra, two superior and two inferior. Consequently, a functional spinal unit has two facet (apophyseal) joints. The role of the facet joint is to direct motion and contribute to weight bearing. Both facet joints are responsible for approximately 30% of weight bearing; the remaining 70% is distributed to the disc. This distribution results, in part, from the spatial orientation of the facet joint (on average 45 degrees from the transverse plane of the vertebral body).

In the sagittal plane, the orientation of the facet joint varies. The superior facets of the C4-C7 vertebra face slightly lateral providing for more axial rotation, whereas the C3 and T1 superior facet orientation is more medial, thereby restricting axial rotation.

An intervertebral disc is present between each vertebra of the lower cervical region. The disc has a discal joint with each of the neighboring vertebrae. The primary role of the disc is to distribute weight across the entire vertebral body. The secondary role is to dictate mobility of the FSU (i.e., the higher the disc, the more mobile the FSU).

B. Ligaments and Joint Capsule

1. The Occipito-Atlanto-Axial Region

Ligaments serve an important role in supporting and stabilizing the head and upper cervical spine. Functionally, the ligaments of the upper cervical spine can be divided into two groups: those that are a continuation of the long paravertebral ligaments (Figure 4.5) and those that are unique to this region (i.e., alar, transverse, apical) (Figure 4.6). From posterior to anterior the ligaments that have counterparts in the lower cervical region are the ligamentum nuchae, posterior atlanto-occipital and atlanto-axial, apophyseal joint capsular ligaments, tectorial membrane, and anterior atlanto-occipital.

The nuchal (back of neck) ligament is a strong supporting structure of the head and neck (Figure 4.6). Attached posteriorly from the T1 spinous process to the occipital protuberance, the nuchal ligament is ideally located to resist the external flexion moment created by the anteriorly located center of mass of the head.

The posterior atlanto-occipital and atlanto-axial membranes run from the posterior rings of the atlas and axis to the foramen magnum. The laxity of these broad membranes allows for a significant amount of rotation at the C1-C2 segment. Below the C2 segment, these ligaments form the thick, strong, and elastic ligamentum flavum (Figure 4.5).

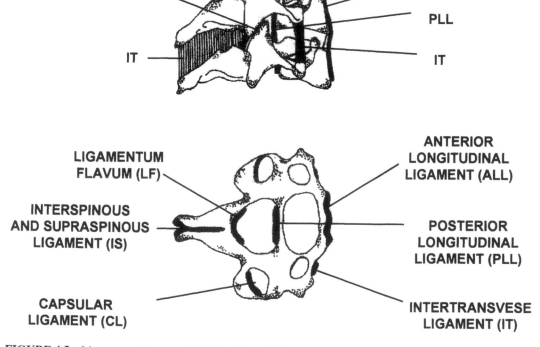

FIGURE 4.5 Ligaments of the cervical spine. (From White, A. A. and Panjabi, M. M., *Clinical Biomechanics of the Spine,* J.B. Lippincott, Philadelphia, 1990, p. 92. With permission.)

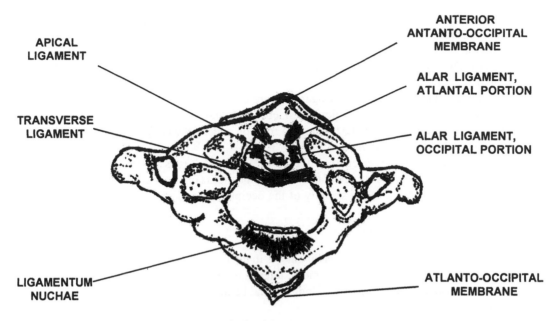

APICAL
LIGAMENT

ANTERIOR
ANTANTO-OCCIPITAL
MEMBRANE

ALAR LIGAMENT,
ATLANTAL PORTION

TRANSVERSE
LIGAMENT

ALAR LIGAMENT,
OCCIPITAL PORTION

LIGAMENTUM
NUCHAE

ATLANTO-OCCIPITAL
MEMBRANE

FIGURE 4.6   Ligaments of the upper cervical spine.

Capsular ligaments serve as the capsule for the apophyseal joints (bilateral joints formed by neighboring facets) (Figure 4.5). The capsular fibers are oriented perpendicular to the facet plane. They are thick, dense and short; however, they allow for an appreciable amount of movement at the apophyseal joint and, consequently, motion at the functional spinal unit (FSU).

The tectoral membrane lies behind the anterior arch of the axis and atlas, immediately posterior to the cruciform ligament complex (specific to the upper cervical region). Proximally, the tectoral membrane attaches to the anterior rim of the foramen magnum, while distally it becomes the posterior longitudinal ligament (Figure 4.5). The broad and strong tectoral membrane reinforces the transverse and alar ligaments and helps prevent upper cervical instability.

The anterior atlanto-occipital membrane, a superior extension of the anterior longitudinal ligament, attaches from the atlas to the occiput (Figure 4.6). Additionally, an extension of the anterior longitudinal ligament also connects from the axis to the atlas (Figure 4.5). The ligament is narrow and translucent and attaches to the vertebral bodies and the discs. It serves as a check for excessive extension at the suboccipital region.

The short upper cervical ligaments are the cruciform ligament complex, alar ligaments, and apical ligament (Figure 4.6). These ligaments have a dual role in the upper cervical spine. Primarily, they assure stability and, secondarily, they contribute to the unique arthrokinematics of the upper cervical region.

The cruciform ligament complex serves an important role in stabilizing the occipito-atlanto-axial region. The cruciform ligament complex lies anterior to the tectoral membrane and contains both horizontal and vertical components. The horizontal component is the transverse ligament, which attaches bilaterally to the posterior aspect of the anterior arch of the atlas (Figure 4.6). The transverse ligament tightly holds the odontoid against the posterior arch of the atlas, preventing pressure from the odontoid on the spinal cord.

Two ligamentous bands form the vertical component of the cruciform ligament complex (Figure 4.6). These bands arise from the transverse ligament and run cranially and caudally. That cross-like arrangement of the transverse ligament and its bands has earned them the name of "cruciform" or "cruciate" ligament complex.

Alar ligaments lie immediately anterior to the cruciform complex. They are bilateral, strong cords running from the lateral aspects of the tip of the dens to the lateral-ventral aspects of the rim of the foramen magnum. At the apex of the odontoid the alar ligaments form an angle of 140 to 180 degrees. Dvorak and Panjabi[8] reported that in approximately 30% of cases the alar ligament has atlantal attachments running from the dens to the posterior aspect of the ventral arch of the atlas.

The atlantal attachments of the alar ligaments are more anterior than the occipital attachments. The alar ligaments restrict occipital flexion, sidebending and excessive rotation between occiput and atlas, and atlas and axis. The restrictions to rotation and sidebending come from the ligament contralateral to the direction of motion.

The final ligament, in this category, is the apical ligament. It runs vertically and attaches from the tip of the dens to the anterior edge of the foramen magnum (Figure 4.6). It is an elastic ligament and may partially contribute to the stability of the occipito-atlantal segment.

2. The Lower Cervical Region

From posterior to anterior there are seven ligaments in the lower cervical spine. They are as follows: supraspinous ligament, interspinous ligament, intertransvese ligament, ligamentum flavum, apophyseal joint capsular ligament, posterior longitudinal ligament, and anterior longitudinal ligament (Figure 4.5).

In the neutral position, ligaments are lax. In the sagittal plane, the ligament located anterior to the axis of rotation is taut in extension (anterior longitudinal ligament), and ligaments located posterior to the axis of rotation are taut during flexion (the remaining six of the ligaments listed above). In sidebending, the ligaments opposite to the side of sidebending are taut, and in rotation all are taut.

C. Spinal Canal, Vertebral Artery, and Upper Cervical Nerve Roots

The vertebral artery holds a prominent place deep in the occipital triangle. It travels from the transverse foramen of the axis laterally to the atlantal transverse foramen. As it exits cranially at the atlas, the vertebral artery turns sharply from lateral to medial (in the transverse plane) and travels on the superior aspect of the posterior arch of the atlas. Approaching midline, it pierces the posterior atlanto-occipital membrane and enters the foramen magnum where it joins the other vertebral artery to form the basilar artery.

The first cervical dorsal ramus, also called the suboccipital nerve, lies between the vertebral artery and the inferior oblique muscle. This nerve innervates the four posterior suboccipital muscles.

The second cervical dorsal ramus is not contained in the occipital triangle. It courses around the caudal border of the inferior oblique muscle. The second cervical dorsal ramus divides into a lateral and medial branch. The medial branch becomes the greater occipital nerve (sensory), which pierces the semispinalis capitus and is a common source of occipital headaches. The lateral branch innervates the "long" posterior cervical muscles (i.e., splenius capitis, longissimus capitis, and semispinalis capitis).

The spinal canal is an osseous ring formed anteriorly by the vertebral body, lateral by the pedicles and posteriorly by adjoining laminae. The size of the canal varies from slightly oval to a triangular shape (Figure 4.4).

The spinal canal contains and protects the spinal cord. The diameter of the spinal canal, based on assessment using clinical x-ray, varies from 24 mm at the C1-C2 to 18 mm at the lower cervical region.[9] The volume of the intrathecal spinal canal decreases with extension, by 1.9 ml, as compared to a flexed position.[10] The cord lengthens in flexion by 10% with elongation being higher at the posterior cord.[11]

III. NORMAL JOINT KINESIOLOGY

A. OSTEOKINEMATICS AND ARTHROKINEMATICS AT THE OCCIPITO-ATLANTO-AXIAL REGION

The C0-C1-C2 region, if treated as one functional spinal unit, has 6 degrees of freedom. The C0-C1 and C1-C2 subunits also have 6 degrees of freedom. This section describes motion in each rotatory, osteokinematic degree of freedom (i.e., flexion, extension, right and left sidebending, and right and left rotation). The linear, arthrokinematic motion will be described only if it is coupled with rotation or it is clinically relevant. Furthermore, each movement pattern and location of its axis of rotation will be discussed, and the muscles activating the movement in this plane and their lever arm will be presented.

Movement pattern in the upper cervical spine is characterized by motion in more than one plane at a time (coupled movement patterns). Those coupled patterns, such as sidebending coupled with rotation, will be described.

1. Flexion and Extension

Flexion and extension occur at the atlanto-occipital and atlanto-axial joints. Since the neutral position in the sagittal plane is not easily identifiable, motion in the sagittal plane is reported as the sum of sagittal movement in both directions. White and Panjabi,[1] in their summary of results from past studies, reported 25 degrees of combined flexion and extension at the atlanto-occipital FSU and 20 degrees at the atlanto-axial FSU.

Flexion at the C0-C1 joints is associated with anterior rolling and posterior gliding of the occipital condyles in relation to the concave atlantal articulations. The reverse takes place with extension. Pure translation, without pre-seated rotation between the occiput and atlas is minimal (i.e., it does not exceed 1 mm).[12] Flexion of the occiput on the atlas is limited by the bony contact between the anterior rim of the foramen magnum and the superior surface of the dens. Extension is limited by connective tissue restraint of the tectorial and atlanto-occipital membranes.

Flexion at the atlanto-axial joint is associated with an inferior glide of the anterior arch of the atlas on the odontoid. During atlantal extension the arch glides superiorly. If the anterior curvature of the dens is sloping posteriorly, some additional extension may be observed (Figure 4.7).

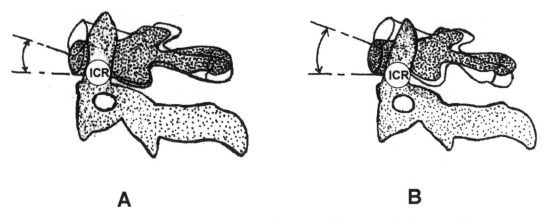

A   **B**

FIGURE 4.7 Location of the instantaneous center of rotation (ICR) in the sagittal plane at the atlanto-axial FSU (A). The curvature of the dens dictates the amount of motion. In (B) the dens is tilted more posteriorly than in (A), allowing for increased motion in the sagittal plane.

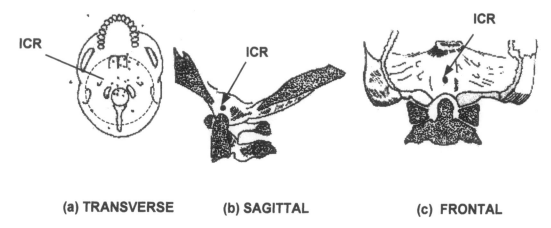

(a) TRANSVERSE   **(b) SAGITTAL**   **(c) FRONTAL**

FIGURE 4.8 Location of the instantaneous center of rotation (ICR) in the (a) transverse, (b) sagittal, and (c) frontal planes for the atlanto-occipital FSU. Note that there are several locations of the ICR in the transverse plane.

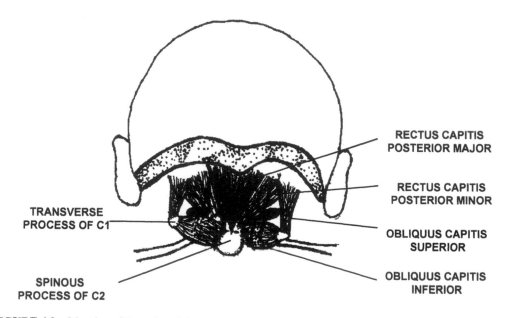

FIGURE 4.9 Muscles of the suboccipital triangle and selected bony landmarks.

Transverse plane translation at the atlanto-axial joint may be as great as, but should not exceed, 4 mm. More than 4 mm of translation is suggestive of instability.[13] Atlanto-axial translation is measured clinically on a radiograph between the anterior border of the dens and the posterior border of the anterior ring of C1. This measure is referred to as the atlanto-dental interval (ADI).

The axis of rotation for flexion and extension at the atlanto-occipital joint is located within the occipital condyles (Figure 4.8). When analyzing the occipital flexion and extension resulting from muscle forces and their lever arms, it becomes quite apparent that the extensors are abundant in number, have longer cross-sectional areas, and have relatively long lever arms (Figure 4.9).

In contrast, the flexors are limited in number, cross-sectional area, and located very close to the axis of rotation. The most laterally placed muscles are considered extensors, by virtue of the relationship of their attachment site to the axis of rotation. However, these muscles (i.e., sterno-cleidomastoid, splenius capitis, rectus capitis lateralis) also have anterior fibers that can act to flex the occiput. This action becomes more pronounced when the occiput is prepositioned in flexion.

TABLE 4.1
Sequence of Motion at the Occipito-Atlanto-Axial Region when Motion Is Initiated as Sidebending of the Occiput to the Right

Sequence	Action
1	Occiput sidebends right
2	Left *occipital* alar ligament becomes taut, resulting in right rotation of the axis
3	Atlas glides to the right, the right *atlantal* alar ligament (if present) becomes taut, causing a reverse glide of the atlas to the left
4	Axis rotated to the right, the resulting C1-C2 motion was left rotation of C1-C2
5	The facet orientation of C0-C1 guides the occiput into opposite rotation to the initiated sidebending

The axis of rotation for flexion and extension at the atlanto-axial joint passes through the dens just above the level of the atlanto-dental articulation (Figure 4.7). With the exception of the rectus capitis posterior minor, all muscles presented in Figure 4.9 are in a position to act on the atlanto-axial joint.

2. Sidebending

Sidebending in the sagittal plane can be initiated at the atlanto-occipital and atlanto-axial joints. Approximately 5 degrees of one-sided movement occurs at each of the two segments. Slight rotation to the opposite side is required to complete the sidebending motion. Thus, this coupled rotation places the sidebending and rotation in the category of coupled motions. This coupled motion results from the shape of the facet joints.

At the atlanto-occipital joint (during sidebending to the right), the right occipital condyle glides medially and anteriorly and the left occipital condyle glides laterally and posteriorly producing left rotation. At the atlanto-axial joint (during sidebending to the right), the inferior facets of the atlas slide off the "apex to apex" position to a lower position. Ultimately the right atlantal facet moves ventrally and the left atlantal facet moves dorsally, producing left rotation.

The axis of rotation for sidebending at the atlanto-occipital joints is aligned through the center of an imaginary arch formed by the occipital condyles in the sagittal plane (Figure 4.8). The axis of rotation for sidebending at the atlanto-axial joints is in the inferior aspect of the odontoid process (Figure 4.8).

Right occipital sidebending results in right rotation of the axis. There is no accompanying atlantal rotation. By convention of nomenclature (i.e., position of superior vertebrae in relation to the inferior vertebrae), the right rotation of the axis is described as left rotation at the atlanto-axial joint. This is another example of coupled motion at the upper cervical spine. The sequence of motion at the occipito-atlanto-axial region when motion is initiated as sidebending of the occiput is presented in Table 4.1.

3. Rotation

Rotation in the transverse plane can be initiated at either the occipito-atlantal or the atlanto–axial joint. One-sided rotation is approximately 5 degrees at the occipito-atlantal joint and 40 degrees at the atlanto-axial joint. To complete the rotation at each FSU, slight sidebending to the opposite side is required. Thus, this coupled sidebending places the sidebending and rotation in the category of coupled motions.

At the atlanto-occipital joint, during rotation to the right, the left occipital condyle glides medially and anteriorly and the right occipital condyle glides laterally and posteriorly, producing a secondary left sidebending. This coupled motion results from the shape of the facet joints.

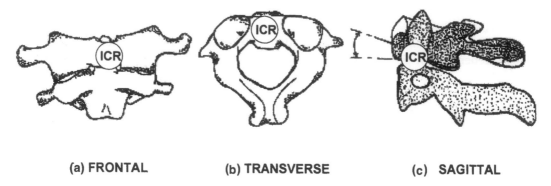

(a) FRONTAL   **(b) TRANSVERSE**   **(c) SAGITTAL**

FIGURE 4.10   Location of the instantaneous center of rotation in the (a) frontal, (b) transverse, and (c) sagittal planes at the atlanto-axial FSU.

At the atlanto-axial joint, rotation to the right is accompanied by sidebending to the left. The inferior facets of the atlas glide off the apex-to-apex position with the superior articular surfaces of the axis. During right rotation, the apex of the left inferior atlantal facet moves anteriorly and medially and the apex of the right inferior atlantal facet moves posteriorly and laterally in relation to the apex of the corresponding superior axial articulations.

The rotation at the atlanto-axial segment is limited by the alar ligaments, which tighten as the rotation progresses. The alar ligaments can be partially released from tension by placing the occiput in a slight opposite (in this example, left) sidebending. Consequently further atlanto-axial rotation is possible. The coupled motion at the atlanto-axial segment is a result of the shape of the facet joints and orientation of the alar ligaments.

The axis of rotation for the atlanto-occipital FSU has a very scattered distribution (Figure 4.8a) and for the atlanto-axial joint is placed vertically in the dens (Figure 4.10c).[14]

B. Osteokinematics and Arthrokinematics at the Lower Cervical Spine

Each cervical FSU has 6 degrees of freedom. The osteokinematic degrees of freedom will be described in relationship to it axis of rotation. Muscles activating the movement in each plane and their lever arms will be presented. Additionally, uniplanar and multiplanar motion will be identified.

1. Flexion and Extension

Flexion and extension occur in the sagittal plane. These rotatory (osteokinematic) motions are coupled with linear (arthokinematic) motions.[15] The linear motions occur at the discal and facet joints. During flexion, the superior vertebra rotates anteriorly. There is a coupled anterior translation of the superior vertebra on the inferior vertebra of the FSU at the discal joint. At the same time, the superior facet surfaces glide superiorly and anteriorly along the plane of the facet joints.

During extension, the superior vertebra rotates posteriorly. There is a coupled posterior translation of the superior vertebra on the inferior vertebra of the FSU at the discal joint. Conjointly, the superior facet surfaces glide inferiorly and posteriorly along the plane of the facet joints.

In a "normal" cervical FSU, the amount of translation does not exceed 2 mm in each direction.[16] Some authors[17,18] discuss tilting of the superior vertebra on the interior vertebra during flexion and extension. This tilt is a descriptive term for rotation of a vertebra about an axis of rotation.

The axis of rotation for flexion and extension at the cervical spine passes though the anterior aspect of the vertebral body of the caudal vertebra of an FSU (Figure 4.11). Of the segments caudal to C2, the C2-C3 segment has the least amount of sagittal motion and C5-C6 has the greatest amount of sagittal motion (Table 4.2).

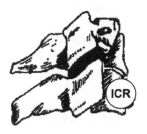
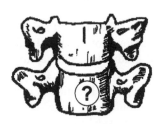
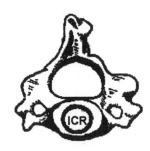

| **(a) SAGITTAL** | **(b) FRONTAL** | **(c) TRANSVERSE** |

FIGURE 4.11 Location of the instantaneous center of rotation in the (a) sagittal, (b) frontal and (c) transverse planes at a typical cervical FSU.

TABLE 4.2
Representative Values of Segmental Range of Motion in the Cervical Spine

FSU	Coupled Flexion/Extension (degrees)	One Side Lateral Bending (degrees)	One Side Axial Rotation (degrees)
C0–C1	25	5	5
C1–C2	20	5	40
C2–C3	10	10	3
C3–C4	15	11	7
C4–C5	20	11	7
C5–C6	20	8	7
C6–C7	17	7	6
C7–T1	9	4	2

Data from White and Panjabi.[1]

This larger amount of motion at the C5-C6 level has been associated with increased incidence of spondylosis at this level.[19] In general, the quantity of the segmental motion at the lower cervical region is dictated by the height of the intervertebral disc and the direction is guided by the orientation and shape of the facet and uncovertebral joints.

2. Sidebending and Rotation

In the lower cervical spine, sidebending and rotation occur conjunctly. That is, when motion is initiated with sidebending, rotation follows; when it is initiated by rotation, it is followed by sidebending.

Sidebending takes place in the frontal plane. This rotatory (osteokinematic) motion is coupled with another osteokinematic motion, i.e., rotation and linear (arthokinematic) motions. The linear motions occur at the discal and facet joints.

The coupled sidebending and rotation are results of the guidance of facet and uncovertebral joints. For example, when a motion is initiated with right sidebending, right rotation of the superior vertebra will follow. This pattern takes place regardless of the position of the FSU in the sagittal plane.

During sidebending to the right, the superior vertebra glides right at the discal joint. The accompanying rotation results from the right inferior facet of the superior vertebra gliding posteriorly and inferiorly while the left glides anteriorly and superiorly along the facet joint surface.

Lysell[6] describes a gradual cranio-caudal decrease in the amount of axial rotation that is associated with lateral bending.

The axis of rotation for sidebending at the cervical spine passes from anterior to posterior in the caudal vertebra of an FSU. The amount of unilateral sidebending ranges from 10 degrees at C2-C3 through the C4-C5 FSU and gradually decreases to less than 5 degrees at the C7-T1 FSU (Table 4.2).

Rotation takes place in the transverse plane. Rotation is coupled with ipsilateral sidebending. The superior vertebra glides at the discal joint to the same side as the rotation and gliding motion, and the facet joints follow the pattern during sidebending.

The axis of rotation for axial rotation at the cervical spine passes vertically through the center of the vertebral body (Figure 4.11c). The amount of unilateral rotation is 2 to 3 degrees at C2-C3 and C7-T1 segments and 5 to 7 degrees at the C3-C4 to C6-C7 segments. This pattern of motion reflects the orientation of the facet joints. The superior facets of the mid-cervical spine face slightly laterally and, therefore, promote greater degrees of rotation.

C. MUSCLES AND THEIR FUNCTION

1. The Occipito-Atlanto-Axial Region

The upper cervical muscles are able to move the occipito-atlas-axis complex independently of the lower cervical spine. The upper cervical muscles (rectus capitis posterior minor and major, and obliquus capitis inferior and superior) are referred to as suboccipital muscles, which structurally form a suboccipital triangle in the posterior aspect of the neck (Figure 4.9). The anterior suboccipital muscles are an extension of the muscles and will be discussed in the section on the lower cervical region below.

Most medially, at the suboccipital triangle, the rectus capitis posterior minor ascends from the posterior arch of the atlas to the occiput. Slightly lateral and posterior, the rectus capitis posterior major ascends from the spinous process of the axis to the occiput. These two muscles are occipital extensors.

The inferio-lateral border of the suboccipital triangle is formed by the obliquus capitis inferior. The obliquus capitis inferior ascends laterally and anteriorly from the spinous process of the axis to the transverse process of the atlas. This muscle has a mechanical leverage for rotation of the atlas on the axis.

The lateral border of the suboccipital triangle is formed by the obliquus capitis superior. The obliquus capitis superior ascends superiorly, posteriorly, and medially from the transverse process of the atlas to the occiput. Contraction of this muscle produces ipsilateral occipital sidebending followed by contralateral occipital rotation.

The muscles attaching to the occipital base act on the suboccipital region (Figure 4.12). They are the muscles described above and those that direct the motion of the lower cervical region (described below).

2. The Lower Cervical Region

The muscles of the lower cervical region protect the cervical spine, interconnect and move the cervical FSU, and connect and move the head, neck, and shoulder regions. Most muscles of the cervical region are capable of contributing to multidirectional motions. However, each muscle has a dominant lever arm for one type of motion. Therefore, the muscles will be presented in functional groups. It is evident, in the cervical spine, that a muscle lying close to an axis of rotation may have its action changed if the muscle's line of pull is changed relative to the axis of rotation. That is, a flexor may become an extensor. The cervical extensors are posterior to the axis of rotation in the sagittal plane (Figure 4.13). The extensors are the trapezius, semispinalis (capitis and cervicis), longissimus, and levator scapulae.

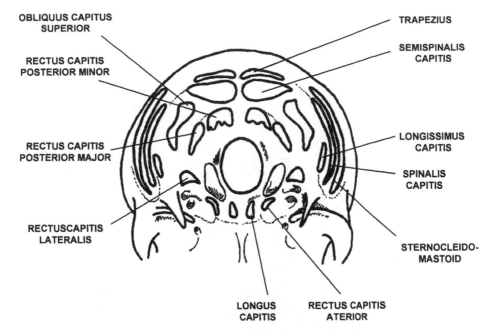

FIGURE 4.12   Muscular attachments to the occipital base. (From Porterfield, J. A. and DeRosa, C., *Mechanical Neck Pain. Perspectives in Functional Anatomy,* W.B. Saunders, Philadelphia, 1995, p. 85. With permission.)

The trapezius lies most superficially and has broad attachments to the occiput, ligamentum nuchae, thoracic spinous processes, spine of scapulae, acromion, and lateral third of the clavicle. The muscle is located far from the center of rotation for the individual FSU (Figure 4.13). Therefore, it has a long lever arm. The long lever arm coupled with broad attachment and substantial cross-sectional area makes this muscle very effective in extension and sidebending.

The splenius capitus (the "bandage" muscle) and cervicis originate from thoracic and cervical spinous processes and ligamentum nuchae and run superior and lateral to the mastoid process (splenius capitis) and posterior tubercle of the cervical transverse process (splenius cervicis), forming a "V" shaped "thin bandage" for the short paravertebral muscles. These muscles have an excellent lever arm for extension, and the lateral attachments also contribute to rotation (Figure 4.13).

The semispinalis capitus and cervicis are in the third layer of posterior cervical muscles. These muscles attach to the occiput and the spinous processes of the cervical vertebrae at and below C2. They are the most effective segmental extensors due to their relatively long lever arm and much larger cross-sectional area (Figure 4.13). The semispinalis muscles serve a critical role in maintaining cervical lordosis.

The longissimus cervicis and capitis are at the same layer as semispinalis, but positioned more lateral. The longissimus cervicis originates from the transverse processes of the upper thoracic spine and attaches to the posterior tubercle of the cervical transverse process. The longissimus capitis runs from upper thoracic transverse processes and attaches to the mastoid process. The longissimii attach closer to the flexion/extension axis of rotation and, consequently, are less powerful extensors than the aforementioned muscles (Figure 4.13). However, they can be effective in sidebending.

The cervical flexors are the longus colii and capitis, rectus capitis anterior and lateralis, infrahyoid, suprahyoid, and sternocleidomastoid. The longus coli lies anteriorly on the vertebral bodies and runs from the upper thoracic vertebrae to the atlas. It attaches to the anterior tubercle of each vertebral body. The longus capitis runs from the anterior tubercle of each vertebral body to the base of the occiput. Both of these muscles are cervical flexors (Figure 4.13).

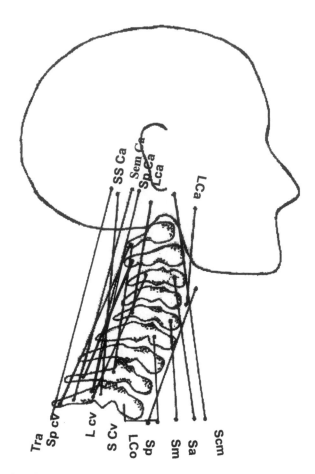

FIGURE 4.13   Sagittal projection of the line of action for cervical musculature. Sternocleidomastoid (Scm), longus capitis (LCa), longus colii (Lco), scalenus anterior (Sa), scalenus medius (Sm), scalenus posterior (Sp), trapezius (Tra), splenius capitis (Sca), splenius cervicis (Sp cv), spinalis capitis (Spi ca), spinalis cervicis (Spi ce), semispinalis capitis (Sem ca), semispinalis cervicis (Sem ce), longissimus capitis (Lca), longissimus cervicis (L cv).

The infrahyoid and suprahyoid are the most anterior neck muscles. They stabilize or move the hyoid bone and do not have any direct influence on the cervical spine. The sternocleidomastoid runs from the sternum and medial aspect of the clavicle to the mastoid process. This muscle has a significant cross-sectional area. Depending on the initial position of the occiput, it can function as a head and neck flexor or extensor (e.g., if the line of action falls behind the atlanto-occipital axis of rotation in the sagittal plane, the sternocleidomastoid will act as an extensor). The secondary motions produced by this muscle are sidebending and contralateral rotation.

Located lateral to the cervical spine (in the frontal plane), the scalene muscles (anterior, middle, and posterior) and levator scapulae act in sidebending. The scalene muscles are positioned lateral to the cervical spine and provide dynamic stability. The scalenes have mechanical leverage for lateral flexion (Figure 4.13). If the anterior scalenes contract bilaterally they can produce cervical flexion.

The levator scapula is described as a lateral flexor of the neck. This muscle originates from the superiomedial border of the scapula and courses superiorly, medially, and anteriorly, attaching to the transverse processes of the foremost cranial vertebrae. It ipsilaterally flexes the cervical spine. The other two movement components produced by the levator scapula are extension and ipsilateral rotation. The cross-sectional area of this muscle is relatively large, which contributes to its torque-producing capabilities.

IV. PATHOKINESIOLOGY: CLINICAL RELEVANCE AND IMPLICATIONS

A. OCCIPITAL-ATLANTAL INSTABILITY

Occipital-atlantal instabilities are mostly of traumatic origin, with more than 1 mm of sagittal plane translation considered abnormal. The patient presentation is very diverse in terms of pain and neurological complaints.

B. OS ODONTOIDEUM AND INSTABILITY

Os odontoideum is a pseudoarthrosis at the base of the odontoid, thought to be of traumatic origin. It is often associated with instability. There may be substantial anterior displacement of the atlas on the axis, including the displacement of the odontoid itself. In those cases surgical fixation may be required.[20]

C. ATLANTO-AXIAL SUBLUXATION OF RHEUMATOID ARTHRITIS ORIGIN

Twenty-three percent of patients with a history of rheumatoid arthritis have atlanto-axial subluxation (i.e., the atlas is displaced in relation to the axis).[21] There are two patterns of subluxations and dislocations at the atlanto-axial joint: translatory and rotatory. These dislocations can be unilateral or bilateral and anterior or posterior. The cause is thought to be attenuation of the transverse ligament. Frequently, patients are asymptomatic.

If symptomatic, the patient typically reports a perception of the "head falling off," hearing a clunking sound with excessive movements, occasional difficulty swallowing, tinnitus, and other symptoms related to the subcranial region.[22] The potential consequences of displacement in this area include quadriplegia and death.

D. COMMINUTED FRACTURE OF THE RING OF C1 (JEFFERSON FRACTURE)

A comminuted fracture of the atlas is often associated with instability and is related to direct trauma such as falling on the head or a heavy object falling on top of the head. Patient presentations vary and may include pain, suboccipital headaches, vertigo, tinnitus, numbness, nausea, or drop attacks. The management of this condition typically requires surgical fixation.

E. CERVICAL SPONDYLOSIS

Cervical spondylosis is a common degenerative process leading to mechanical neck pain. It is thought that the process begins at the intervertebral disc and subsequently involves other structures, such as the apophyseal and uncovertebral joints. The degenerative process may become symptomatic at any stage of presentation.

Symptoms may be placed in one of four categories: neck pain, neck pain with proximal referral, radicular pain, and myelopathy. The neck pain, neck pain with proximal referral, and upper extremity radicular pain can be caused by several cervical structures containing nociceptors, including the disc, nerve root sleeve, facet joints, and ligaments.

In patients with spondylolytic disease, exacerbated pain is related more to changes in the foraminal size and nerve root motion, rather than to changes in size of herniated discs.[23] In cervical spondylitic myelopathy, the cervical cord is compromised in the spinal cord as a result of degenerative changes of the cervical spine. It is the most serious consequence of cervical intervertebral disc degeneration and the most common cervical spinal cord disorder after middle age.[24,25] Narrowing of the spinal canal, also referred to as spinal stenosis, is another form of spondylosis. The management of patients with spondylosis is most often conservative, but occasionally it requires surgical intervention.

F. ACCELERATION INJURY

Acceleration injury is a descriptive term for the mechanism of injury that is associated with rapid acceleration and deceleration. Symptoms from acceleration injuries may include headache, vertigo, and fatigue, as well as neck pain. This type of injury may involve several structures in addition to the cervical musculoskeletal system (i.e., the temporomandibular joints, esophagus, trachea, and central nervous system). Hyperextension injuries tend to be more disruptive to the musculosketal system than the hyperflexion injuries,[26] as they produce high sheer and tensile forces on the cervical spine.

V. SUMMARY AND CONCLUSIONS

The cervical region structurally and functionally has two distinct regions: the upper (C0-C2) and lower (C2-T1) cervical regions. Unique ligaments in the upper cervical region are capable of both limiting and guiding motion (alar ligament). Additionally, the transverse orientation and the unique rounded shape at the facet joints substitute for the lack of an intervertebral disc. Finally, while the upper cervical spine consists of only two FSUs, it produces 50% of the available cervical rotation. The lower cervical spine, consisting of five FSUs, provides the remaining amount of rotation. The lower cervical spine also has intervertebral discs, facet joints, and uncovertebral joints that enhance and guide mobility. Both regions have coupled motions when sidebending or rotation is initiated first.

The common pathokinematic conditions that affect the cervical spine are generally of a traumatic, systemic, or degenerative nature. Pathologies of traumatic origin vary significantly in the extent of injury. Systemic conditions may relate to ligamentous laxity (rheumatoid arthritis) or impaired ossification (os odontoideum). Degenerative changes are commonly related to spondylosis, stenosis, joint arthrosis, or disc injury.

REFERENCES

1. White, A. A. and Panjabi, M. M., *Clinical Biomechanics of the Spine,* J.B. Lippincott, Philadelphia, 1991.
2. Shapiro, R., Youngberg, A. S., and Rothman, S. L., The differential diagnosis of traumatic lesions of the occipito-atlanto-axial segment, *Radiol. Clin. North Am.,* 11, 505, 1973.
3. Dvorak, J. et al., Biomechanics of the craniocervical region: the alar and transverse ligaments, *J. Orthop. Res.,* 6, 452, 1988.
4. Werne, S., Studies in spontaneous atlas dislocation, *Acta Orthop. Scand.,* 23, 35, 1957.
5. Dreyer, S. J. and Boden, S. D., Natural history of rheumatoid arthritis of the cervical spine, *Clin. Orthop. Rel. Res.,* 366, 98, 1999.
6. Lysell, E., Motion in the cervical spine, *Acta Orthop. Scand. (Suppl.),* 123, 1, 1969.
7. Clausen, J. D. et al., Uncinate processes and Luschka joints influence the biomechanics of the cervical spine: quantification using a finite element model of the C5-C6 segment, *J. Orthop. Res.,* 15, 342, 1997.
8. Dvorak, J. and Panjabi, M. M., Functional anatomy of the alar ligaments, *Spine,* 12, 183, 1987.
9. Eisomont, F. J. et al., Cervical sagittal spinal canal size in spine injury, *Spine,* 9, 663, 1984.
10. Holmes, A. et al., Changes in cervical canal spinal volume during in vitro flexion-extension, *Spine,* 21, 1313, 1996.
11. Qing, Y., Dougherty, L., and Margulies, S. S., In vivo human cervical spinal cord deformation and displacement in flexion, *Spine,* 23, 1677, 1998.
12. Wiesel, S. W. and Rothman, R. H., Occipital atlantal hypermobility, *Spine,* 4, 187, 1979.
13. White, A. A. et al., Biomechanical analysis of clinical stability in the cervical spine, *Clin. Orthop.,* 109, 85, 1975.
14. Hiroshi, L. et al., Three-dimensional motion analysis of the upper cervical spine during axial rotation, *Spine,* 18, 238, 1993.

15. Amevo, B., Instantaneous axis of the typical cervical motion segments. I. An empirical study of technical errors, *Clin. Biomech.*, 6, 31, 1991.
16. Panjabi, M. M. et al., Three dimensional load displacement curves of the cervical spine, *J. Orthop. Res.*, 4, 152, 1986.
17. Jones, M. D., Cineradiographic studies of the normal cervical spine, *Calif. Med.*, 93, 293, 1960.
18. Kapandji, I. P., *The Physiology of Joints,* Vol. 3, Churchill Livingstone, New York, 1982.
19. White, A. A. et al., Relief of a pain by anterior cervical spine fusion for spondylosis. A report of 65 patients, *J. Bone Joint Surg. [Am.]*, 55, 525, 1973.
20. Blauth, M. et al., Operative oder konservative Behandlung der Pseudaarthrose des Dens axis. Wie gefahrlich ist es, eine Denspseudarthrose nichr zu stabilisieren? (Operative versus non operative treatment of odontoid non unions. How dangerous is it not to stabilize a non union of the dens?), *Chirurgie.*, 70, 1225, 1999.
21. Neva, M. H., Kaarela, K., and Kauppi, M., Prevalence of radiological changes in the cervical spin — a cross sectional study after 20 years from presentation of rheumatoid arthritis, *J. Rheumatol.*, 27, 90, 2000.
22. Grieve, G. P., *Common Vertebral Joint Problems*, 2nd edition, Churchill Livingstone, New York, 1988.
23. Muhle, C., Exacerbated pain in cervical radiculopathy at axial rotation, flexion, extension, and coupled motions of the cervical spine, *Invest. Radiol.*, 33, 279, 1998.
24. Lundsford, L. D., Bissonette, D. J., and Zorub, D. S., Anterior surgery for cervical disc disease. II. Treatment of cervical spondylotic myelopathy in 32 cases, *J. Neurosurg.*, 53, 12, 1980.
25. Wilberger, J. E. and Chedid, M. K., Acute cervical spondylotic myelopathy, *Neurosurgery,* 22, 145, 1988.
26. Macnab, I., Acceleration injuries of the cervical spine, *J. Bone Joint Surg. [Am.]*, 46, 1797, 1964.

5 Kinematic MRI of the Cervical Spine

Jari O. Karhu and Seppo K. Koskinen

CONTENTS

I. INTRODUCTION

Diagnostic imaging is routinely performed for the cervical spine using magnetic resonance imaging (MRI). However, common abnormalities that affect this anatomic region are undetected using conventional "static view" MRI techniques. The primary reason for this is that the cervical spine is typically imaged with the patient's neck in a comfortable, neutral position; however, certain disorders are "position-dependent." Thus, to improve the diagnostic yield of MRI, it may be necessary to assess the cervical spine using a kinematic MRI procedure.[1-3] Kinematic MRI is capable of showing the relationship among the odontoid, foramen magnum, spinal cord, and other related anatomic structures as the patient's cervical spine is moved through a given range of motion.

The use of kinematic MRI contributes to a more thorough evaluation of the cervical spine in normal subjects and in patients with abnormalities secondary to trauma, cervical spondylotic disease, and rheumatoid arthritis, as well as with other conditions.[1-22] Furthermore, kinematic MRI may provide critical information for staging disorders and planning conservative or surgical treatments of the cervical spine.[16,19]

0-8493-0807-0/01/$0.00+$.50
© 2001 by Frank G. Shellock

This chapter presents the technical and clinical aspects of kinematic MRI of the cervical spine. Examples of normal and abnormal findings are presented, as well as the clinical applications of kinematic MRI to assess specific disorders.

II. TECHNIQUE

A. POSITIONING DEVICES AND RADIOFREQUENCY COILS

Because of the multidirectional motion of the cervical spine, the use of a positioning device that enables movement in a controlled, repeatable manner is crucial for the performance of the kinematic MRI examination. Obviously, positioning devices must be constructed of nonferromagnetic components and designed with a thorough understanding of cervical spine biomechanics.

Special positioning devices are available for kinematic MRI of the cervical spine that permit flexion and extension, sidebending, rotation, or a combination of movements (Figure 5.1).[1-6] Devices designed for flexion and extension studies of the cervical spine can be used in conventional high-field-strength MR systems but may not accomplish a full range of motion for all patients. For example, the typical maximum range of motion that may be achieved using these positioning devices for kinematic MRI of the cervical spine in a high-field-strength MR system is approximately 50° of flexion to 30° of extension.[4] By comparison, a special positioning device developed for kinematic MRI studies performed in an open MR system (0.23 Tesla) permits a full range of motion in multiple directions.[5] Notably, newer "wide-bore," high-field-strength MR systems do have sufficient space for flexion and extension examinations of the cervical spine.

The complex anatomy of the cervical spine requires that the kinematic MRI examination be performed using a radiofrequency (RF) surface coil to obtain adequate signal-to-noise for imaging.

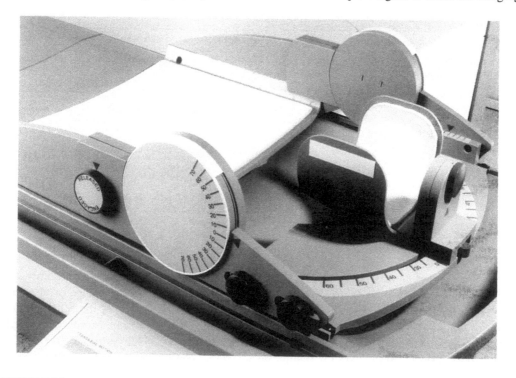

FIGURE 5.1A   Example of a positioning device used for kinematic MRI of the cervical spine. This device is made from MR compatible materials (Picker Nordstar Inc., Helsinki, Finland). Note that this unique device permits movements of the cervical spine in three different ranges of motion: (1) flexion and extension, (2) sidebending, and (3) rotation.

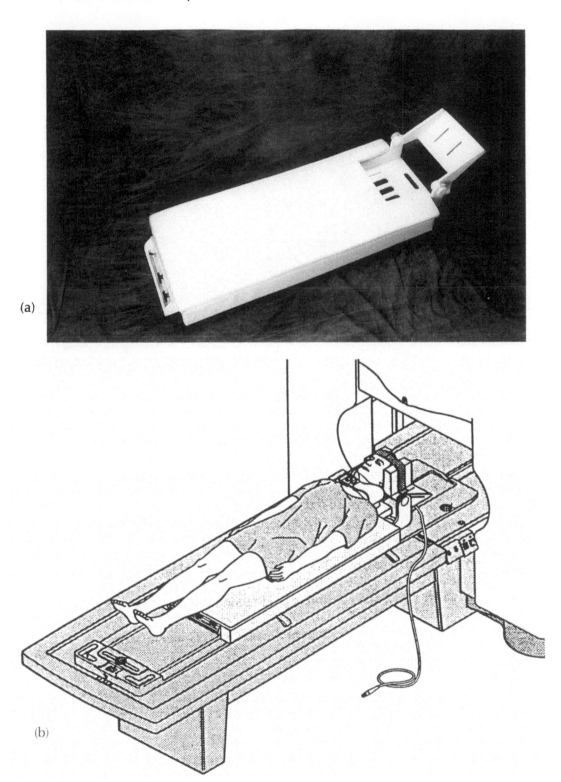

FIGURE 5.1B Positioning device (a) designed for incremental positioning of the cervical spine from flexion to extension (CHAMCO, Inc., Cocoa, FL). Several different types of surface coils may be utilized with this positioning device. (b) Schematic showing the positioning device with a subject prepared for kinematic MRI of the cervical spine using an open MR system. Note the flexible, wrap-around RF coil.

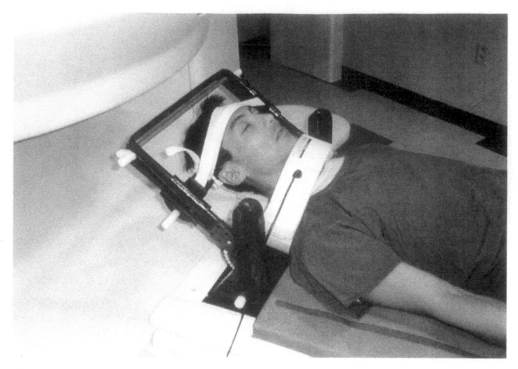

FIGURE 5.1C   Positioning device designed for incremental positions of the cervical spine from flexion to extension (General Electric Medical Systems, Milwaukee, WI). This device supports and stabilizes the subject's head and neck during the kinematic MRI examination. A circumferential, receive-only RF surface coil is typically used to facilitate the kinematic MRI procedure using this positioning device.

A variety of RF coil configurations has been used for kinematic MRI studies, including dual 5-inch, receive-only, circular surface coils; flexible, wrap-around coils; and posterior neck coils.[1-22] The RF coil configuration must be a size and shape to be acceptable for use with the particular positioning device that is utilized for the kinematic MRI procedure. Furthermore, since high-resolution MR images of the cervical spine are frequently needed in addition to the kinematic MRI examination, it is advantageous to use the same RF coil equipment to eliminate the need to reposition the patient and unnecessarily lengthen the overall imaging procedure.

B. THE MAGNETIC RESONANCE SYSTEM: SUPINE VS. UPRIGHT, SEATED POSITIONING

Kinematic MRI of the cervical spine was originally accomplished using conventional, "tunnel-shaped" MR systems. However, the use of an "open"-configured MR system offers advantages that include better access to the patient and the ability to image the cervical spine in positions that cannot be accomplished using conventional MR systems. Whether using a conventional or open-configured MR system, the patient is typically imaged while in a supine position. Therefore, the resulting forces acting on the cervical spine for the kinematic MRI procedure are not similar to those experienced during activities of daily living.

Recently, it has been possible to perform kinematic MRI of the cervical spine with the patient in an upright, seated position using a vertically opened MR system (0.5 Tesla Signa SP, General Electric Medical Systems, Milwaukee, WI).[7] Because images are acquired rapidly using this MR system (e.g., 1 to 10 seconds per image) and the section location can be selected relative to the cervical spine using specialized hardware and software, positioning and movement of the cervical spine can be controlled by muscular action rather than externally applied positioning devices. The use of the vertically opened MR system for kinematic MRI of the cervical spine is believed to

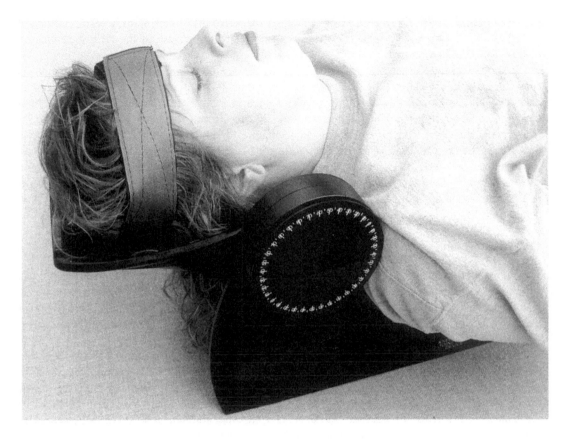

FIGURE 5.1D A newly developed positioning device designed for kinematic MRI of the cervical spine (CHAMCO, Inc., Cocoa, FL).

permit a more physiologic, functional assessment because gravity adds forces (e.g., from the weight of the head and associated supporting musculature) that are not applied with the patient in a supine position. However, the clinical impact of using a supine vs. an upright, seated position for the kinematic MRI examination of the cervical spine is currently unknown.

C. IMAGING PARAMETERS AND PROTOCOL

A variety of pulse sequences and protocols has been used for kinematic MRI of the cervical spine.[1-21] For example, T1-weighted, T2-weighted spin-echo, T2-weighted fast spin-echo, gradient echo, fast gradient echo, and echo planar imaging parameters reportedly have been used for this procedure. However, T2-weighted, fast spin-echo imaging parameters selected to produce a "myelographic effect" are considered to be optimal for most kinematic MRI examinations.

The selection of specific imaging parameters for kinematic MRI is based on the desired image contrast and resolution necessary to assess the suspected cervical spine abnormality or disorder. Additionally, the temporal resolution of the imaging parameters must be considered with respect to the type of kinematic MRI procedure that is used. Kinematic MRI may be conducted using either an incremental, passive positioning or an active movement (i.e., dynamic) technique.

The incremental passive positioning technique involves gradual movement and sequential MR imaging through a specific range of cervical spine motion. Virtually any type of pulse sequence may be applied for the incremental, passive positioning technique. However, kinematic MRI conducted using an active movement (i.e., dynamic) technique typically requires the use of fast gradient echo or echo planar imaging methods. While ultra-fast, half-Fourier acquisition, single-shot turbo spin-echo (HASTE) sequence can be utilized for active movement studies, results compared to fast or "turbo" spin-echo sequences have been problematic because of the lack of delineation of the anatomical structures.[3,22]

It should be noted that, using the incremental, passive positioning technique to evaluate the cervical spine causes stretching of noncontractile elements and assesses the anatomic range of motion.[23] This kinematic examination typically results in a larger movement pattern and is more likely to uncover hypermobility compared with the use of an active movement technique.[24,25] Conversely, the use of the active movement technique for kinematic MRI of the cervical spine determines the "physiologic" range of motion for the patient. Regardless of the technique selected for use, the kinematic MRI examination of the cervical spine must be carried out with extreme care in patients with rheumatoid arthritis and other inflammatory processes of the spine, such as psoriatic arthropathy, ankylosing spondylitis, and systemic lupus erythematosus. Instability associated with these conditions can result in cord compression.

1. Imaging Plane

The major movements of the cervical spine that can be assessed using kinematic MRI techniques are flexion and extension (sagittal plane), sidebending (frontal or coronal plane), and rotation (axial plane) (Figures 5.2 and 5.3). If an abnormality is seen on a mid-sagittal plane image, obliqued axial plane images may be obtained through the area of affected anatomy, in the coronal plane during sidebending, and in the axial plane during rotation.

In addition, the cervical spine has coupled or complex motion in other planes of movement than the primary movement. One of the most important of these coupled motions is unilateral rotation of segments C2-Th1 and contralateral rotation of segments C0-C2, which are associated with sidebending[26-28] (Figure 5.4). There is also unilateral transverse gliding movement of the atlas associated with sidebending (Figure 5.5).[5] In general, the imaging plane used for the kinematic MRI procedure must be selected in consideration of the suspected pathology or condition that is present.

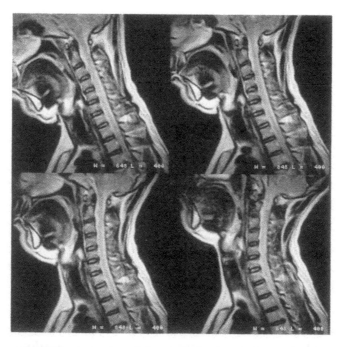

FIGURE 5.2 Kinematic MRI examination of the cervical spine performed in a healthy subject showing flexion (top left), neutral (top right), and extension (bottom left and right). Mid-sagittal plane image obtained using the incremental, passive positioning technique.

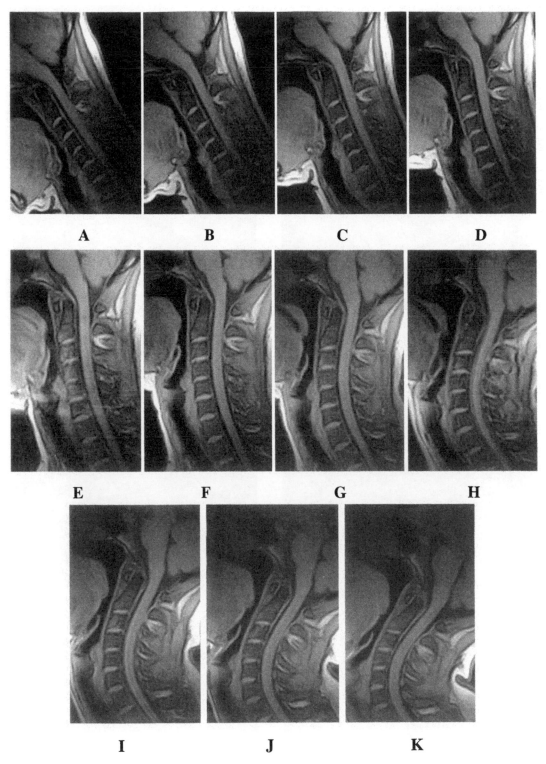

FIGURE 5.3 Kinematic MRI of the cervical spine performed in a normal subject during (A) 50° flexion, (B) 40° flexion, (C) 30° flexion, (D) 20° flexion, (E) 10° flexion, (F) neutral position, (G) 10° extension, (H) 20° extension, (I) 30° extension, (J) 40° extension, and (K) 50° extension. This kinematic MRI study was performed using an incremental, passive positioning technique.

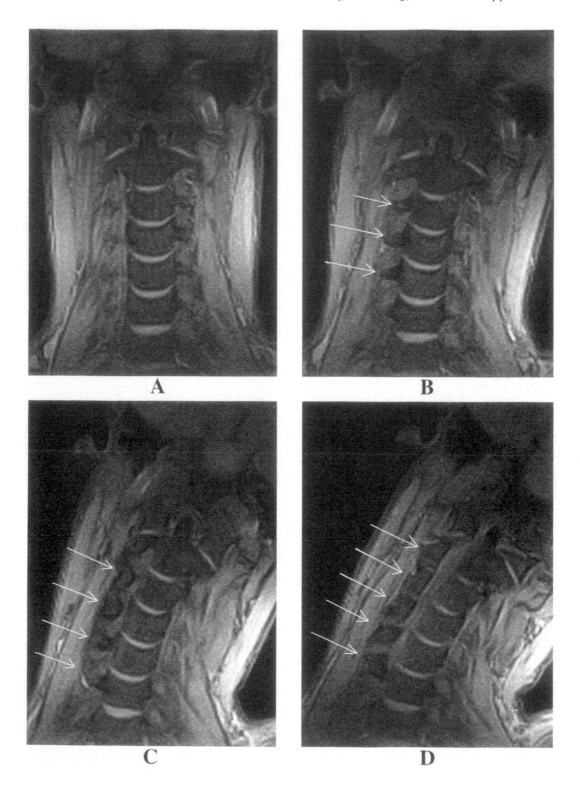

FIGURE 5.4   Kinematic MRI of the cervical spine during sidebending to the left in a normal subject: (A) neutral position, (B) 15° sidebending (C), 30° sidebending, and (D) 45° sidebending. Note the increasing combined rotation to the right in the lower cervical spine associated with these movements (arrows).

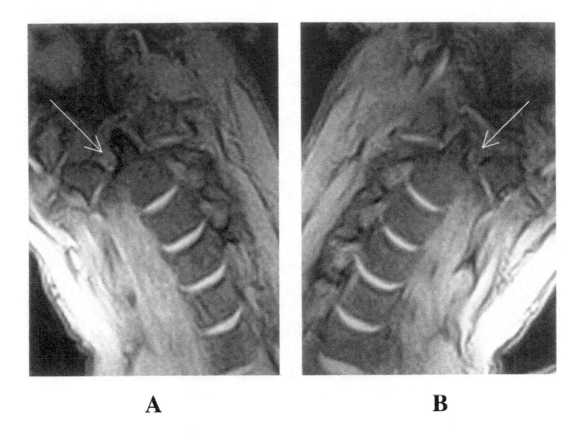

A   **B**

FIGURE 5.5   Kinematic MRI of the cervical spine during sidebending by a normal subject. Sidebending of (A) 45° to the right and (B) 45° to the left. Note the transversal unilateral gliding movement of the atlas shown as widening of the gap between massa lateralis of the atlas and dens (arrow).

D. ASSESSMENT OF KINEMATIC MRI EXAMINATIONS

Knowledge of normal cervical spine anatomy, motion patterns, and ranges of motion forms the basis for interpreting kinematic MRI examinations of the cervical spine. Notably, kinematic MRI studies are usually analyzed qualitatively because quantitative parameters tend to have only limited diagnostic value. If detailed quantitative analysis is needed, one should be aware that presently there are no exact values for the normal and pathological findings.[24-29]

For certain cervical spine movement patterns, however, values have been derived using MRI as well as other imaging modalities (Tables 5.1 to 5.6). Clinical methods using commercially available electronic goniometers have been used to analyze either active or passive three-dimensional normal ranges of motion for the entire cervical spine *in vivo* (Table 5.1).[23,26,28,29] When age and gender-related passive motions of the cervical spine were studied, some significantly decreased motion differences were found between various age groups within gender. However, rotation in the atlanto-axial joint (C1-C2) for the maximally flexed position of the neck did not decrease with age.[23] Therefore, previously determined values for cervical spine movements may be used to guide the evaluation of kinematic MRI examinations.

1. Sagittal Plane Motion

Most studies of cervical spine kinematics have used conventional plain film radiographs and motion analysis of flexion and extension movement, most of which occur from C3-C7.[24,25,27,30,31] The most prominent range of flexion and extension takes place at the level of C4-C5 and C5-C6 segments;

TABLE 5.1
Three-Dimensional Motion of the Cervical Spine *in Vivo*

Type of Movement	Subject Age	Sex	Flexion/Extension	Lateral Bending	Axial Rotation	Ref.
Passive	20–29	m	153	101	184	23
		f	149	100	182	
	30–39	m	141	95	175	
		f	156	106	186	
Passive	26.7	m	61[a]	47[b]	146	29
		f	60[a]	45[b]	165	
Active	25.9	m&f	122	88	144	28
Active	32	m&f	140	91	153	26

[a] Measured as flexion only.
[b] Measured as lateral bending to the right only.

TABLE 5.2
**Sagittal Flexion/Extension Segmental Motion
of the Cervical Spine**

	Dvorak 88[a]		Penning[a]	Ordway[a]	Muhle[b]
	Active	Passive	—	Active	—
C0-C1	—	—		25	—
C1-C2	12	15	30	12	—
C2-C3	10	12	12	13	11
C3-C4	15	17	18	17	12
C4-C5	19	21	20	19	15
C5-C6	20	23	20	19	19
C6-C7	19	21	15	17	20

[a] Measured using conventional radiographs.
[b] Measured using kinematic MRI.

however, some motion occurs at the occipito-atlantal joint (C0-C1) (Table 5.2).[8,24,27,31] Additionally, findings have shown that cervical protrusion and retraction are associated with flexion and extension movements of the cervical spine.[31]

Retraction consists of lower cervical extension and upper cervical flexion, whereas protrusion consists of upper cervical extension and lower cervical flexion. Only retraction takes C0-C1 and C1-C2 to their full end-range of flexion and only protrusion takes C0-C1 and C1-C2 to their full end-range of extension.[31]

Using cineradiography (i.e., fluoroscopy), Hino et al.[32] demonstrated that the normal cervical spine showed a well-regulated stepwise flexion motion pattern that initiated at C1-C2 and transmitted to the lower segments with time lags. A different order for the onset of flexion was observed between the normal and pathologic cervical spine. In patients with rheumatoid arthritis who had anterior atlanto-axial subluxation, C1-C2 motion initiated significantly earlier than C2-C3 motion. In patients with subaxial segmental instability, motion in the unstable segments preceded that in the intact segments.[32]

The minimum space needed for the cervical cord at the C1-C2 level, measured as the diameter of the bony spinal canal (posterior atlantodental interval) using conventional radiography, is 13 to

14 mm.[33-35] In an *in vitro* study of the volume of the intrathecal cervical spinal canal at the level of the segments C2-C7, the volume reduced 1.9 ml in the extension position when compared with the flexion position.[36] This change in volume is caused by decrease of the length and width of the spinal canal during extension. Notably, this change is likely to be greater in the cervical spine than elsewhere in the spine.

2. Rotation

The greatest intervertebral motion in the spine is axial rotation at C1-C2, of which 75% is constituted by the so-called "neutral zone."[37] The special movements of the upper cervical spine (occiput-C2) are enabled by unique design of the articulations and stabilizing ligaments, of which the most important are the alar and transversal ligaments and the tectorial membrane. Rotation can be assessed in either the neutral, flexed, or extended positions. During maximal flexion of the cervical spine, the segments C3-C7 become locked and the rotation occurs almost entirely in the upper cervical spine.[23]

Computed tomography (CT) has been used to evaluate the segmental rotation of the cervical spine. The mean range of rotation of the eight segments between occiput and thoracic spine in normal subjects is presented in Table 5.3.[38,39]

TABLE 5.3
Normal Values of Unilateral Segmental Rotation of the Cervical Spine Assessed Using Functional CT

	Penning	Dvorak
C0-C1	1	2.8
C1-C2	40.5	41.5
C2-C3	3	—
C3-C4	6.5	—
C4-C5	6.8	—
C5-C6	6.9	—
C6-C7	5.4	—
C7-Th1	2.1	—
C0-Th1	72.2	—
C2-Th1	30.7	30.8

Rotational hypermobility of the upper cervical spine is suspected to be caused by soft tissue damage, especially by traumatic lesion of the contralateral alar ligament.[39-41] A rotation at C0-C1 of more than 7° and at C1-C2 of more than 54° indicates hypermobility[41] and a rotation at C1-C2 of less than 29° indicates hypomobility. A right-left difference of more than 5° at C0-C1 and more than 8° at C1-C2 is considered pathological[39] (Figure 5.6). Hypermobile rotation in the upper cervical spine has also been found to be associated with contralateral paradoxical motion. That is, the lower (C1 or C2) vertebra rotates more out of the neutral position than the upper segment (occiput or C1).[40]

3. Kinematic MRI and Segmental Motion Analysis

As previously indicated, there have been few detailed studies of normal motion of the cervical spine using kinematic MRI. In an investigation utilizing segmental kinematic MRI analysis between 50° flexion and 30° extension, there was increased motion at the lower segments, with the greatest motion being observed at the C6-C7 level.[8] This distribution of segmental motion differs slightly

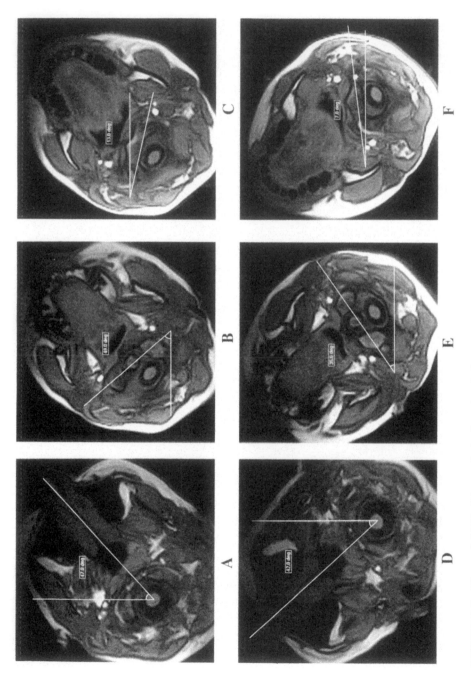

FIGURE 5.6 Kinematic MRI of the cervical spine using the incremental, passive positioning technique (axial plane). This examination shows hypomobility of the atlanto-axial joint during rotation to the right. There also is a pathological left-right difference at the same level. In addition, there is paradoxal rotation of the atlas in relation to the occiput during rotation to the left (atlas rotates 2° more than occiput) and associated atlanto-occipital hypermobility on the right side. This condition may be caused by injury of the left alar ligament. (A) Occiput rotates 47° to the left, (B) atlas rotates 49° to the left, and (C) axis rotates 13° to the left. (D) Occiput rotates 42° to the right, (E) atlas rotates 35° to the right, and (F) axis rotates 7° to the right.

from that obtained in previous studies using conventional plain film radiography (Table 5.2). Nevertheless, kinematic MRI yields data on segmental motion of the cervical spine comparable to those obtained using flexion and extension radiographs.

To date, kinematic MRI has been used to evaluate not only flexion and extension, but also rotation and sidebending of the occipito-atlanto-axial complex in asymptomatic subjects[5] (Figures 5.2, 5.3, 5.4, 5.5 and 5.7). Segmental motion of the upper cervical spine obtained from healthy normal subjects in three planes using kinematic MRI is presented in Tables 5.4 to 5.6.

4. Position-Related Changes in the Cervical Spinal Canal and Cord

When the cervical spinal canal is evaluated using kinematic MRI, both bony and soft tissue borders of the canal must be taken into consideration because the narrowing of the canal is often caused by pathological soft tissue (Figure 5.8). Normally the diameter of the cervical spinal canal and the cerobrospinal fluid space is at its widest in the craniovertebral junction, which is appropriate considering the wide range of motion of the structures of the region.

Using kinematic MRI, the diameter of the normal cervical spinal canal at the level of the atlas has been reported to be approximately 15 mm.[54] The mean diameter of the cord at the C1-C2 level has been reported to be 7.2 to 7.7 mm.[8,15] This value decreased gradually in the caudal direction, where it was observed to be 6.6 mm at C7.[8]

The cervicomedullary angle (i.e., the angle between the lines drawn along the anterior aspects of the cervical cord and medulla) is an effective measure of cord distortion. With the cervical spine in a neutral position, the cervicomedullary angle is normally 135° to 175°[42] and there are significant differences between angles in flexion, neutral, and extension positions of the cervical spine.[30,54]

The length of the cervical spinal canal increases approximately 1.2 cm (approximately 10%) more during flexion than during extension, resulting in stretching and increase in axial tension of the cord, which follows the shortest route through the spinal canal and displaces anteriorly.[9,27] The greatest elongation takes place on the posterior surface of the cord.[27,43]

Detailed physiologic changes and differences in the diameter of the cervical cord and the surrounding subarachnoid space (between 50° flexion and 30° extension at the level of segments C2-C7) have been demonstrated using kinematic MRI.[8] The sagittal diameter of the cervical cord reduces up to 14% in flexion and increases up to 15% in extension when compared with the neutral position.

During flexion, the ventral subarachnoid space is 12 to 43% narrower and the dorsal subarachnoid space is 21 to 89% wider than in the neutral position, depending on the level. The greatest reduction in the size of the ventral subarachnoid space takes place at C4-C7. In extension there is only a small degree of widening of the ventral subarachnoid space (maximum of 9%). Because of the shortening of the cervical spinal canal, thickening of the cord, and folding of the ligamenta flava, the whole subarachnoid space is smallest in extension and the diameter of the dorsal subarachnoid space decreases up to 17%.[8]

III. CLINICAL APPLICATIONS

Kinematic MRI of the cervical spine has been used to evaluate patients with cervical instabilities, rheumatoid arthritis, and cervical spondylotic disease, as well as other abnormalities and disorders.[1-4,6,9-22]

A. Instability

When patients with distortion injury of the cervical spine were examined, 17 out of 50 patients had ligamentous instabilities and disc protrusions diagnosed only by means of kinematic MRI.[12] Kinematic MRI has also been applied to evaluate a patient diagnosed with os odontoideum. This is the most common

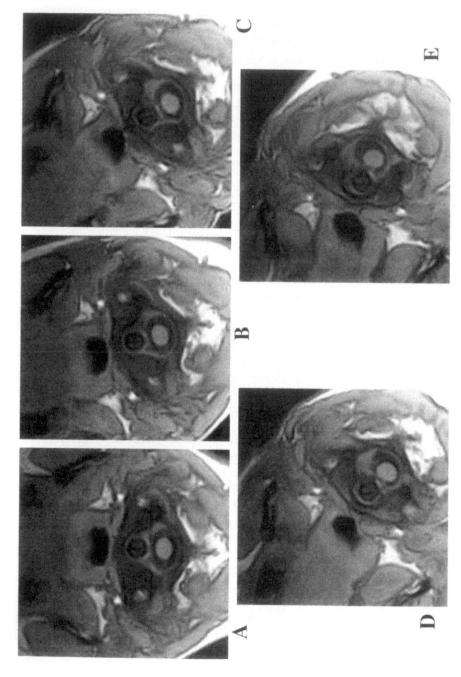

FIGURE 5.7 Kinematic MRI of the cervical spine during rotation to the right in a normal subject. The examination was performed using an incremental, passive positioning technique. (A) neutral position, (B) 20° rotation, (C) 40° rotation, (D) 60° rotation, and (E) 80° rotation.

TABLE 5.4
Mean Motion Between Segments C0-C1, C1-C2, and C0-C2

Flexion and Extension(°)		Mean[a]	ROM[b] f 50	Angle of the Positioning Device											ROM[b] e 50
				f 50	f 40	f 30	f 20	f 10	f/e 0	e 10	e 20	e 30	e 40	e 50	
C0-C1	F	12	4	15 (5)	13 (4)	12 (4)	12 (4)	11 (4)	11 (4)	11 (5)	12 (7)	11 (6)	10 (8)	11 (6)	0
	M	16	3	20 (4)	18 (5)	18 (5)	19 (6)	18 (5)	16 (5)	16 (6)	14 (7)	15 (4)	13 (5)	13 (4)	-3
	M&F	14	4	17 (5)	16 (5)	15 (6)	16 (6)	14 (6)	14 (5)	14 (6)	13 (7)	13 (6)	12 (7)	12 (5)	-2
C1-C2	F	-8	5	-4 (9)	-5 (8)	-4 (8)	-6 (7)	-8 (8)	-9 (9)	-11 (8)	-10 (8)	-10 (9)	10 (7)	-11 (7)	-2
	M	-14	2	-12 (4)	-11 (7)	-11 (6)	-12 (7)	-14 (7)	-15 (6)	-15 (6)	-15 (7)	-1	-16 (7)	-19 (7)	-4
	M&F	-11	4	-8 (8)	-8 (8)	-7 (8)	-9 (7)	-11 (8)	-12 (8)	-13 (7)	-13 (8)	-13 (8)	-13 (8)	-15 (8)	-3
C0-C2	F	4	9	11 (8)	8 (8)	9 (10)	6 (9)	3 (10)	2 (12)	0 (12)	2 (13)	1 (13)	1 (13)	0 (11)	-2
	M	2	6	7 (5)	8 (7)	7 (7)	7 (7)	4 (8)	2 (7)	1 (9)	0 (10)	-1 (8)	-3 (8)	-6 (6)	-7
	M&F	3	8	9 (7)	8 (7)	8 (8)	7 (8)	3 (9)	2 (10)	1 (10)	1 (12)	0 (10)	-1 (11)	-3 (9)	-4

Note: Motion range from 50° flexion (f) to 50° extension (e) in women (F, n = 10), men (M, n = 10), and genders combined (M&F, n = 20). The more positive/less negative the value is, the more flexion there is between segments. The more negative/less positive the value is, the more extension there is between segments. The direction of motion at each level is indicated by the change of the value: increasing value indicates flexion and decreasing value indicates extension.

[a] The mean is calculated from all positions from 50° flexion to 50° extension.

[b] ROM (range of motion) f/e 50 is the difference between 50° flexion or extension and zero-position (f/e 0).

From Karhu, J. O. et al., Kinematic MRI of the upper cervical spine using a novel positioning device, *Spine*, 24(19), 2046, 1999. With permission.

TABLE 5.5
Mean (SD) Motion between Segments C0-C1, C1-C2, and C0-C2

Lateral Bending (°)		Mean left[a]	-45	-30	-15	0	15	30	45	Mean right[a]
					Angle of the Positioning Device					
C0-C1	F	-3 (3)	-5 (2)	-3 (3)	-1 (2)	0 (2)	2 (3)	3 (2)	4 (3)	3 (3)
	M	-3 (3)	-4 (3)	-3 (3)	-2 (2)	0 (1)	1 (2)	2 (2)	3 (2)	2 (2)
	M&F	-3 (3)	-4 (3)	-3 (3)	-1 (2)	0 (2)	1 (2)	2 (2)	3 (2)	2 (2)
C1-C2	F	-1 (3)	-2 (2)	-1 (3)	-1 (3)	1 (2)	2 (2)	2 (2)	4 (2)	2 (2)
	M	-2 (3)	-3 (2)	-2 (3)	-1 (3)	0 (1)	-1 (2)	1 (2)	2 (2)	1 (2)
	M&F	-2 (3)	-3 (2)	-1 (3)	-1 (3)	0 (2)	1 (3)	1 (2)	3 (2)	2 (2)
C0-C2	F	-4 (3)	-7 (3)	-4 (3)	-2 (3)	1 (2)	3 (3)	4 (3)	8 (3)	5 (3)
	M	-4 (3)	-6 (3)	-4 (3)	-3 (3)	-1 (2)	0 (2)	3 (2)	5 (2)	3 (3)
	M&F	-4 (3)	-7 (3)	-4 (3)	-2 (3)	0 (2)	2 (3)	4 (2)	6 (3)	4 (3)

Note: Mean motion in women (F, n = 10), men (M, n = 10), and genders combined (M&F, n = 20) in lateral bending from 45° to the left to 45° to the right. Negative values indicate motion to the left.

[a] Mean is calculated from all positions (from 15° to 45°) to each direction.

From Karhu, J. O. et al., Kinematic MRI of the upper cervical spine using a novel positioning device, *Spine*, 24(19), 2046, 1999. With permission.

TABLE 5.6
Mean (SD) Rotational Difference (Segmental Motion) between C0-C1, C1-C2, and C0-C2

Rotation (°)		Mean left[a]	-80	-60	-40	-20	0	20	40	60	80	Mean right[a]
						Angle of the Positioning Device						
C0-C1	F	-4 (4)	-5 (3)	-6 (3)	-4 (4)	-1 (2)	2 (1)	2 (2)	3 (2)	3 (2)	4 (3)	3 (2)
	M	-3 (3)	-5 (3)	-5 (2)	-3 (3)	0 (3)	1 (2)	0 (3)	2 (3)	4 (2)	4 (2)	2 (3)
	M&F	-4 (3)	-5 (3)	-6 (3)	-4 (4)	0 (3)	1 (2)	1 (2)	2 (2)	3 (2)	4 (3)	3 (3)
C1-C2	F	-28 (7)	-34 (4)	-32 (3)	-27 (4)	-17 (4)	0 (3)	15 (4)	28 (4)	35 (3)	37 (3)	29 (9)
	M	-31 (8)	-39 (3)	-36 (4)	-30 (4)	-20 (4)	-1 (3)	16 (4)	30 (4)	36 (3)	40 (4)	30 (10)
	M&F	-29 (8)	-36 (4)	-34 (4)	-28 (4)	-19 (4)	-1 (3)	15 (4)	29 (4)	36 (3)	38 (4)	29 (10)
C0-C2	F	-31 (9)	-39 (4)	-38 (4)	-30 (4)	-18 (3)	2 (3)	17 (3)	31 (4)	38 (3)	40 (3)	32 (10)
	M	-34 (10)	-44 (1)	-41 (3)	-33 (5)	-20 (5)	0 (4)	16 (5)	31 (3)	40 (4)	44 (6)	33 (12)
	M&F	-33 (10)	-41 (4)	-39 (4)	-32 (5)	-19 (4)	1 (4)	16 (4)	31 (3)	39 (4)	42 (5)	32 (11)

Note: Mean difference in women (F, n = 10), men (M, n = 10), and genders combined (M&F, n = 20) from 80° to the left to 80° to the right. Negative values indicate motion to the left.

[a] Mean is calculated from all positions (from 20° to 80°) to each direction.

From Karhu, J. O. et al., Kinematic MRI of the upper cervical spine using a novel positioning device, *Spine*, 24(19), 2046, 1999. With permission.

form of odontoid anomaly and is associated with atlanto-axial instability.[13] Additionally, instability due to post-traumatic pseudoarthrosis of the odontoid can be evaluated using kinematic MRI of the cervical spine (Figure 5.9). In pediatric patients with occipito-cervical anomalies and instabilities (e.g., Down's syndrome), performing kinematic MRI during flexion and extension of the cervical spine has been reported to be useful in the assessment of spinal cord compression secondary to hypermobility.[14]

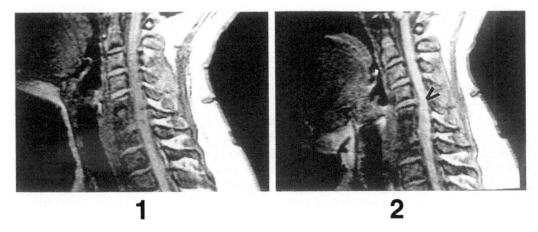

1 **2**

FIGURE 5.8 Kinematic MRI examination of the cervical spine showing neutral (1) and flexion (2) performed using the incremental, passive positioning technique (sagittal plane; fast spoiled gradient echo pulse sequence). There is a narrowing of the cord seen during flexion (2, arrow head) that is not apparent with the cervical spine in a neutral position.

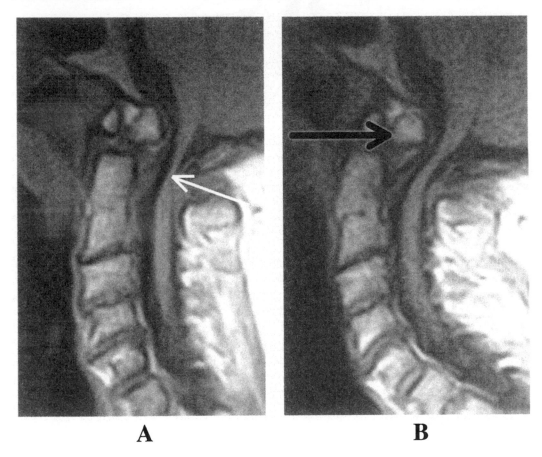

A **B**

FIGURE 5.9 Kinematic MRI of the cervical spine performed using the incremental, passive positioning technique. This patient has post-traumatic unstable pseudoarthrosis of the dens: (A) neutral position, note pathologically narrow cord (thin white arrow); (B) extended position, posterior dislocation of the tip of the dens (thick black arrow).

B. Cervical Spondylotic Disease

Degenerative changes of the cervical spine, including loss of disc height, disc protrusion or herniation, foraminal stenosis, osteophytic formation, hypertrophy and buckling of the ligamentum flavum, and spondylolisthesis with possible segmental instability, may result in radicular compression or cervical myelopathy. Cervical myelopathy is the most serious complication of cervical spondylosis and the most common acquired cause of spinal cord dysfunction.

The pathophysiology of myelopathy involves the combination of a developmentally narrow spinal canal, progressive spondylosis, dynamic changes of the cervical spinal canal, and progressive ischemia.[44] Compared with the use of conventional plain film radiography, myelography, CT-myelography, and static MRI techniques, the use of kinematic MRI provides additional information in patients with advanced stages of degenerative disease of the cervical spine by enabling evaluation of the spinal stenosis and maximum point of cord encroachment related to spinal movements.[19]

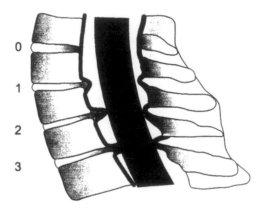

FIGURE 5.10   Schematic representation of the four-grade classification system used to categorize spinal stenosis based on static and dynamic findings seen on kinematic MRI in patients with different stages of cervical spondylotic myelopathy. Grade 0, normal width of the spinal canal; grade 1, partial obliteration of the anterior or posterior subarachnoid space or both; grade 2, complete obliteration of the anterior or posterior subarachnoid space or both; and grade 3, anterior or posterior cord impingement or both ("pincer effect"). (From Muhle, C. et al., Classification system based on kinematic MR imaging in cervical spondylitic myelopathy, *Am. J. Neuroradiol.*, 19, 1763, 1998. With permission.)

A four-grade classification system has been developed for spinal stenosis, based on static and dynamic findings in kinematic MRI in patients with different forms of cervical spondylotic myelopathy[10] (Figure 5.10). In extension, kinematic MRI shows an increased prevalence of functional cord impingement from both anterior and posterior aspects (i.e., the "pincer effect") and cord encroachment at multiple segments in patients with progressing stages of degenerative disease (Figure 5.11). In contrast, during flexion, there is cord decompression in many patients with cervical spinal stenosis.[10,11] In patients with cervical disc herniation or cervical spondylotic disease, exacerbated pain at provocative maneuvers is related more to changes in the foraminal size and to nerve root motion than to changes in the size of herniated discs.[20]

C. Rheumatoid Arthritis

Functional disorders of the cervical spine are often present in patients with rheumatoid arthritis.[33-35,42,45-52] Kinematic MRI is well suited to diagnose and stage the severity of these abnormalities[6,15-18] (Figures 5.12 to 5.16). In patients with rheumatoid arthritis or other inflammatory diseases, the kinematic MRI study should be performed using gadolinium enhancement (see Figure 5.15).

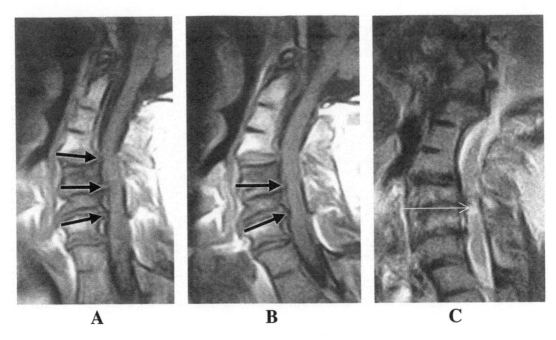

A   **B**   **C**

FIGURE 5.11 Kinematic MRI of the cervical spine obtained in a patient with severe degenerative spondy-lotic disease of the cervical spine. The spinal canal is stenotic from the C4-C5 level to the C7-Th1 level. There is grade 3 stenosis (pincer effect) at the level of the C4-C5, C5-C6, and C6-C7 intervertebral discs (black arrows). Additionally, (A) flexion and (B) extension obtained using T1-weighted pulse sequence shows signal intensity changes. (C) Extension obtained using T2 weighted pulse sequence. At the C5-C6 level, there is an area of increased signal in the cord, indicating cervical myelopathy.

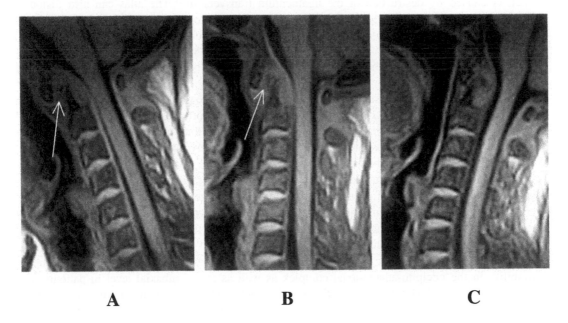

A   **B**   **C**

FIGURE 5.12 Kinematic MRI of the cervical spine obtained in a patient with rheumatoid arthritis and unstable atlanto-axial subluxation (arrow). There is an eroded dens and moderate pannus tissue. (A) Flexion: there is moderate anterior atlanto-axial subluxation, but posteriorly there is a wide enough cerebrospinal fluid space and the spinal canal is not stenotic. (B) Neutral: atlanto-axial subluxation is still present in the neutral position. (C) Extension: the atlas is located in its normal position.

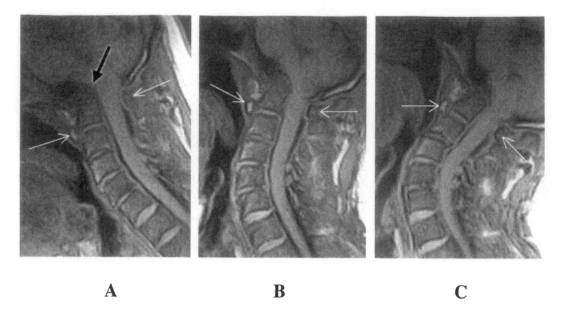

A   B   C

Figure 5.13   Kinematic MRI of the cervical spine obtained in a patient with rheumatoid arthritis and severe vertical subluxation of the upper cervical spine. Anterior and posterior arches of the atlas (white arrows) are located at the level of the lower endplate of the axis and markedly eroded dens protrudes into the foramen magnum. (A) Flexion, with compression and steep angulation in the junction of the medulla and the cord (black arrow); (B) neutral; (C) extension.

The most common abnormality in the rheumatoid cervical spine is atlanto-axial subluxation, which is caused by destruction of the ligamentum transversum.[45] The atlas can also dislocate posteriorly, laterally, rotationally, or vertically. Typically the progression of cervical disease starts from isolated, unstable atlanto-axial subluxation, leads to destruction of the dens and the bilateral occipito-atlanto-axial joint complex, and eventually results in vertical subluxation (superior migration of the odontoid). This is the second most common deformity of the rheumatoid cervical spine (Figure 5.13).[47,48]

Development and progression of vertical subluxation is usually associated with a decrease in atlanto-axial subluxation.[47,48] The third common type of abnormality of the region is subaxial subluxation (Figure 5.14), which is often multisegmental.[48] In long-term rheumatoid arthritis, the compression of the upper cervical cord or medulla is caused by either atlanto-axial subluxation, the mass effect of the periodontoid inflammatory pannus tissue, or a combination of these factors.

The stability of the rheumatoid cervical spine is usually assessed with lateral radiographs in neutral, flexion, and extension positions. Static view MR images are used to evaluate the craniovertebral junction of the rheumatoid patient with spinal cord compression symptoms because of their ability to directly demonstrate the dens erosion, the pannus, the obliteration of the cerebrospinal fluid space, and possible impingement of the cord.

In addition to these static factors, kinematic MRI is able to show the degree of vertebral instability in the occipito-atlanto-axial complex as well as at the subaxial level in patients with rheumatoid arthritis.[6] However, conventional radiographs, which are obtained with the patient in an upright, seated position, tend to be more precise in assessing the exact magnitude of atlanto-axial subluxation.[54]

If quantitative evaluation is needed, several measurements can be included in the interpretation of the kinematic MRI of the rheumatoid cervical spine. Atlanto-axial subluxation can be measured reliably as the anterior atlantodental interval, that is, the distance between anterior arch of the atlas and the dens, or as the posterior atlantodental interval, the distance between the dens and posterior

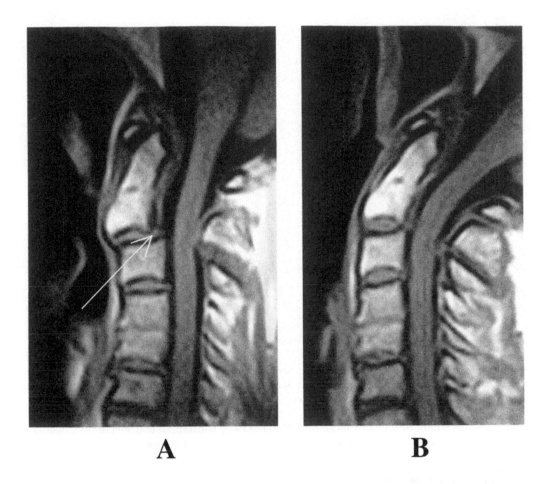

A   **B**

Figure 5.14   Kinematic MRI of the cervical spine performed in a patient with systemic lupus erythematosus and subaxial instability of the segment C2-C3. Subluxation of C2 (arrow) is evident in flexion (A), but not in extension (B).

arch of the atlas. Normal values for the anterior atlantodental interval obtained from conventional radiography (less than 3 mm) can be applied also to the kinematic MRI examination.[46]

Although atlanto-axial subluxation of 9 mm or more seen on conventional radiographs has been found to be associated with the risk of cord compression,[49] the magnitude of atlanto-axial subluxation by itself does not correlate with clinical symptoms and signs or severity of the disease.[45,50,51] Using kinematic MRI with the cervical spine in flexion, a diameter of the cervical spinal canal of 10 mm or less,[15] a diameter of the cord of 6 mm or less,[15] and cervicomedullary angle of less than 135°[42] have been shown to correlate with myelopathy.

Vertical subluxation can be evaluated quantitatively in the mid-sagittal plane by measuring the cranial migration distance. That is, the distance between the posterocaudal corner of the axis and the line drawn between the basion and the opisthion (foramen magnum line). Additionally, this may be accomplished by assessing directly the position of the tip of the dens relative to this line or to the line drawn from the hard palate to the opisthion (Chamberlain-line) (Figure 5.13).

Normally, the odontoid peg is located below the foramen magnum line and commonly below or just tangent to the Chamberlain-line, but occasionally also a few millimeters above it.[53] The mean cranial migration distance in normal subjects ranges from 38.7 to 40 mm[5,15] and there is a difference between genders.[5] If a cranial migration distance of 31 mm or less is measured and there is severe pain present, operative fusion should be considered.[15] In the subaxial cervical spine,

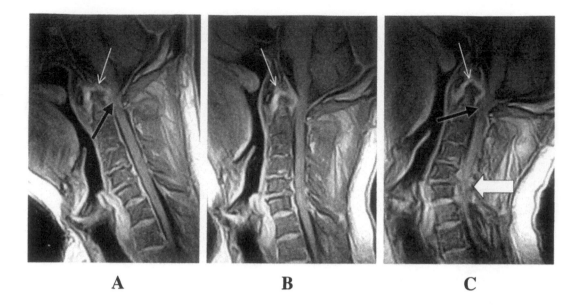

A   **B**   **C**

Figure 5.15   Kinematic MRI of the cervical spine obtained in a patient with rheumatoid arthritis using the contrast enhanced technique. Enhancement of the inflammatory pannus tissue is seen around the dens (white arrow). (A) Flexion: the cord compression (black arrow) is caused by the pannus and atlanto-axial subluxation. (B) Neutral position. (C) Extension: the compression and the distortion of the cord (black arrow) is even more evident than in flexed. There is also subaxial spinal stenosis at the C5-C6 level (white block arrow).

vertebral displacement of 2 mm or more is considered to be substantial and severe myelopathy has been found to be associated with a mean anterior displacement of 3 mm.[52]

D. THERAPEUTIC CONSIDERATIONS AND FUTURE APPLICATIONS

Kinematic MRI of the cervical spine can influence the therapeutic or intraoperative management of patients with spondylotic myelopathy and radiculopathy associated with spinal stenosis.[19] Furthermore, this diagnostic procedure is considered to be particularly useful in the planning of stabilization and decompressive operations of the rheumatoid upper cervical spine.[6,15-17]

For example, von Schnarkowski et al.[12] reported that 2 of 17 trauma patients with ligamentous instabilities and disc protrusions diagnosed by kinematic MRI of the cervical spine were treated by operative spinal fusion. A patient with unstable os odontoideum and compression of the cord demonstrated in the flexion position seen on kinematic MRI also underwent surgery.[13]

In another study, Weng and Haynes[14] reported that, for pediatric patients with various occipito-cervical anomalies and instabilities, flexion and extension kinematic MRI views were found to be useful in selecting appropriate patients for a stabilization operation. Pediatric patients with evidence of cord compression as demonstrated on kinematic MRI had neurologic manifestations and underwent surgery. Alternatively, flexion and extension kinematic MRI views of the cervical spine may allow arthrodesis to be avoided when there is no evidence of cord impingement.

Comparison studies of the cervical spine in the supine and upright, seated positions may improve our understanding of the functional dynamics of normal and abnormal intervertebral discs. "Weight bearing" images of the spine may prove useful in determining the significance of protruding discs, as well as in patients with rheumatoid arthritis clinically suspected of having myelopathy due to instability of the cervical spine or superior migration of the odontoid process or both (Figure 5.16). Further studies on post-traumatic soft tissue pathology manifested as hypermobility during upper cervical spine rotation or as cervical spine instability in flexion and extension positions are also needed.

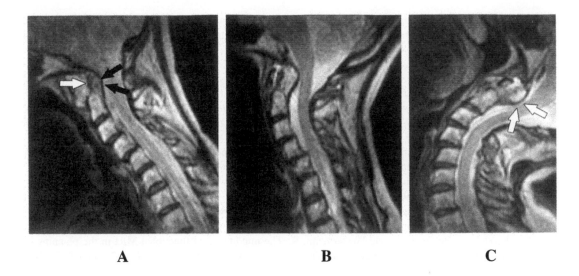

A   B   C

FIGURE 5.16 Kinematic MRI of the cervical spine obtained in a patient with rheumatoid arthritis using the upright, seated positioning technique. (A) Flexion: the anterior arch of C1 is anteriorly displaced (atlanto-axial subluxation) relative to the eroded dens (white arrow). Synovitis and fluid (black arrows) surround the dens. Less severe anterior subluxation is present at several subaxial levels. There is no spinal cord compression. (B) Neutral: the subluxations have improved. The fluid and synovitis around the dens changes shape with the atlanto-axial movement. (C) Extension: the alignment is now normal at most levels. The fluid and synovitis now bulge posteriorly to the dens (arrows).

IV. SUMMARY AND CONCLUSIONS

The application of kinematic MRI of the cervical spine is a crucial step toward improving our understanding of this important anatomic area. Findings from recent studies indicate that this specialized imaging procedure improves diagnostic accuracy for certain spinal disorders. Obviously, the appropriate use of kinematic MRI procedures will ultimately have a direct impact on patient care and surgical planning, eventually leading to improved patient management and decreased healthcare costs.

REFERENCES

1. Shellock, F. G., Kinematic MRI of the joints, *Seminars Musculoskeletal Radiol.,* 1, 143, 1997.
2. Shellock, F. G., Kinematic MRI of the joints, in *Magnetic Resonance Imaging in Orthopaedics and Rheumatology,* 2nd edition, Stoller, D. W., Ed., Lippincott-Raven, Philadelphia, 1996.
3. Muhle, C. et al., Comparison of T2-weighted turbo-spin echo sequence and ultra-fast HASTE sequence in the diagnosis of cervical myelopathies and spinal stenoses against static and kinematic MRI of the cervical spine, *RÖFO,* 5, 467, 1997.
4. Muhle, C. et al., Kinematic MRI in degenerative cervical spine changes, *RÖFO,* 163(2), 148, 1995.
5. Karhu, J. O. et al., Kinematic MRI of the upper cervical spine using a novel positioning device, *Spine,* 24, 2046, 1999.
6. Allmann, K.-H. et al., Functional MRI of the cervical spine in patients with rheumatoid arthritis, *Acta Radiol.,* 39, 543, 1998.
7. Smith, S. D., Upright and supine kinematic cervical spine MR imaging, *Society for Magnetic Resonance Technologists, Sixth Annual Meeting Syllabus,* International Society for Magnetic Resonance in Medicine, Berkeley, CA, 1997, p. 5.
8. Muhle, C. et al., Biomechanical aspects of the subarachnoid space and cervical cord in healthy individuals examined with kinematic magnetic resonance imaging, *Spine,* 23, 556, 1998.

9. Koschorek, F., Jensen, H.-P., and Terwey, B., Dynamic evaluation of cervical spinal cord by magnetic resonance imaging: improvement of indication for surgical treatment of chronic cervical myelopathy, *Magn. Reson. Imag.*, 4, 421, 1986.

10. Muhle, C. et al., Classification system based on kinematic MR imaging in cervical spondylitic myelopathy, *Am. J. Neuroradiol.*, 19, 1763, 1998.

11. Muhle, C. et al., Dynamic changes of the spinal canal in patients with cervical spondylosis at flexion and extension using magnetic resonance imaging, *Invest. Radiol.*, 33, 444, 1998.

12. von Schnarkowski, P. et al., Functional MRI of the cervical spine after distortion injury, *RÖFO*, 4, 319, 1995.

13. Hughes, T. B., Richman, J. D., and Rothfus, W. E., Diagnosis of os odontoideum using kinematic magnetic resonance imaging, *Spine*, 24, 715, 1999.

14. Weng, M. S. and Haynes, R. J., Flexion and extension cervical MRI in a pediatric population, *J. Pediatr. Orthop.*, 16, 359, 1996.

15. Dvorak, J. et al., Functional evaluation of the spinal cord by magnetic resonance imaging in patients with rheumatoid arthritis and instability of upper cervical spine, *Spine*, 14, 1057, 1989.

16. Krödel, A., Refior, H. J., and Westermann, S., The importance of functional MRI in the planning of stabilizing operations on the cervical spine in rheumatoid patients, *Arch. Orthop. Trauma Surg.*, 109, 30, 1989.

17. Bell, G. R. and Stearns, K. L., Flexion-extension MRI of the upper rheumatoid cervical spine, *Orthopedics*, 14, 969, 1991.

18. Roca, A., Bernreuter, W., and Alarcon, G., Functional MRI should be included in the evaluation of the cervical spine in patients with rheumatoid arthritis, *J. Rheumatol.*, 20, 1485, 1993.

19. Muhle, C. et al., Kinematic MR imaging in surgical management of cervical disc disease, spondylosis and spondylotic myelopathy, *Acta Radiol.*, 40, 146, 1999.

20. Muhle, C. et al., Exacerbated pain in cervical radiculopathy at axial rotation, flexion, extension, and coupled motions of the cervical spine, *Invest. Radiol.*, 33, 279, 1998.

21. Shellock, F.G., Sullenberger, P., Mink, J. H., Deutsch, A., Horrigan, J., Bloze, A., and Hashoian, R., MRI of the cervical spine during flexion and extension: development and implementation of a new technique, *J. Magn. Reson. Imag.*, WIP, S21, 1994.

22. Duerinckx, A. J. et al., MR imaging of cervical spine motion with HASTE, *Magn. Reson. Imag.*, 17, 371, 1999.

23. Dvorak, J. et al., Age and gender related normal motion of the cervical spine, *Spine*, 175, 393, 1992.

24. Dvorak, J. et al., Functional radiographic diagnostics of the cervical spine: flexion/extension, *Spine*, 13, 748, 1988.

25. Dvorak, J. et al., Clinical validation of functional flexion/extension radiographs of the cervical spine, *Spine*, 18, 120, 1993.

26. Ålund, M. and Larsson, S. E., Three dimensional analysis of neck motion, *Spine*, 15, 87, 1990.

27. Penning, L., Normal movements of the cervical spine, *Am. J. Roentgen.*, 130, 317, 1978.

28. Feipel, V. et al., Normal global motion of the cervical spine: an electrogoniometric study, *Clin. Biomech.*, 14, 463, 1999.

29. McClure, P., Siegler, S., and Nobilini, R., Three-dimensional flexibility characters of the human cervical spine in vivo, *Spine*, 23, 216, 1998.

30. Dvorak, J. et al., In vivo flexion/extension of the normal cervical spine, *J. Orthop. Res.*, 9, 828, 1991.

31. Ordway, N. R. et al., Cervical flexion, extension, protrusion, and retraction, *Spine*, 24, 240, 1999.

32. Hino, H. et al., Dynamic motion analysis of normal and unstable cervical spines using cineradiography, *Spine*, 24, 163, 1999.

33. Kawaida, H. et al., Magnetic resonance imaging of upper cervical disorders in rheumatoid arthritis, *Spine*, 14, 1144, 1989.

34. Boden, S. D. et al., Rheumatoid arthritis of the cervical spine. A long-term analysis with predictors of paralysis and recovery, *J. Bone Joint Surg. [Am.]*, 75, 1282, 1993.

35. Zeidman, S. M. and Ducker, T. B., Rheumatoid arthritis. Neuroanatomy, compression and grading of deficits, *Spine*, 19, 2259, 1994.

36. Holmes, A. et al., Changes in cervical canal spinal volume during in vitro flexion-extension, *Spine*, 21, 1313, 1996.

37. Panjabi, M. et al., Three-dimensional movements of the upper cervical spine, *Spine*, 13, 726, 1988.

38. Penning, L. and Wilmink, J. T., Rotation of the cervical spine, a CT study in normal subjects, *Spine*, 12, 732, 1987.

39. Dvorak, J., Hayek, J., and Zehnder, R., CT-functional diagnostics of the rotatory instability of upper cervical spine. II. An evaluation on healthy adults and patients with suspected instability, *Spine*, 12, 726, 1987.

40. Antinnes, J. A. et al., The value of functional computed tomography in the evaluation of soft-tissue injury in the upper cervical spine, *Eur. Spine J.*, 3, 98, 1994.

41. Dvorak, J. et al., Functional diagnostics of the cervical spine using computer tomography, *Neuroradiology*, 30, 132, 1988.

42. Bundschuh, C. et al., Rheumatoid arthritis of the cervical spine: surface-coil MR imaging, *Am. J. Roentgen.*, 151, 181, 1988.

43. Qing, Y., Dougherty, L., and Margulies, S. S., In vivo human cervical spinal cord deformation and displacement in flexion, *Spine*, 23, 1677, 1998.

44. Fehlings, M. G. and Skaf, G., A review of the pathophysiology of cervical spondylotic myelopathy with insights for potential novel mechanism drawn from traumatic spinal cord injury, *Spine*, 23, 2730, 1998.

45. Rana, N. A., Natural history of atlanto-axial subluxation in rheumatoid arthritis, *Spine*, 14, 1054, 1989.

46. Rana, N. A. et al., Atlanto-axial subluxation in rheumatoid arthritis, *J. Bone Joint Surg. [Br.]*, 55, 458, 1973.

47. Casey, A. et al., Vertical translocation: the enigma of the disappearing atlantodens interval in patients with myelopathy and rheumatoid arthritis. I. Clinical, radiological and neuropathological features, *J. Neurosurg.*, 87, 856, 1997.

48. Reiter, M. F. and Boden, S. D., Inflammatory disorders of the cervical spine, *Spine*, 23, 2755, 1998.

49. Weissman, B. N. et al., Prognostic feature of atlantoaxial subluxation in rheumatoid arthritis patients, *Radiology*, 144, 745, 1982.

50. Castro, S. et al., Cervical spine involvement in rheumatoid arthritis: a clinical neurologic and radiological evaluation, *Clin. Exp. Rheumatol.*, 12, 367, 1994.

51. Reijnierse, M. et al., The cervical spine in rheumatoid arthritis: relationship between neurologic signs and morphology on MRI and radiographs, *Skeletal Radiol.*, 25, 113, 1996.

52. Yonezawa, T. et al., Subaxial lesions in rheumatoid arthritis, *Spine*, 20, 208, 1995.

53. Smoker, W. R. K., Craniovertebral junction: normal anatomy, craniometry and congenital anomalies, *Radiographics*, 14, 255, 1994.

54. Karhu, J. O., Unpublished observations, 2000.

Part III

Ankle

6 The Ankle and Foot: Functional Anatomy and Kinesiology

Susan Mais Requejo

CONTENTS

0-8493-0807-0/01/$0.00+$.50
© 2001 by Frank G. Shellock

I. INTRODUCTION

The ankle and foot belong to one of the most complex regions of the body. These joints, like other major joints in the lower extremity, participate in load bearing and provide stability. In addition, the ankle and foot must be mobile to adapt to changes of the weight-bearing surfaces.

The ankle and foot complex meets these unique requirements through interactions of its 26 bones (28 with sesamoids) that form 25 component joints (Figure 6.1).[1,2] These joints include the proximal and distal tibiofibular joints, the ankle joint, the subtalar joint, the talonavicular and calcaneocuboid joints (transverse tarsal joints), five tarsometatarsal joints, five metatarsalphalangeal joints, and nine interphalangeal joints. This chapter will discuss the ankle, subtalar, and transverse tarsal joints with regard to functional anatomy, normal kinematics, and pathokinesiology.

II. FUNCTIONAL ANATOMY

A. OSSEOUS STRUCTURES AND ARTICULATING SURFACES

1. The Ankle

The ankle joint consists of the articulations between the distal tibia and the talus (tibiotalar), and the talus and fibula (talofibular) (Figure 6.2). The distal tibia and fibula create a deep socket, or "mortise," for the convex talus. The function of the ankle is dependent on this mortise which maintains joint integrity and allows for the transmission of force from the foot to the shank. The fibula bears approximately 10% of the body weight and functions primarily as a pincer of the mortise and attachment site for muscle.[1]

The distal tibiofibula joint consists of the fibrous union of the concave tibia and convex fibula (Figure 6.2). This joint is considered a syndesmosis joint, bound by ligaments with no synovial membrane.[2] The bones actually do not come into contact, but are separated by fibroadipose tissue.

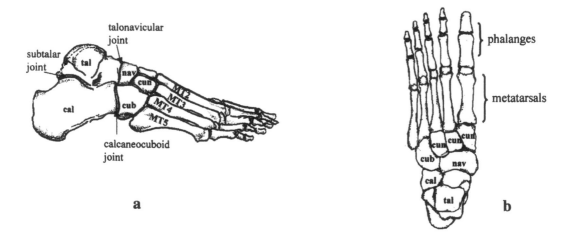

FIGURE 6.1 Schematic view of the bones of the ankle and foot. cal, calcaneous; tal, talus; cub, cuboid; cun, cuneiform; nav, navicular; MT, metatarsal. (a) Lateral view; (b) dorsal view.

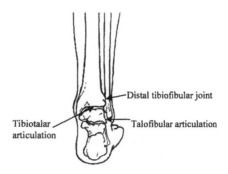

FIGURE 6.2   Posterior view of the ankle joint consisting of the tibiotalar and talofibular articulations. Also shown is the distal tibiofibular joint.

The dorsal surface of the talus (trochlea) is usually wedge shaped, with the anterior portion wider than the posterior.[3] The lateral articulating surface of the talus is large and relatively flat and articulates with a reciprocally shaped surface of the fibula. The smaller medial facet articulates with the distal surface of the tibia.

2.   The Subtalar Joint

The subtalar joint consists of articulations between the inferior talus and superior calcaneous (Figure 6.1). While there is a noted variability in the number of facets, most anatomy texts identify three: posterior, middle, and anterior.[4,5]

These plane articulations are divided functionally into two separate chambers: posterior and anterior.[6] The posterior chamber is formed by the articulation between the posterior concave facet of the talus and the larger convex posterior facet of the calcaneous, and is surrounded by a joint capsule. It is also referred to as the talocalcaneal joint.

The anterior chamber is formed by the inferior convex facets of the talus with the superior concave middle and anterior facets of the calcaneous.[6] Because this joint shares a joint capsule with the talonavicular joint, it is often referred to as the talocalcanealnavicular joint.[7] This joint is considered the functional link between the rearfoot and the midfoot.[1]

Anterior to the posterior facet (dividing the two chambers) is a deep groove that separates the anterior and middle facets from the posterior facet. This funnel shaped tunnel is called the tarsal canal.[4] The larger lateral end extends anterior to the fibula to a palpable space called the sinus tarsi. Medially, the smaller end lies posterior to the medial malleolus, just above the sustentaculum tali, a bony projection on the calcaneous. Notably, there are ligaments that run the entire length of the canal, completely dividing the two chambers of the subtalar joint.

3.   The Midtarsal Joint

The midtarsal joint is also referred to as the transverse tarsal joint, or Chopart's joint.[8] It is formed by two articulations: the talonavicular and the calcanealcuboid joints (Figure 6.1). The two joints transect the foot horizontally and form an s-shaped joint when viewed from above. The talonavicular joint consists of a convex talar head and a concave navicular bone. In contrast, the calcaneous is concave and the cuboid is convex. This reciprocal shape restricts motion somewhat at the calcaneal cuboid joint, as compared with the more mobile ball-and-socket shape of the talonavicular joint.[1]

The talonavicular joint is structurally linked to the subtalar joint through a shared joint capsule and supporting ligaments and is referred to as the talocalcaneonavicular joint.[7] Therefore, motion of the mobile talus on the calcaneous is simultaneously reflected as motion of the talus on the navicular.

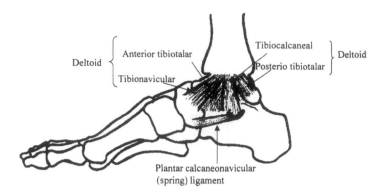

FIGURE 6.3 Medial view of the foot and ankle. The primary ligament providing stability to resist eversion is the large fan shaped deltoid ligament. It consists of the tibionavicular, tibiocalcaneal, and tibiotalar portions which blend together. Providing stability for the talocalcaneonavicular joint is the spring ligament which runs from the sustentaculum tali of the calcaneous to the inferior navicular, supporting the head of the talus.

B. Ligaments and Joint Capsule

1. The Ankle

The ankle is one of the most congruent joints in the body. It is able to withstand extremely high forces with little nontraumatic arthritis.[1] Stability of the ankle joint is dependent on the articular joint surfaces, the integrity of the ligaments, and the actions of the supporting muscles.

The strong ligaments between the tibia and fibula help to maintain the stable mortise of the ankle joint. The most important stabilizer of the distal tibiofibular joint is the crural tibiofibular interosseus ligament, which runs obliquely between the tibia and fibula.[1] Other supporting structures include the anterior and posterior tibiofibular ligaments and the interosseous membrane.[2]

Two other major ligaments that further maintain the mortise are the medial and lateral collateral ligaments. Medial joint stability is provided by the strong medial collateral ligament, the deltoid ligament (Figure 6.3). This ligament has both superficial and deep fibers and provides resistance to eversion.[7] It arises from the medial malleolus and fans out to attach to the navicular, talus, and calcaneous, forming the tibionavicular, tibiotalar, and tibiocalcaneal portions (Figure 6.3). Forces that would distract the medial side of the joint often avulse the medial malleolus before the deltoid ligament tears.[1]

Lateral joint stability is provided by the lateral collateral ligament (LCL) (Figure 6.4). The LCL is separated into three separate bands and is responsible for restricting inversion. The anterior talofibular ligament (ATFL) is a flat band that arises from the distal fibula extending anteromedially to the neck of the talus (Figure 6.4). The ATFL is the weakest and most commonly injured.[1,9] Plantarflexion of the ankle further predisposes the ATFL to injury as it becomes aligned more vertically, making it the primary supporting structure on the lateral side (Figure 6.5).[9]

The calcaneal-fibular ligament is a strong round cord that passes from the tip of the fibular malleolus to the calcaneus (Figure 6.4). The posterior talofibular ligament is a thick, strong band that runs horizontally from the posterior fibular fossa to the talus (Figure 6.4). This ligament is the strongest of the collaterals and is rarely torn in isolation.[1,9]

2. The Subtalar Joint

The subtalar joint is a very stable joint that is supported by the extremely strong talocalcaneal ligaments. The talocalcaneal ligaments all span from the talus to the calcaneous to support the joint. The interosseous ligament, which lies within the tarsal canal, is the chief talocalcaneal

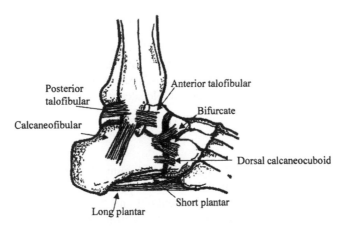

FIGURE 6.4 Lateral view of the foot and ankle. Ligaments that provide stability of the ankle joint are separated into three separate bands and are responsible for restricting inversion. These include the anterior talofibular ligament, calcaneofibular ligament, and posterior talofibular ligament. Ligaments providing stability to the calcanealcuboid articulation of the midtarsal joint include the lateral band of the bifurcate ligament, the dorsal calcaneocuboid, and the short and long plantar ligaments.

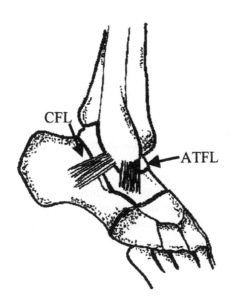

FIGURE 6.5 Plantarflexion of the ankle predisposes the anterior talofibular ligament (ATFL) to injury. Observe how it becomes aligned more vertically, making it the primary supporting structure on the lateral side.

ligament.[1,7] This ligament, is composed predominantly of collagen fibers and contains many proprioceptive nerve endings, important in providing position sense of the ankle.

The interosseus ligament is composed of anterior and posterior bands.[7] The anterior band runs from the calcaneous (in an anterior-lateral direction) to insert just inferior to the talar neck.[7] The posterior band travels from the posterior facet of the calcaneous anterior to the talus.

The cervical ligament is just lateral to the interosseus ligament (within the tarsal canal) and attaches from the upper surface of the calcaneous to the inferior-lateral aspect of the neck of the talus.[10] Some authors consider this ligament as part of the interosseus ligament.[7] The extrinsic calcaneofibular ligament and the tibiocalcaneal part of the deltoid ligament also cross the subtalar joint, providing stability.[11] Additional reinforcement is provided by the posterior and lateral talo-calcaneal ligaments.[1,7]

Both ligaments and bones contribute significantly to stability of the subtalar joint. Subtalar inversion is limited primarily by the lateral collateral ankle, interosseous and cervical ligaments, and the sustentaculum tali abutting the medial talus.[1,9] Eversion is primarily limited by the tibio-calcaneal portion of the deltoid ligament, medial talocalcaneal ligament, and the lateral process of the talus striking the calcaneous.[9]

3. The Midtarsal Joint

Several ligaments provide support to the midtarsal joint (Figure 6.4). The calcanealcuboid articulation is supported by the lateral band of the bifurcate ligament (also known as the calcaneocuboid ligament), the dorsal calcaneocuboid and the short (calcaneocuboid) and long plantar ligaments.[1] The long plantar ligament is a thick strong band that extends from the plantar surface of the calcaneous to the plantar surface of the cuboid bone (deep fibers) and fibers that extend from the calcaneus to the proximal ends of the second through fifth metatarsal bones (superficial fibers).[7]

Medially, the spring (plantar calcaneonavicular) ligament is the primary support for both the transverse tarsal and the talocalcaneonavicular joints (Figure 6.3).[7] Supporting the medial head of the talus, the spring ligament runs from the sustentaculum tali inserting on the inferior navicular. On the lateral side of the talus, the medial band of the bifurcate ligament (lateral calcaneonavicular ligament) also supports the talus. Besides the ligaments, additional support is provided by extrinsic muscles of the foot that pass medial and lateral to the midtarsal joint, as well as intrinsic muscles inferiorly.[1]

III. NORMAL JOINT KINEMATICS

A. Principles of Motion

The primary motions in the ankle and foot take place in the three orthogonal planes (Figure 6.6).[7] Movements in the sagittal plane are plantarflexion and dorsiflexion. The frontal plane movements are inversion and eversion, and transverse plane movements are abduction and adduction.

Dorsiflexion is the motion where the foot approximates the tibia and plantarflexion is movement of the foot downward, away from the tibia (Figure 6.6). Dorsiflexion and plantarflexion occur around a frontal plane axis in the sagittal plane.[7] Inversion is the motion when the medial border

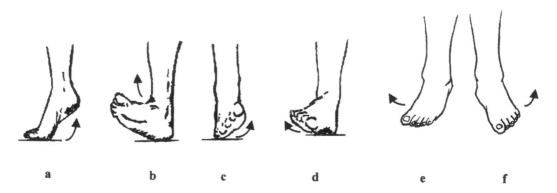

a   b   c   d   e   f

FIGURE 6.6 Movement of the foot in the sagittal plane, (a) plantarflexion and (b) dorsiflexion. Movement of the right foot in the frontal plane, (c) inversion and (d) eversion. Movement of the foot in the transverse plane, (e) adduction and (f) abduction. (Adapted from Hoppenfield, S., *Physical Examination of the Spine and Extremities.* Appleton-Century-Crofts, Norwalk, CT, 1976, p. 223. With permission.)

of the foot becomes elevated and the lateral border depressed.[7] Eversion is the motion when the medial border of the foot becomes depressed and the lateral border elevated.[7] Inversion and eversion occur about the longitudinal/sagittal axis in the frontal plane. Adduction is an inward movement of the foot, while abduction is an outward movement of the foot.[7] Abduction and adduction occur about a vertical axis in the transverse plane.[7]

The ankle, subtalar, and midtarsal joints all have separate axes of rotation, that are not exactly perpendicular to any of the three cardinal planes.[7] The amount of movement in each plane is dependent on the location of the axis relative to the cardinal planes. For example, the ankle axis lies very close to the frontal plane and most of the motion occurs as plantarfexion and dorsiflexion. However, because it is not precisely perpendicular to the frontal plane, slight motion in the other two planes may be observed.

B. OSTEOKINEMATICS

1. The Ankle

Typically, the ankle is considered to have a single oblique axis with the primary motions of plantarflexion and dorsiflexion in the sagittal plane.[3,12] However, early investigators demonstrated that the axis of rotation changed continuously during ankle motion.[13,14] Furthermore, Barnett and Napier[15] and Hicks[16] described two separate axes of rotation: one for plantarflexion and one for dorsiflexion. Inman[3] originally proposed a single axis as passing just distal to the tips of the medial and lateral malleoli. The axis is tilted down 10 degrees from the horizontal plane (Figure 6.7a) and rotated laterally 20 to 30 degrees with respect to the knee axis (Figure 6.7b).[16] This oblique axis results in triplanar motion accounting for slight motion of the ankle out of the sagittal plane. The average range of motion at the ankle is 20 degrees dorsiflexion and 50 degrees of plantarflexion.[7,18]

2. The Subtalar Joint

Motion at the subtalar joint occurs primarily between the talus and the calcaneus. Manter[19] identified a single axis of rotation resulting in one degree of freedom. He described the axis as extending

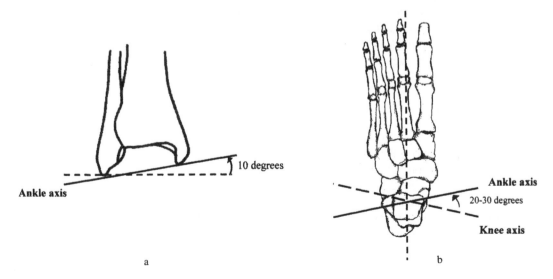

FIGURE 6.7 Axis of rotation of the ankle joint. In a neutral position of the ankle joint, the axis passes approximately through the tips of the malleoli. (a) As the fibula extends further distally the axis is tipped down 10 degrees in the frontal plane. (b) As the fibula is more posterior than the tibia the axis is rotated laterally. Relative to the knee axis, the ankle axis is rotated posteriorly 20 to 30 degrees in the transverse plane.

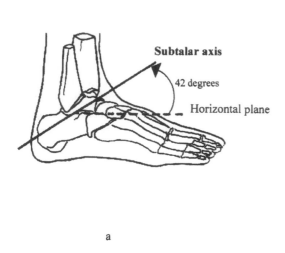

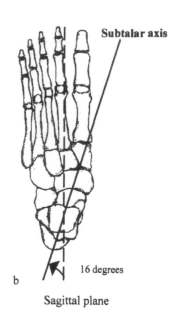

FIGURE 6.8 Simplified axis of rotation of the subtalar axis in (a) Lateral view: sagittal plane. The axis rises 42 degrees from the horizontal. (b) Top view: transverse plane. The axis is oriented 16 degrees from the midline of the foot.

42 degrees superior from the horizontal plane and 23 degrees medially from the long axis of the foot (Figure 6.8). However, Inman[3] reported a wide range of individual variation in this orientation with deviations in the horizontal plane ranging from 20 to 68 degrees and deviations from the longitudinal axis ranging from 4 to 47 degrees.

Because the axis of the subtalar joint is oblique to all three cardinal planes, motion occurs in the frontal, sagittal, and transverse planes (triplanar motion). Motion in these three planes occurs simultaneously and is referred to as either pronation or supination. Pronation is described as being a combination of dorsiflexion, eversion, and abduction of the foot, while supination consists of plantarflexion, inversion, and adduction of the foot.[1,6] However, the primary motion that occurs at the subtalar joint is inversion and eversion, which takes place in the frontal plane. Investigators have identified the average amount of motion at the subtalar joint as 18.7 degrees inversion and 12.2 degrees eversion.[20]

3. The Midtarsal Joint

Manter[19] identified two joint axes in the midtarsal joint, a longitudinal and an oblique axis. The longitudinal axis projects antero-dorsal at an angle of 16 degrees and is directed medially 9 degrees (Figure 6.9). The second axis is described as oblique and is projected up from the floor anteriorly and dorsally at angles of 52 degrees and 57 degrees, respectively (Figure 6.10). The resultant motion at this axis is also triplanar, producing pronation and supination. The primary components of motion at the longitudinal axis is inversion/eversion and at the oblique axis is abduction/adduction and dorsiflexion/plantarflexion.[1]

Mann and Inman[21] have described the two axes of the midtarsal joint in relationship to foot function. Because these two axes are positioned in the frontal plane with the superior axis through the talus and the inferior through the calcaneous, the two axes become parallel when the calcaneous is everted and the subtalar joint is pronated. This allows for more motion between the midtarsal bones (Figure 6.11). However, when the calcaneous is inverted and the subtalar joint supinated, the two axes converge, significantly restricting motion at the midtarsal joint. Notably, this movement

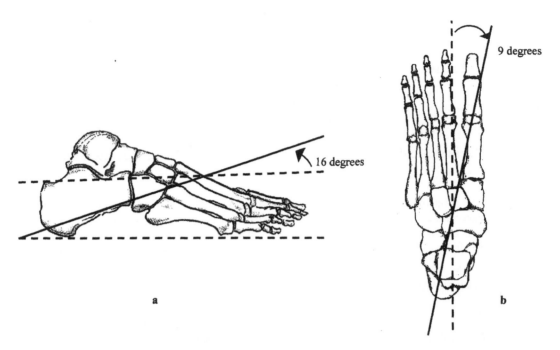

FIGURE 6.9 Longitudinal axis of rotation of the transverse tarsal joint. (a) Lateral view: sagittal plane. The axis rises 16 degrees from the horizontal. (b) Top view: transverse plane. The axis is oriented 9 degrees medially from the midline of the foot.

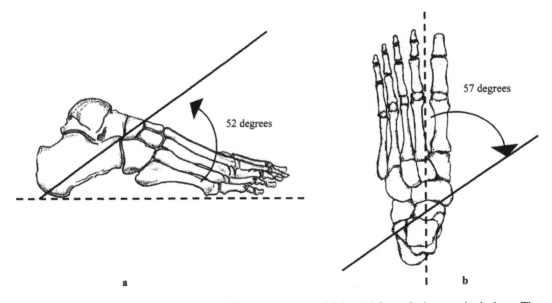

FIGURE 6.10 Oblique axis of rotation of the transverse tarsal joint. (a) Lateral view: sagittal plane. The axis rises 52 degrees from the horizontal. (b) Top view: transverse plane. The axis is oriented 57 degrees medially from the midline of the foot.

pattern is essential during gait, when the foot needs to be more mobile in early stance and then more rigid in terminal stance.

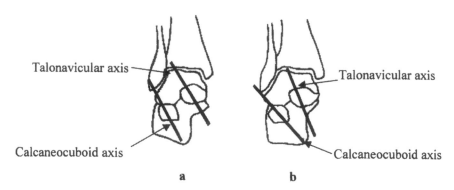

FIGURE 6.11   Anteroposterior view of the transverse tarsal joints. The anterior articulation of the talar head and the calcaneous are shown with the orientation of the talonavicular and the calcaneocuboid axes. (a) When the hindfoot is everted, these axes are parallel so more motion in the transverse tarsal joints is permitted. (b) When the hindfoot is inverted, the axes are divergent so there is less motion in the transverse tarsal joints.

C. ARTHROKINEMATICS

1. The Ankle

Motion of the ankle occurs primarily in the tibiotalar and fibulotalar articulations. A few degrees of motion also occur at the distal tibiofibular joint to accommodate the change of shape of the talus during dorsiflexion and plantarflexion. Sammarco and colleagues[14] used multiple roentgenographic exposures and determined the instant centers of rotation and displacement of the ankle joint contact points. During motion from full dorsiflexion to full plantarflexion, they found all of the instant centers of rotation were located within the talus. There was distraction of the contact points at the beginning of the motion, followed by gliding, and ending with compression of the joint surface at the end of plantarflexion. They proposed that the distraction and compression at extreme range may play an important role in the needed lubrication of the joint.

Barnett and Napier[15] reported a difference in the radius of curvature of the talar facets, with the lateral talar facet being larger than the medial. Therefore, during dorsiflexion, the fibula has to glide anteriorly to accommodate the larger lateral facet.[1] This greater excursion of the fibula results in internal rotation of the lower leg in weight bearing dorsiflexion and external rotation during plantarflexion.[1]

In order to maintain contact with the talus, the fibula must also rotate laterally along its long axis during dorsiflexion and medially during plantarflexion, which is reflected in motion at the tibiofibular joints.[15] The fibula also may glide superiorly during dorsiflexion to accommodate the wider portion of the talus.[1]

2. The Subtalar Joint

The subtalar joint is typically described as a gliding joint.[2,7] In general, during pronation, the talus glides medially with respect to the calcaneous and during supination the talus glides laterally.[7] Thus, the talus is easily palpated on its lateral aspect during supination and medially during pronation.

However, the actual movement is more complex. As the posterior facet of the talus is concave, movement of the talus is accompanied by a slide in the same direction (concave surface moving on a stationary convex surface). However, the anterior and middle facets are convex, causing a slide in the opposite direction. Therefore, the talus glides in a complex twisting motion.

Manter[19] compared the subtalar joint to a screw, in which the talus rotates on a stationary calcaneous. The right foot behaves like a right handed screw and the left foot, a left handed screw.

There is also a small amount of forward translation (1.5 mm for each 10 degrees of rotation) of the talus along the axis during pronation that is thought to reverse during supination.[19]

3. The Midtarsal Joint

The midtarsal joint is the functional articulation between the hindfoot (talus and calcaneous) and the midfoot (navicular and cuboid). These articulations have been described as "plane" or "gliding" joints. In supination, Kapandji[7] described the movement of the bones as follows: the navicular glides medially and inferiorly on the head of the talus while the cuboid glides on the calcaneous in the same direction. In pronation, these movements are reversed.

D. Muscular Actions

Muscles that function at the ankle, subtalar, and midtarsal joints are contained in the three muscular compartments of the lower leg: (1) anterior, (2) posterior, and (3) lateral (Figure 6.12).[2] The tibia, fibula, and interrosseus membrane separate the anterior and posterior compartments. The lateral compartment is separated from the other two by the intermuscular septum, which projects laterally from the fibula.

With reference to the ankle, muscles that cross anterior to the ankle joint function as dorsiflexors, whereas muscles that cross posteriorly are plantarflexors. Muscles that originate in the lateral compartment and cross the subtalar joint axis laterally function as evertors. Muscles that are medial to the subtalar joint axis are considered invertors.

Because no muscle attaches directly to the talus, none of the muscles of the lower leg function exclusively at the ankle. Consequently, muscles that have action on the ankle joint also have action at the subtalar joint. Therefore, if a muscle crosses posterior to the ankle axis of rotation, but medial to the subtalar axis, it will be a plantarflexor and an invertor (i.e., the tibialis posterior muscle) (Figure 6.13).[22]

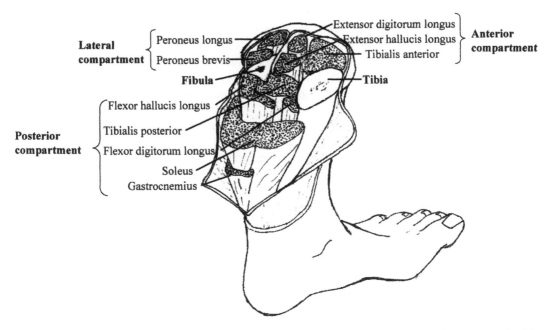

FIGURE 6.12   Cross section of all muscles that function at foot and ankle. The muscles are contained in three muscular compartments of the lower leg: (1) anterior, (2) posterior, and (3) lateral. The tibia, fibula, and interrosseus membrane separate the anterior and posterior compartments. The lateral compartment is separated from the other two by the intermuscular septum. (Adapted from Thompson, C. and Floyd, R. T., *Manual of Structural Kinesiology,* 12th edition, Mosby Year Book, St. Louis, 1994, p. 150. With permission.)

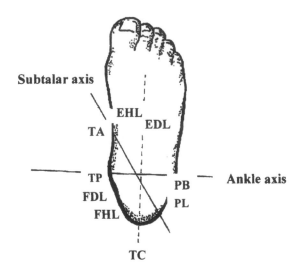

FIGURE 6.13 Line of pull of the extrinsic muscles relative to the ankle and subtalar axes. EDL, Extensor digitorum longus; EHL, extensor hallucis longus; FDL, flexor digitorum longus; FHL, flexor hallucis longus; PB, peroneus brevis; PL, peroneus longus; TA, tibialis anterior; TC, tendocalcaneous; TP, tibialis posterior. Muscles anterior to the ankle axis function as dorsiflexors, muscles posterior to the ankle axis as plantarflexors. Muscles medial to the subtalar axis function as invertors, while muscles lateral will function as evertors. (Adapted from Mann, R., Biomechanics of the foot, in *Atlas of Orthoses: Biomechanical Principles and Application*, 2nd edition, American Academy of Orthopedic Surgeons, Eds., C.V. Mosby, St. Louis, 1985, p. 120. With permission.)

Muscles of the anterior compartment that dorsiflex the ankle include the tibialis anterior, extensor digitorum longus, and extensor hallucis longus (Figure 6.14). These muscles are bound anteriorly at the ankle joint by strong bands of deep fascia, the extensor retinaculum. In addition to being a dorsiflexor, the tibialis anterior also inverts the subtalar joint (Figure 6.13). In contrast, the extensor digitorum longus and extensor hallucis longus cross lateral to the subtalar axis and are evertors of the subtalar joint. The tibialis anterior is the primary dorsiflexor of the ankle. It has a good leverage and a greater cross-sectional area than all the toe extensors combined.[23]

The lateral compartment is formed by the lateral surface of the fibula, the anterior and posterior intermuscular septum, and the crural fascia. The muscles contained in the lateral compartment are the peroneus longus (PL) and peroneus brevis (PB) (Figure 6.14). These two muscles also cross posterior to the ankle axis of rotation, which results in additional plantarflexion capability (Figure 6.13). The tendons of the PL and PB run in the same sheath proximal to the lateral malleolus, and are separated distally as the peroneus longus runs under the cuboid. The PB passes posterior to the distal fibula and attaches to the base of the fifth metatarsal. The PL remains posterior and lateral to the PB tendon and makes three turns as it descends into the foot: at the tip of the lateral malleolus, around the trochlear process of the calcaneous, and sharply around the lateral aspect of the cuboid. Finally, it inserts into the base of the first metatarsal and medial cuneiform.[2] These distal attachments result in the ability of the PL to depress the first ray, aiding stability during walking.[24]

Eversion of the subtalar joint is controlled primarily by the peroneal muscles. The peroneus longus, having a greater cross-sectional area, has the greatest torque-producing capability for eversion. The muscles that control inversion include the tibialis posterior, tibialis anterior, flexor digitorum longus, flexor hallucis longus, and soleus (Figure 6.13). The much larger size of the soleus (5 times larger than the tibialis posterior) makes it the most significant invertor, even though the tibialis posterior has twice the lever arm.[25]

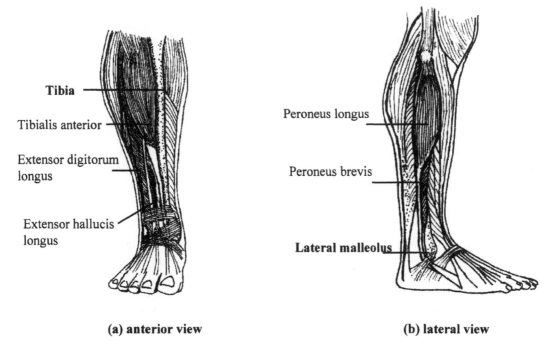

(a) anterior view   **(b) lateral view**

FIGURE 6.14   (a) Muscles of the anterior compartment that dorsiflex the ankle include the tibialis anterior (TA), extensor digitorum longus (EDL), and extensor hallucis longus (EHL). (b) The muscles contained in the lateral compartment are the peroneus longus (PL) and peroneus brevis (PB). Both muscles evert the subtalar joint and are weak plantarflexors of the ankle.

The posterior compartment is the largest of the three compartments. The muscles in the posterior compartment are further divided into superficial and deep groups by a transverse intermuscular septum. The superficial group, which includes the gastrocnemius, soleus, and plantaris, forms a powerful muscle group whose primary function is plantarflexion (Figure 6.12). The deep muscles of the posterior compartment include the tibialis posterior, flexor digitorum longus, and flexor hallucis longus (Figure 6.12). All muscles in the posterior compartment have the capability to plantarflex the ankle and all invert the subtalar joint.[22]

Plantarflexion of the ankle is performed almost excusively by the triceps surae. The gastocnemius and soleus have a large cross-sectional area (43 cm compared to 33 cm for all the other plantarflexors combined).[23] Also, the tendocalcaneous is furthest away from the ankle axis (approximately 5 cm) (Figure 6.13).[22] Other muscles that also pass posterior to the axis of rotation do not have as great a lever arm and are not as effective as plantarflexors. The tendons of tibialis posterior and the peroneal muscles lie close to the malleoli, and the flexor digitorm longus only slightly farther back. The flexor hallucis longus has somewhat better leverage, as its tendon runs under the sustentaculum tali.[23]

The primary muscles that cross the midtarsal joint include the tibialis posterior and peroneus longus. These two tendons cross each other on the bottom of the foot to give a "sling like" support to the midtarsal joint.[23]

E. JOINT FUNCTION DURING GAIT

1. The Ankle

The normal pattern of ankle motion during gait has been studied extensively and has been well summarized by Perry.[24] The foot and ankle function to meet the three demands during gait: shock absorption, stability, and progression. At initial contact (heel strike), the ankle is in a neutral position and rapidly plantarflexes until the foot is flat. The pretibial muscles (primarily tibialis anterior) work eccentrically to control lowering of the foot.

As the body weight is transferred over the stationary foot, the motion rapidly changes to dorsiflexion. The posterior calf muscles work eccentrically to control the forward movement of the tibia and provide stability of the lower limb. In terminal stance, progression of the limb is facilitated by heel rise with continued ankle dorsiflexion. Transfer of body weight over the forefoot necessitates a demand for strong soleus and gastrocnemius action (80% of maximum capacity).[24] The ankle then rapidly returns to a plantarflexed position, reaching a maximum of 20 degrees at the preswing phase.

Plantarflexion continues during initial swing and then reverses again to a neutral ankle in midswing. It maintains this position to clear the foot through the rest of swing. The pretibial muscles are active throughout swing to hold the foot in a dorsiflexed position.

2. The Subtalar Joint

During a weight-bearing activity such as gait, the mobility of the subtalar joint is essential to transfer the rotary motion of the lower extremity to the foot.[26] As the foot itself does not rotate on the ground, motion within the subtalar joint exists to transfer this rotation. Mann[22] referred to the subtalar joint as a "mitered hinge" connecting the leg to the foot. For example, at the beginning of stance the calcaneus everts and the talus internally rotates. However, since the talus cannot rotate within the mortise, it takes the tibia and fibula with it, causing lower leg internal rotation. In contrast, during late stance, the calcaneous inverts while the talus rotates laterally. Again the talus cannot rotate laterally and consequently carries the tibial and fibula into external rotation. In essence, the talus is an extension of the tibia in the sagittal and transverse planes. This function of the subtalar joint is critical for dampening the rotational forces imposed by body weight while the foot remains in contact with the ground.

The foot makes contact with the ground in a slightly inverted position relative to the resting position of the subtalar joint. The foot immediately everts, or pronates, to absorb the shock of loading.[27] Using three-dimensional analysis, Reischl and co-workers found peak pronation to occur at 26.8% of stance.[28] The muscles responsible for controlling this motion are the invertor muscles of the ankle, the tibialis posterior and anterior, and soleus, which are working eccentrically.[24]

During late stance, advancement of the body over the supporting limb requires stability of the entire foot. To meet this demand, the subtalar joint reverses its everted position to more inversion. McPoil and Cornwall[20] reported that the subtalar joint does not return to a fully inverted position during stance, as previously accepted, but instead supinates to the resting subtalar stance position. This supination action of the subtalar joint stabilizes the midtarsal joint and allows a rigid lever for toe off. The muscles responsible for providing this stability at the subtalar joint are the soleus muscle, continued action of the tibialis posterior, and increased action of the toe flexors.[24] The average range of motion at the subtalar joint during gait has been reported as 4 to 6 degrees of inversion and eversion.[20,27]

3. The Midtarsal Joint

During gait, the axes of the midtarsal joints are parallel in early stance to absorb the weight of the body at initial contact and allow the foot to become a mobile adapter to the ground. During mid to late stance, it is desirable for the foot to become more rigid in preparation for toe off; thus, the axes of the midtarsal joint converge, thereby providing increased stability.[24]

Dynamic support of the midtarsal joint is provided primarily by tibialis posterior.[24,29] Other muscles contributing to stability include flexor digitorum longus, flexor hallucis longus, and the intrinsic foot muscles.[1] The plantar fascia also offers passive stability to the midtarsal joint in terminal stance and preswing.[24]

IV. PATHOKINESIOLOGY: CLINICAL RELEVANCE AND IMPLICATIONS

The ankle and foot complex is commonly injured due to the diverse demand for both stability and mobility. Specific pathologies are generally the result of direct trauma and repetitive stress syndromes, as well as anatomic deformities and malalignment. The incidence of ankle and foot injuries varies depending on the age and activity level. For example, in a large group of male marine recruits who were followed through training, the most frequent site of musculoskeletal injury was the ankle/foot region, which accounted for 34.3% of the injuries.[30]

The disability resulting from lesions of the ankle and foot can be further worsened as a result of altered mechanics of gait leading to stress in more proximal joints. Specific injuries common at the foot and ankle include the following: collateral ligament sprains, impingement syndromes, tendon injuries, osteochondral defects, and sinus tarsi syndrome.

A. COLLATERAL LIGAMENT SPRAINS AND TEARS

Sprains of the ankle involve the lateral collateral ligament approximately 85% to 95% of the time.[31] Surgical exploration of acute ankle sprains has indicated that 60% to 70% of injuries are midsubstance tears to the anterior talofibular ligament (ATFL) followed by a 20% incidence of combined ATFL/calcaneofibular ligament (CFL) injury.[3] The remaining 10% of sprains are injuries to the syndesmosis, deltoid ligament, isolated CFL, or posterior talofibular ligament (PTFL) or subtalar ligamentous injuries.[31,32]

According to the American Foot and Ankle Society, a grade I ankle sprain is commonly described as a mild injury to the lateral ankle ligament with minor swelling and tenderness, and slight or no loss in function.[32] The ankle remains stable and normal activity is possible, but will most likely be painful. Pathology is believed to be limited to at most a partial tear of ATFL and a minor strain to the CFL.

A grade II injury is a moderate ankle injury with diffuse swelling, tenderness, and difficulty weight bearing. Functional activity is significantly limited and the ankle is partly unstable. A partial to complete injury to the ATFL and a partial tear of the CFL result in a mildly positive anterior drawer but a negative tilt (angular displacement of the talus in the mortise).[32]

A grade III ankle sprain is a severe ligament injury, usually with complete rupture of the ATFL and CFL. Weight bearing is not tolerated, and there is marked swelling and tenderness. Both anterior drawer and talar tilt tests are both clinically and radiologically positive. Injury to the PTFL is rarely present and does not present with a clinically significant injury pattern.[32]

1. Etiology and Mechanism of Injury

Lateral ankle sprains are much more common due to the increased range of motion available in inversion. Also, the medial deltoid ligament is much stronger than all the lateral ligaments combined.[33] Most ankle sprains occur in a plantarflexed position, which is inherently more unstable due to the decreased bony fit of the talus. During plantarflexion, the ATFL is also in a more vertical position, functioning as the primary resistance to inversion, thus resulting in more injuries (Figure 6.5). The CFL is most commonly injured in dorsiflexion and inversion. However, CFL tears are rare as an isolated injury and are more often associated with an ATFL tear.[32]

Lateral ligamentous injuries often occur with the foot fixed on the ground in a supinated position, with concurrent external rotation of the tibia.[33] As the foot twists medially, relative to the lower leg, there is a predictable sequence of torn structures. The first structure damaged is the ATFL, followed by the anterolateral capsule, and then the distal tibiofibular ligament.[33] Progressive inversion stress may likely tear the CFL.[33] Finally, the PTFL may rupture, which is associated with ankle dislocation. During this severe injury, there may also be concurrent distal lateral malleolus avulsion, medial malleolar fracture, and/or talar neck compression fracture.

Initially following a lateral ankle sprain, swelling is limited to the lateral ankle and there is tenderness over the ATFL and possibly the CFL. Soon after, the swelling often becomes diffuse, and localization of tenderness may be difficult.[33] Passive inversion and end range plantarflexion will reproduce the pain.

Diagnostic imaging is helpful in differentiating a lateral ankle sprain from the following: talar dome fracture, distal fibula fracture, and Jones fracture (fifth metatarsal).[32,33] Other differentials include peroneal tendon dislocation, midfoot sprain, and achilles tendon rupture. Differentiation between tenderness over the lateral collateral ligaments versus the inferior tibiofibular ligament can rule out a syndesmotic sprain.

B. ANKLE IMPINGEMENT SYNDROMES

1. Soft Tissue Impingement

Most patients with ankle sprains recover completely; however, a few have persistent pain as a result of soft tissue impingement. The hypertrophied synovial tissue or scarring of the ATFL can become entrapped in the anterolateral gutter of the ankle. It is reported that impingement occurs primarily in the superior portion of the ATFL. This may also be associated with chondral lesions in the talus and/or the fibula.[32]

These patients complain of chronic ankle pain and often report a history of remote or recurrent inversion ankle sprains.[34] There may be swelling, with or without instability. There is often local tenderness over the lateral gutter and intermittent swelling. Pain with dorsiflexion of the ankle is the most provocative test, because the hypertrophic tissue can become entrapped in this position.[32,34]

Another less common type of soft tissue impingement is talar impingement by the anteroinferior tibiofibular ligament. Bassett et al. hypothesized that following a severe sprain, the ATFL has increased laxity which causes the talar dome to protrude more anteriorly.[35] Then, during dorsiflexion, the distal fasicle of the anteroinferior tibiofibular ligament impinges on the talus.[34,35] Symptoms include persistent or intermittent pain and tenderness in the region of the anterior inferior tibiofibular ligament and the anterolateral aspect of the talus. Symptoms are typically aggravated with dorsiflexion and relieved with plantarflexion.[35]

2. Osseus Impingement

Osseus impingement occurs most commonly in the anterior or posterior aspect of the ankle. Symptoms associated with anterior impingement are elicited with dorsiflexion, and posterior impingement with plantarflexion.[36,37] Causes of anterior impingement include a traction exotosis on the talus as well as osteophytes, which can occur on the anterior lip of the tibia.[38] Repetitive and forced dorsiflexion placing traction on the anterior capsule is the proposed mechanism of injury.[38] Incidence rates for anterior impingent have been reported as 45% in football players and 59% of dancers.[38,39] Posterior impingement is most commonly associated with an anatomic variant on the posterior talus or an os trigonum (an abnormal secondary ossification center on the lateral tubercle of the talus).[37,38] This syndrome is most commonly seen in runners, soccer and football players, and ballet dancers.[37] The mechanism of injury is thought to be forceful and/or repetitive plantarflexion.[38] Subsequent pain and swelling in the posterior ankle occurs when the accessory bone is pinched between the tibia and calcaneous.[40]

C. PERONEAL TENDON DYSFUNCTION

Peroneal tendon subluxation and tenosynovitis are common pathologies of the peroneal tendons and may be acute or chronic. Acute subluxation of the tendons is rare and occurs most commonly in athletic activities such as skiing, soccer, or basketball.[41] Chronic injury is more common and is often due to tendon degeneration of the peroneus longus or brevis.

1. Etiology and Mechanism of Injury

An acute subluxation is caused by a sudden, forceful passive dorsiflexion of the everted foot with a sudden strong reflex contraction of the peroneal muscles.[42] The strong and sudden contraction of the peroneals causes the retinaculum to tear or to strip subperiosteally from its fibular insertion.[41] Acute peroneal injuries may also occur concurrently with an ankle sprain, where both lateral ligaments and the superior retinaculum are stretched or torn concurrently.[43] Bassett and Speer[44] have also postulated that during an inversion trauma, a split lesion of the peroneus brevis can occur without injury of the superior retinaculum.

An acute subluxing peroneal tendon is frequently unrecognized and misdiagnosed as an ankle sprain. The patient usually describes a traumatic injury with associated lateral swelling and ecchymosis which is often associated with a popping or snapping sound.

Predisposing factors for chronic subluxation include insufficiency of the peroneal retinaculum and variations in the retromalleolar sulcus, such as a flat, shallow, or convex groove.[45] Chronic injury of the peroneus longus tendon (PLT) is often due to tendon degeneration and longitudingal splitting. [43] PLT tendinosis and tearing is more common in sedentary, middle-aged individuals who attempt vigorous activity.[46] Co-existing conditions, such as diabetes mellitus, also can contribute to degeneration of the tendon.[46]

There is a frequent association between peroneus brevis tendon tendonopathy and chronic ankle laxity.[44,47,48] Bonnin and co-workers[48] have proposed that the peroneus brevis tendon is impinged against the posterolateral edge of the malleolus. In chronic laxity, the repetition of abnormal varus and anterior drawer leads to excessive stress of the tendon as it is wedged between the lateral malleolus and peroneus longus. Continued friction can lead to degeneration and tendonopathy.[47,48]

Patients will most often complain of pain behind the fibula and above the joint line. This differentiates it from the pain of a lateral ankle sprain, which is in front of the ankle along the anterior talofibular ligament. There is also swelling and tenderness posterior to the lateral malleolus. Provocative tests include passive inversion and resisted eversion with a dorsiflexed ankle.[41]

D. POSTERIOR TIBIAL TENDON DYSFUNCTION

Posterior tibial tendon dysfunction (PTTD) is acknowledged as a common cause of acquired flat foot in middle-aged and geriatric patients.[49-52] Despite its high incidence, PTTD often remains an elusive and overlooked diagnosis. PTTD represents a spectrum of impairments, ranging from isolated medial ankle pain and swelling to a rigid flat foot deformity.[52,53] The cause of PTTD is varied and may result from a peritendinitis or a partial or complete rupture of the tendon.

1. Etiology and Mechanism of Injury

Factors associated with PTTD include the following: age related degenerative changes, pre-existing tenosynovitis, and acute traumatic rupture.[54] Predisposition to PTTD includes hypertension, obesity, diabetes, steroid exposure, and inflammatory arthrides.[54-56] Frey and Shereff[57] have identified another factor in developing PTTD, an area of hypovascularity in the tendon posterior and distal to the medial malleolus. These authors have speculated that the sharp turn the tendon takes around the distal medial malleolus predisposes it to decreased blood flow and degeneration.

Upon surgical exploration of PTTD there are varying degrees of degenerative changes within the tendon. Funk and co-workers[50] identified four distinct types of lesions in patients: group I had a complete avulsion of the posterior tibial tendon from the navicular bone; group II had a midsubstance rupture just distal to the medial malleolus; group III had a longitudinal tear without a rupture; and group IV had synovitits around the tendon without any signs of tendon disruption. Often there is abundant synovial inflammation around the tendon, although there can also be significant tendon degeneration without tenosynovitis.[52]

Patients most often complain of gradual pain and swelling on the medial aspect of the ankle and the onset of flatfoot deformity.[51] The mechanism of injury is often not clearly known, as some patients can recall a certain acute incidence of trauma, while others cannot.[50] Pain is elicited upon palpation of the posterior tibial tendon and often with resistance of plantarflexion and inversion. However, palpation of the tendon during contraction may not be a reliable indicator of an intact or disrupted tendon.[50] Flattening of the longitudinal arch is common with weight bearing.

Posterior tibial tendon function is evaluated by having the patient perform a heel rise. The ability to invert the calcaneous is often absent and repeated heel rise is difficult without pain and or fatigue.[52] Range of motion at the ankle joint is not usually restricted, but subtalar motion may be limited depending on the severity. In the more severe cases, subtalar inversion may even be ankylosed. Also, in the later stages of PTTD, forefoot adduction may be lost and a forefoot varus relative to the rearfoot can become fixed.[51-53]

E. OSTEOCHONDRAL DEFECTS

The term *osteochondral defect* is used to describe the separation of a fragment of articular cartilage, with or without the subchondral bone.[59] Other terms that are synonymous include *osteochondritis dissecans*, *transchondral fracture*, and *osteochondral fracture*.[59] In the ankle, osteochondral lesions of the talus are an uncommon but therapeutically significant problem.[60]

Osteochondral defects result from a shearing, rotatory, or impact force that acts tangentially across the surface of the talus.[38] The cause is primarily trauma (acute or chronic repetitive), but idiopathic causes also have been reported.[32] Both medial and lateral lesions of the talus are common. Lateral lesions are produced when a stress causes the anterolateral aspect of the talar dome to impact the fibula.[32] It is thought that the lateral lesions are more shallow and tend to occur secondary to trauma. Medial lesions tend to be deeper and more posterior and are often associated with osteonecrosis.[32] The medial lesion typically results when the posteriormedial talar dome impacts the tibial articular surface.

Osteochondral defects are often associated with severe ankle sprains. Common symptoms include pain, intermittent swelling, stiffness, and locking secondary to loose bodies in the ankle joint.[32,38] The patient usually reports medial or lateral joint tenderness and decreased range of ankle motion. Palpation of the talar dome in plantarflexion elicits pain.

F. SINUS TARSI SYNDROME

Sinus tarsi syndrome is inflammation within the sinus tarsi secondary to trauma or overuse.[61] The sinus tarsi is the oval space between the talus and the calcaneous and is continuous with the tarsal tunnel. The sinus tarsi and tarsal canal are filled with fatty tissue, subtalar ligaments, a branch of the posterior tibial artery, bursa, and nerve endings.[62] Sinus tarsi syndrome is characterized by chronic diffuse pain on the lateral aspect of the foot increased by palpation over the lateral aspect of the sinus tarsi. Pain is often provoked with supination.[63]

Chronic ankle sprains have been reported as a common cause of sinus tarsi syndrome.[61] Arthroscopic reports indicate scarring and synovial inflammation in the lateral talocalcaneal recess.[64] Some authors, however, contend that talocalcaneal instability, possibly with a tear of the interosseus ligament, is the cause of this dysfunction.[65] Inflammatory processes such as rheumatoid arthritis and gout are also associated with this clinical entity.[61,65]

V. SUMMARY AND CONCLUSIONS

Multiple bones of the ankle and foot contribute to both mobility and stability. Although the joints of the ankle and foot are discussed separately, they act as a functional unit with contributions from each individual joint. The foot and ankle have two primary functions: (1) propulsion, where the complex is more rigid, and (2) shock absorption, when the complex is more flexible. Normal movement of all joints of the ankle and foot provide range of motion to allow functional mobility as well as stability.

Knowledge of the normal anatomy and biomechanics of the foot and ankle is essential in understanding the pathokinesiology of injury. In the future, kinematic MRI of the ankle and foot should further facilitate our understanding of the normal function and biomechanics of this complex region. Furthermore, dynamic imaging may provide a unique diagnostic tool for the multiple pathologies associated with the ankle and foot.

REFERENCES

1. Norkin, C. C. and Levangie, P. K., *Joint Structure and Function*, F.A. Davis, Philadelphia, 1992, chap. 12.
2. Moore, K. and Dalley, A., *Clinically Oriented Anatomy*, Lippincott, Williams & Wilkins, Philadelphia, 1999, chap. 5.
3. Inman, V. T., *The Joints of the Ankle*, Williams & Wilkins, Baltimore, MD, 1976.
4. Sarrafian, S. K., *Anatomy of the Foot and Ankle: Descriptive, Topographic, Functional*, 2nd edition, J. B. Lippincott, Philadelphia, 1993.
5. Agur, A. M. R., *Grant's Atlas of Anatomy*, 9th edition, Williams & Wilkins, Baltimore, 1991, chap. 5.
6. Rockar, P. A., The subtalar joint: anatomy and joint motion, *J. Orthop. Sports Phys. Ther.*, 21, 361, 1995.
7. Kapandji, I. A., *The Physiology of the Joints, Vol II, The Lower Limb*, Churchill Livingstone, New York, 1970.
8. Sammarco, J. G., Biomechanics of the foot, in *Basic Biomechanics of the Skeletal System*, Nordin, M. and Frankel, V. H., Eds., Lea & Febiger, Philadelphia, 1989, chap. 9.
9. Patel, D. V. and Warren, R. F., Ankle sprain: clinical evaluation and current treatment concepts, in *Disorders of the Heel, Rearfoot, and Ankle*, Ranawat, C. and Positano, R., Eds., Churchill Livingstone, New York, 1999, chap. 23.
10. Smith, J. W., The ligamentous structures of the canalis and sinus tarsi, *J. Anat.*, 92, 612, 1958.
11. Sarrafian, S. K., Biomechanics of the subtalar joint, *Clin. Orthop.*, 290, 17, 1993.
12. Singh, A. K., Starkweather, K. D., Hollister, A. M., Jatana, S., and Lupichuk, A. G., Kinematics of the ankle: a hinge axis model, *Foot Ankle*, 13, 439, 1992.
13. Lundberg, A., Svensson, O., Nemeth, G., and Selvik, G., The axis of rotation of the ankle joint, *J. Bone Joint Surg.*, 71B, 94, 1989.
14. Sammarco, G. J., Burstein, A. H., and Frankel, V. H., Biomechanics of the ankle: a kinematic study, *Orthop. Clin. North Am.*, 4, 75, 1973.
15. Barnett, C. H. and Napier, J. R., The axis of rotation of the ankle joint in man: its influence upon the form of the talus and the mobility of the fibula, *J. Anat.*, 86, 1, 1952.
16. Hicks, J., Mechanics of the foot. I. The joints, *J. Anat.*, 87, 345, 1953.
17. Frankel, V. H. and Nordin M., Biomechanics of the ankle, in *Basic Biomechanics of the Skeletal System*, 2nd edition, Nordin, M. and Frankel, V. H., Eds., Lea & Febiger, Philadelphia, 1989, chap. 8.
18. American Academy of Orthopedic Surgeons, *Joint Motion: Method of Measuring and Recording*, American Academy of Orthopedic Surgeons, Chicago, 1965.
19. Manter, J., Movements of the subtalar and transverse tarsal joints of the human foot, *Anat. Rec.*, 80, 397, 1941.
20. McPoil, T. G. and Cornwall, M. W., Relationship between neutral subtalar joint position and pattern of rearfoot motion during walking, *Foot Ankle*, 15, 141, 1994.
21. Mann, R. A. and Inman, V. T., Phasic activity of intrinsic muscles of the foot, *J. Bone Joint Surg.*, 46A, 469, 1964.
22. Mann, R., Biomechanics of the foot, in *Atlas of Orthoses: Biomechanical Principles and Application*, 2nd edition, American Academy of Orthopedic Surgeons, Eds., C.V. Mosby, St. Louis, 1985, p. 112.
23. Smith, L. K., Weiss, E. L., and Lehmkuhl, L. D., *Brunnstrom's Clinical Kinesiology*, F.A. Davis, Philadelphia, 1996, chap. 10.
24. Perry, J., *Gait Analysis: Normal and Pathological Function*. Slack, Thorofare, NJ, 1992, chap. 4.
25. Perry, J., Anatomy and biomechanics of the hindfoot, *Clin. Orthop.*, 177, 9, 1983.

26. Donatelli, R. A., *The Biomechanics of the Foot and Ankle,* 2nd edition, F.A. Davis, Philadelphia, 1996, chap. 1.

27. Wright, D. G., DeSai, S. M., and Henderson, W. H., Action of the subtalar joint and ankle-joint complex during the stance phase of walking, *J. Bone Joint Surg.,* 46A, 361, 1964.

28. Reischl, S. F., Powers, C. M., Rao, S., and Perry, J., Relationship between foot pronation and rotation of the tibia and femur during walking, *Foot Ankle Int.,* 20, 513, 1999.

29. Thordarson, D. B., Schmotzer, H., Chon, J., and Peters, J., Dynamic support of the human longitudinal arch: a biomechanical evaluation, *Clin. Orthop.,* 316, 165, 1995.

30. Almeida, S. A., Williams, K. M., Shaffer, R. A., and Brodine, S. K., Epidemiological patterns of musculoskeletal injuries and physical training, *Med. Sci. Sports Exerc.,* 31, 1176, 1999.

31. Birrer, R. B. and Dellacorte, M. P., Sports medicine, in *Common Foot Problems in Primary Care,* 2nd edition, Birrer, R. B., Dellacorte, M. P., and Grisafi, P. J., Eds., Hanley & Belfus, Philadelphia, 1998, chap. 14.

32. Lewis, J. E. and Marymount, J. V., Ankle arthroscopy and sports related injuries, in *Orthopaedic Knowledge Update: Foot and Ankle 2,* Mizel, M. S., Miller, R. A., and Scioli, M. W., Eds., American Academy of Orthopedic Surgeons, Rosemont, IL, 1998, chap. 4.

33. Safran, M. R., Benedetti, R. S., Bartolozzi, A. R., and Mandelbaum, B. R., Lateral ankle sprains: a comprehensive review. I: Etiology, pathoanatomy, histopathogenesis and diagnosis, *Med. Sci. Sports Exerc.,* 31, S429, 1999.

34. Farooki, S., Yao, L., and Seeger, L. L., Anterolateral impingement of the ankle: effectiveness of MR imaging, *Radiology,* 207, 357, 1998.

35. Bassett, F. H., Gates, H. S., Billys, J. B., Morris, H. B., and Nikolaou, P. K., Talar impingement by the anteroinferior tibiofibular ligament, *J. Bone Joint Surg.,* 72A, 55, 1990.

36. Ogilvie-Harris, D. J., Mahomed, N., and Demaziere, A., Anterior impingement of the ankle treated by arthroscopic removal of bony spurs, *J. Bone Joint Surg. [Br.],* 75, 437, 1993.

37. Brown, G. P., Feehery, R. V., Jr., and Grant, S. M., Case study: the painful os trigonum syndrome, *J. Orthop. Sports Phys. Ther.,* 22, 22, 1995.

38. Pavlov, H., Potter H., Ditchek J., and Schneider, R., Imaging of the hindfoot and ankle, in *Disorders of the Heel, Rearfoot, and Ankle,* Ranawat, C. and Positano, R., Eds., Churchill Livingstone, New York, 1999, chap. 2.

39. Kleiger, B., Anterior tibiotalar impingement syndromes in dancers, *Foot Ankle,* 3, 69, 1982.

40. Johnson, R. P., Collier, B. D., and Carrera, G. F., The os trigonum syndrome: use of bone scan in the diagnosis, *J. Trauma,* 24, 761, 1984.

41. Safran, M. R., O'Malley, D., Jr., and Fu, F. H., Peroneal tendon subluxation in athletes: new exam technique, case reports, and review, *Med. Sci. Sports Exerc.,* 31, S487, 1999.

42. Earle, S. A., Moritz, J. R., and Tapper, E. M., Dislocation of the peroneal tendons of the ankle: an analysis of 25 ski injuries, *Northwest Med.,* 71, 108, 1972.

43. Khoury, N. J., El-Khoury, G. Y., Saltzman, C. L., and Kathol, M. H., Peroneus longus and brevis tendon tears: MR imaging evaluation, *Radiology,* 200, 833, 1996.

44. Bassett, F. H. D. and Speer, K. P., Longitudinal rupture of the peroneal tendons, *Am. J. Sports Med.,* 21, 354, 1993.

45. Edwards, M., The relation of the peroneal tendon to the fibula, calcaneous and cuboidieum, *Am. J. Anat.,* 42, 213, 1928.

46. Sammarco, G. J., Peroneal tendon injuries, *Orthop. Clin. North Am.,* 25, 135, 1994.

47. Munk, R. L. and Davis, P. H., Longitudinal rupture of the peroneus brevis tendon, *J. Trauma,* 16, 803, 1976.

48. Bonnin, M., Tavernier, T., and Bouysset, M., Split lesions of the peroneus brevis tendon in chronic ankle laxity, *Am. J. Sports Med.,* 25, 699, 1997.

49. Dellacorte, M. P., Caruso, R., and Grisafi, J., The geriatric foot, in *Common Foot Problems in Primary Care,* 2nd edition, Birrer, R. B., Dellacorte, M. P., and Grisafi, P. J., Eds., Hanley & Belfus, Philadelphia, 1998, chap. 11.

50. Funk, D. A., Cass, J. R., and Johnson, K. A., Acquired flat foot deformity secondary to posterior tibial tendon pathology, *J. Bone Joint Surg. [Am.],* 68, 95, 1986.

51. Geideman, W. M. and Johnson, J. E., Posterior tibial tendon dysfunction, *J. Orthop. Sports Phys. Ther.,* 30, 68, 2000.

52. Katchis, S. D., Posterior tibial tendon dysfunction, in *Disorders of the Heel, Rearfoot and Ankle,* Ranawat, C. S. and Positano, R. G., Eds., Churchill Livingstone, New York, 1999, chap. 29.

53. Smith, C. F., Anatomy, function, and pathophysiology of the posterior tibial tendon, *Clin. Pod. Med. Surg.,* 16, 399, 1999.

54. Sin, S. L., Berkman, A. R., and Lee, T. H., Tendon problems of the foot and ankle, in *Orthopaedic Knowledge Update: Foot and Ankle 2,* Mizel, M. S., Miller, R. A., and Scioli, M. W., Eds., American Academy of Orthopedic Surgeons, Rosemont, IL, 1998, chap. 20.

55. Michelson, J., Easley, M., Wigley, F. M., and Hellmann, D., Posterior tibial tendon dysfunction in rheumatoid arthritis, *Foot Ankle Int.,* 16, 156, 1995.

56. Myerson, M., Solomon, G., and Shereff, M., Posterior tibial tendon dysfunction: its association with seronegative inflammatory disease, *Foot Ankle,* 9, 219, 1989.

57. Frey, C. and Shereff, M. N. G., Vascularity of the posterior tibial tendon, *J. Bone Joint Surg. [Am.],* 72, 884, 1990.

58. Abboudi, J. and Kupcha, P., Supination lag as an indication of posterior tibial tendon dysfunction, *Foot Ankle Int.,* 19, 570, 1998.

59. Tol, J. L., Struijs, P. A., Bossuyt, P. M., Verhagen, R. A., and van Dijk, C. N., Treatment strategies in osteochondral defects of the talar dome: a systematic review, *Foot Ankle Int.,* 21,119, 2000.

60. Hepple, S., Winson, I. G., and Glew, D., Osteochondral lesions of the talus: a revised classification, *Foot Ankle Int.,* 20, 789, 1999.

61. Martin, T. P., Current trends in foot and ankle imaging, in *Orthopaedic Knowledge Update: Foot and Ankle 2,* Mizel, M. S., Miller, R. A., and Scioli, M. W., Eds., American Academy of Orthopedic Surgeons, Rosemont, IL, 1998, p. 324.

62. Beltran, J., Munchow, A. M., Khabiri, H., Magee, D. G., McGhee, R. B., and Grossman, S. G., Ligaments of the lateral aspect of the ankle and sinus tarsi: an imaging study, *Radiology,* 177, 455, 1990.

63. Louweren, J. W. K. and Snijders, C. J., Lateral ankle instability: an overview, in *Disorders of the Heel, Rearfoot and Ankle,* Ranawat, C. S. and Positano, R. G., Eds., Churchill Livingstone, New York, 1999, p. 349.

64. Meyer, J. M. and Lagier, R., Post-traumatic sinus tarsi syndrome. An anatomical and radiological study, *Acta Orthop. Scand.,* 48, 121, 1977.

65. Kjaersgaard-Andersen, P., Soballe, K., Andersen, K., and Pilgaard, S., Sinus tarsi syndrome: presentation of seven cases and review of the literature, *J. Foot Surg.,* 28, 3, 1989.

7 Kinematic MRI of the Ankle

Michael R. Terk

CONTENTS

I. INTRODUCTION

The ankle is best assessed by magnetic resonance imaging (MRI) by using a combination of standard, high-resolution static MRI methods and kinematic MRI techniques.[1-3] Although kinematic MRI of other joints is well established, relatively little has been written about the application of this technique to the ankle, despite the initial description in 1990 by Shellock and Mandelbaum.[1] Unfortunately, kinematic MRI of the ankle has not become a common part of the diagnostic imager's armamentarium of clinical studies. This omission is somewhat surprising, particularly since the ankle is prone to a variety of derangements that might best be evaluated by such a unique diagnostic method.

Kinematic MRI of the ankle is no more difficult to accomplish than kinematic MRI of the patellofemoral joint, perhaps easier because of the limited space requirements, and certainly, far easier than kinematic MRI of the shoulder. It is also not for the rarity of impairment that ankle kinematic MRI has not gained in interest, since up to 12% of athletic injuries are to the ankle.[1]

Although a large variety of ankle pathologies and conditions can be effectively demonstrated by static MRI techniques,[2,3] it is reasonably clear that abnormalities that are position-dependent and may be only detectable transiently (e.g., impingement syndromes, peroneal tendon subluxation) lend themselves to evaluation by kinematic MRI.[1-8] Other proposed clinical applications for kinematic MRI of the ankle include assessment of tibio-talar rotation, evaluation of partial tears of the tendons and ligaments, and determination of loading areas of the talar dome.[4]

Perhaps the paucity of literature regarding kinematic MRI of the ankle is simply a reflection of the tremendous demand for clinical imaging of other musculoskeletal articulations. Alternatively, researchers' interests may not yet have turned to this fruitful area for investigation. It is this author's hope that this chapter might stimulate additional interest in this potentially exciting area. With the growing interest in MRI-assisted orthopedic examinations, it appears likely that greater interest in kinematic MRI of the ankle will follow.

0-8493-0807-0/01/$0.00+$.50
© 2001 by Frank G. Shellock

In this chapter, the technical and clinical aspects of kinematic MRI of the ankle will be presented. There will be a discussion of the kinematic MRI technique, the basic pulse sequences employed, and speculation about pulse sequences yet to be applied. Obviously, the choice of techniques and imaging parameters and configuration of the MR system will affect the performance of the examination. These factors will also be discussed. Examples of normal and abnormal anatomy and findings will be presented, as well as the clinical applications of kinematic MRI techniques to specific clinical syndromes.

II. TECHNIQUE

A. POSITIONING DEVICES AND RADIOFREQUENCY COILS

A variety of positioning devices has been developed for use in kinematic MRI of the ankle (Figure 7.1). These devices have certain requirements in common: they must be compatible with the magnetic field environment (i.e., lacking ferromagnetic parts in their construction); they must allow a reproducible range of motion; and they must control the movement of the ankle. In some situations, application of a load or stress may be desirable. Finally, the device used for kinematic MRI of the ankle must contain sufficient provisions for patient comfort and joint stability to facilitate acquisition of the MR images.

The positioning device used in this author's experience is relatively simple (Figure 7.1). It is constructed of polyvinyl chloride (PVC) with a hinged footplate to which the foot is held in place using Velcro straps, thereby allowing an axis center of rotation. An arm component is attached with a visible scale that can be moved by the MR system operator for passive ankle motion, or may be used to apply a counter force (i.e., for stress views). Other positioning devices for kinematic MRI of the ankle have been described, most notably by Hinterman and Nigg[6] for use in *in vitro* applications and by Muhle et al.[7] for use in *in vivo* applications.

The small size and complex anatomy of the ankle make high-resolution kinematic MR views essential for optimal examination of this joint.[1-3] Therefore, the positioning apparatus must be able to incorporate the proper radiofrequency (RF) coil to permit the signal-to-noise necessary for MRI of the ankle. RF coils shown to be useful for kinematic MRI of the ankle include dual 5-inch, flexible, circular (circumferential), and dedicated-extremity RF coils. Optimally, a positioning device should permit the acquisition of static views, high-resolution MRI views, and kinematic MRI studies without the need for an equipment change.[1,4,5,8]

B. THE MAGNETIC RESONANCE SYSTEM

The choice of the MR system configuration raises an issue of interest. Ankle anatomy and motion, being limited in size and extent, do not require particularly wide bore or "open" MR system configurations. For example, for studies of simple ankle plantarflexed and dorsiflexed positions, standard MR sytems such as conventional high-field-strength MR systems are suitable for kinematic MRI of the ankle. Of note is that a standard "closed-configured" MR system was first used for kinematic MRI of the ankle.

If, on the other hand, one wishes to study axial loading as might occur with weight bearing, a different configuration would be needed. Several such MR systems do exist, with vertical openings primarily intended for interventional MR procedures, but easily adaptable to kinematic MRI procedures.[15]

Obviously, open MR systems offer some advantages that include better access to the patient for physical examination and manipulation. As the concept of the MR-guided orthopedic examination advances, open MR systems may provide more practical applications for the ankle and other joints.

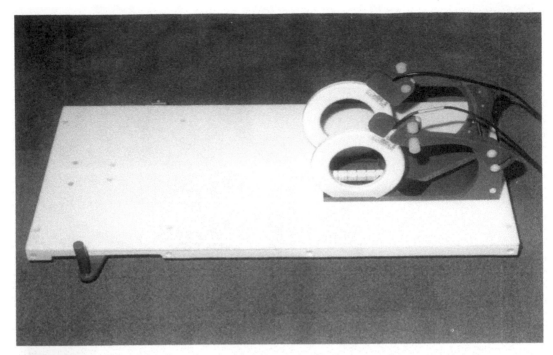

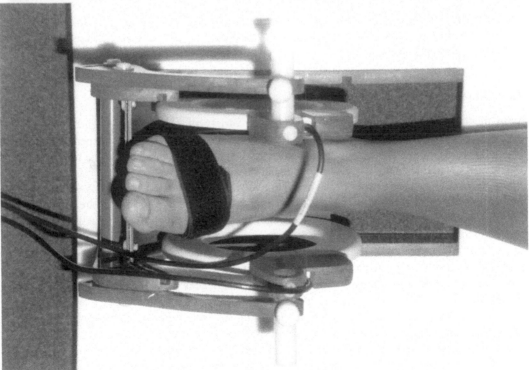

FIGURE 7.1A Example of a positioning device used for kinematic MRI of the ankle. The device has a handle to guide the positions of the ankle (Captain Plastic, Seattle, WA). This device is constructed to allow the fixation of two 5-inch circular coils to each side of the ankle. Overall view (top) and close up view (bottom) of the positioning device. The close up view shows the subject's ankle strapped to the positioning device by a Velcro strap.

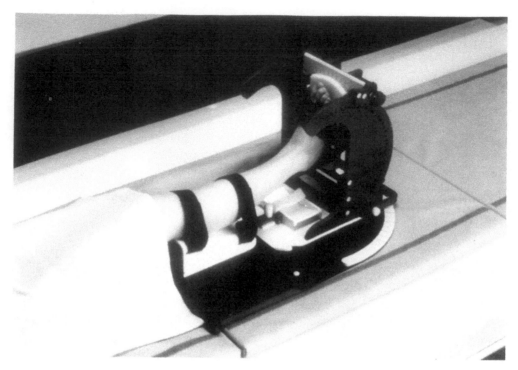

FIGURE 7.1B   A positioning device designed to allow single or combined incremental positions of the ankle (General Electric Medical Systems, Milwaukee, WI). This positioning device is typically used with a circumferential, receive-only surface coil.

C. IMAGING PARAMETERS AND PROTOCOL

With the rapid development of instrumentation, a variety of MR pulse sequences can be used successfully. The available sequences can be grouped into three categories, depending primarily on the speed of image acquisition desired for the kinematic MRI procedure. The oldest and most universally available method is the incremental, passive positioning method.[1,4,5] Using this technique, the ankle is moved from dorsiflexed, to neutral, to plantarflexed positions with a predetermined number of movement increments made during which static MR images are obtained.

T1-weighted or spin density-weighted images provide good anatomical visualization and may be obtained in a relatively rapid manner if some compromises are made to resolution and/or signal to noise. With the reduction of inter echo spacing, T1-weighted fast spin echo images have become practical with substantial reductions in acquisition time or increases in resolution (Figures 7.2 to 7.4). Gradient echo and spoiled gradient echo pulse sequences may also be used if greater speed is required.

The second general method is termed active-movement, dynamic, or "real-time" kinematic MRI. This technique uses fast imaging pulse sequences such that the motion does not need to be completely stopped during the acquisition of images.[4] Two types of pulse sequences are typically used for this application: fast gradient recalled echo in the steady state (GRASS) and single shot, fast spin echo techniques. The fast GRASS sequences employ very short repetition times (TR) as well as short echo times (TE). Notably, these fast pulse sequences have been used to perform kinematic MRI studies of the ankle without the need for a positioning device.

Muhle et al. reported the use of an "ultra-fast" pulse sequence for kinematic MRI, with promising results.[7] This rapid pulse sequence involves acquisition of multiple phase encoded echoes that are obtained with each repetition. Only half the data to fill k-space is required with a computer

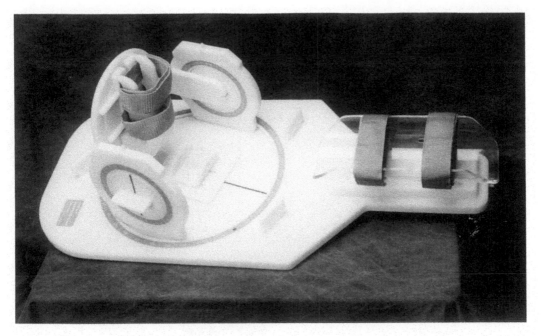

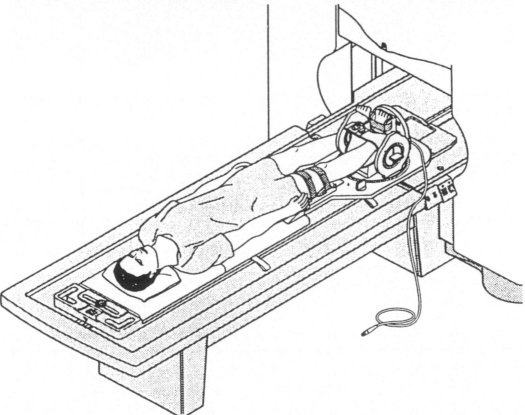

FIGURE 7.1C   A positioning device designed to allow single or combined incremental positions of the ankle (top) (CHAMCO, Inc., Cocoa, FL). (bottom) Schematic showing the positioning device, a flexible surface coil, and a subject prepared for kinematic MRI of the ankle using an open MR system. Several different types of surface coils may be utilized with this positioning device.

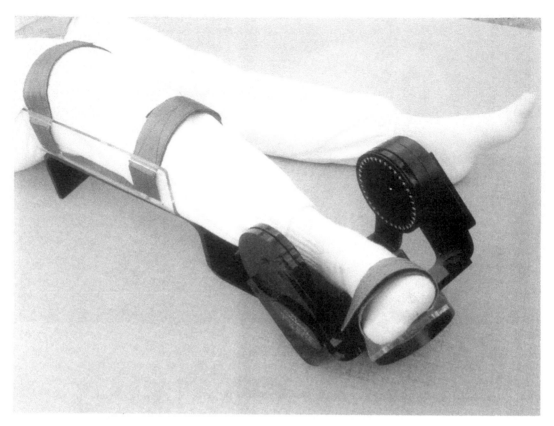

FIGURE 7.1D   A newly developed positioning device designed to allow single or combined incremental positions of the ankle for kinematic MRI examinations (Chamco, Cocoa, FL).

generating calculations of the missing data. While there tends to be slight blurring with this imaging method, this limitation is less severe as inter echo spacing times are reduced.

There is a reduction in resolution and contrast when some of these rapid pulse sequences are employed. However, such protocols offer the great advantage of sufficient imaging speed for kinematic MRI procedures that may require continuous muscle contractions associated with ankle movements for a more physiological examination. As MRI technology evolves more rapid pulse sequences, the reality of MR fluoroscopy may be achieved, providing true real-time, kinematic MRI.

Regardless of the imaging technique used to acquire the MR images, viewing the resulting kinematic MRI examination is facilitated using the MR system software to create a cine-loop (i.e., paging images selected from a given section location).[1,4,5] Although not real-time, this method can produce the impression of repetitive motion and is particularly useful when reviewing multiple images obtained from different imaging planes for the kinematic MRI procedure.

A final alternative for the kinematic MRI study of the ankle is to retrospectively analyze imaging data. As described by Udupa et al.,[9] this method employs an analysis of the more complex supination and pronation motions at the subtalar joint using three-dimensional MRI reformations. Hirsch et al.[10] used a similar method to study the ankle.

1. Section Locations and Imaging Planes

There is controversy as to whether motion at the ankle joint needs to be defined by single axis or by multiple axes.[9] Because motion may be more complex than a simple hinge axis, misregistration of section locations may occur when direct kinematic MRI is performed. Misregistration also occurs with a single axis of imaging. With any single axis positioning device, anatomic structures anterior

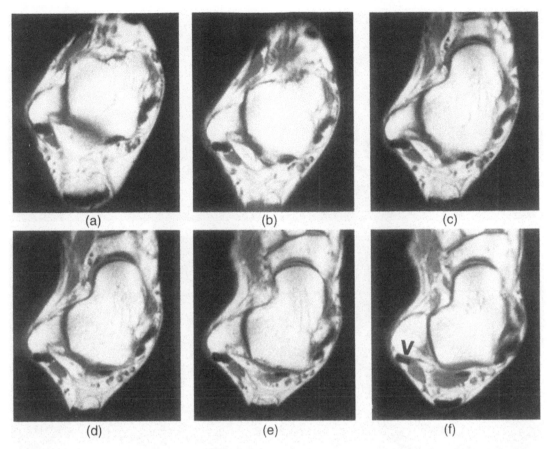

FIGURE 7.2 Kinematic MRI of the ankle performed using axial plane imaging (T1-weighted, spin echo) with passive, incremental movements from plantarflexion, to neutral, to dorsiflexion positions (a to f). Note the flattening of the peroneus brevis as it is compressed between the posterior surface of the fibula and the peroneus longus (f, arrow head)

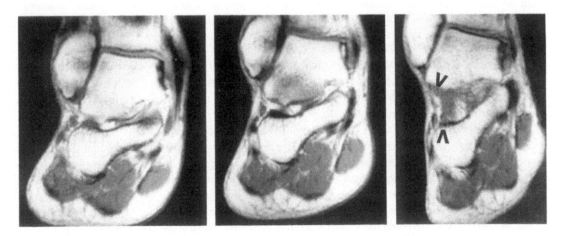

FIGURE 7.3 Kinematic MRI of the ankle performed using coronal plane imaging (T1-weighted, spin echo) with the joint in eversion (right), neutral (center), and inversion (left) positions. Motion is occurring at the subtalar joint. It is evident from the images that, at this level, eversion is limited by contact between the lateral talus and calcaneus, while with inversion, greater motion is possible because of a more medial axis of rotation (arrow heads).

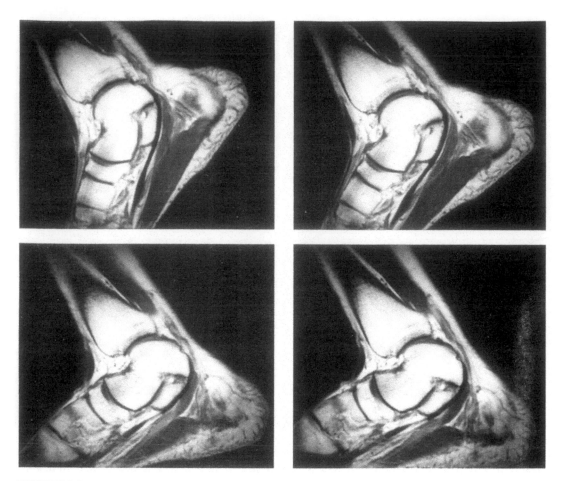

FIGURE 7.4 Kinematic MRI of the ankle performed using sagittal plane imaging (T1-weighted, spin echo). There are successive movements from maximum plantarflexion (left, upper image), to partial plantarflexion (right, upper image), to neutral (right, lower image), to dorsiflexion positions (left, lower panel). This is a normal kinematic study showing smooth, even movement as the talus rotates beneath the tibia in association with the various incremental positions. Potential anterior impingement or osseous impingement syndromes typically can be seen between the anterior tibia and talus using this kinematic MRI procedure.

to the axis of rotation will appear to move to a more inferior section location with plantarflexion of the ankle. Conversely, posterior structures will appear in progressively more superior locations with plantarflexion. Clearly, the opposite situation applies with dorsiflexion of the ankle. Although the change in registration may result from the off axis motion, it may also occur as a result of gross changes in the subject's position.

Regardless of the cause, some correction needs to be made for relative changes to the imaging plane during kinematic MRI of the ankle. The most direct solution to this problem is to obtain multiple section locations incremented along the axis of imaging. The resulting section locations can then be matched for a single anatomical reference and then combined together in the cine-loop display to provide the proper kinematic MRI examination of the ankle. Obviously, this correction requires multiple section locations to be acquired, usually resulting in longer image acquisition times. Alternatively, one could use oblique section locations, altering the angle with each positional change of the ankle.

A more elegant approach to obtain the proper section location to view the area of interest is to actively track an anatomical structure and to correct selection of the section location from returning positional data. For example, Melchert et al. used a pneumatic-electrical device attached to the joint to measure skin-muscle shifting.[13]

Dumoulin et al.[14] also addressed this problem using an MR signal source that could be detected with determination of its position in the MR system, thereby permitting selection of the desired section location. While this so-called "tracking device" was originally intended for interventional MR applications, Pearle et al.[15] applied this method to track joint motion for kinematic MRI procedures.

Among the inherent advantages of MRI is its ability to image in multiple planes. This feature is effectively applied to kinematic MRI examinations, allowing axial, sagittal, coronal, and oblique plane imaging (Figures 7.2 to 7.4). The appropriate plane can be selected based on the anatomic structure or the pathologic feature being evaluated. For example, the axial plane should be selected for investigation of peroneal tendon subluxation because this would best show abnormal motion, while the sagittal plane might better demonstrate anterior impingement or osseous syndromes with plantarflexion and dorsiflexion movements of the ankle. Alternatively, if inversion and eversion motions are to be studied (e.g., for assessment of subtalar instability or assessment of lateral and medial soft tissues), the coronal plane of imaging tends to be the most suitable.

III. CLINICAL APPLICATIONS

A. Tendon Dysfunction

Peroneal tendon dysfunction has been related to a number of anatomical variations. Hypertrophy of the peroneal tubercle, as well as anatomic variations in the fibular and retromalleolar groove, has been associated with the development of stenosing tenosynovitis.[16-19] Absence or insufficiency of the peroneal retinaculum may also predispose the peroneal tendons to dislocation or subluxation. Acute dislocation of the peroneal tendons is relatively rare, usually encountered in violent, passive dorsiflexion of the foot. Rupture of the peroneal tendons is normally encountered in overuse syndromes, typically in athletes.[19]

Chronic subluxation of the peroneal tendons can be disabling, particularly if tendon pathology is also present.[21,22] The incidence of peroneal tendon subluxation is on the rise due to an increase in recreational sports activities and an additional awareness of the abnormality. Although lateral joint pain and tenderness are characteristic in patients with peroneal tendon dysfunction, other associated injuries may produce identical symptoms.[21,22]

Historically, peroneal tendon subluxation was initially described by Monteggia in 1803.[20] Since that time, this condition has received relatively little attention in the medical, and particularly the diagnostic imaging, literature.

The peroneal tendon complex is comprised of the peroneus longus and brevis tendons, which are ensheathed by a common synovial membrane. The tendon and sheath bundle course through a fibro-osseous canal, composed primarily of the superior peroneal retinaculum and the undersurface of the distal fibular tip.

The normal kinematic function of the peroneal tendons is dependent on the integrity of several elastic structures, especially the superior peroneal retinaculum, and a morphologically adequate retromalleolar groove. The soft tissue structures and the retromalleolar groove serve to maintain the peroneal tendons in a stable position during movements of the ankle.[1] A normal kinematic study of the peroneus longus and brevis tendons shows the tendons in a fixed position relative to the retromalleolar groove of the lateral malleolus during dorsiflexed, neutral, and plantarflexed positions of the ankle.

In the case of peroneal tendon subluxation, the positional abnormality may be transient and not observable with static imaging techniques. There are two main anatomical abnormalities that predispose these tendons to subluxation: (1) a deficiency of the peroneal retinaculum and (2) a convex or shallow posterior surface of the fibula forming the peroneal groove.[21] While these abnormalities are, at times, detectable with static imaging, they are frequently difficult to image or, if present, may not be related to symptomatic subluxation. It is the very transient nature of peroneal subluxation that makes kinematic MRI of the ankle a useful examination in the detection of this condition.[8]

Partial tears of the peroneal tendons have been well described and are said to frequently take the form of longitudinal tears or "splits."[19] The ability of MRI to detect the split has been well documented; however, the predisposing factor is frequently obscure, occurring in the absence of obvious anatomical abnormality.[19] It has been hypothesized that repetitive compression of the peroneus brevis against the fibula by the peroneus longus may play a role. This effect is shown in Figure 7.2, where such compression can be seen as flattening of the peroneus brevis in images obtained with progressive dorsiflexion movements of the ankle.

Alternatively, abnormal subluxation of the peroneus longus as a result of retinacular insufficiency creates a "rubbing effect" on the peroneus brevis and predisposes this structure to tendonopathy. Retinacular deficiency may also cause abnormal motion, resulting in peroneous longus tendonopathy (Figure 7.5).

The presence of peroneal tendon subluxation may have associated serious sequellae. If this abnormality is not repaired or treated in the early stages following injury, there is a poor long-term prognosis. Therefore, a rapid and accurate diagnosis of this condition is critical for appropriate patient management.

Although the peroneal tendons have received modest attention with kinematic MRI, other tendons have been less appreciated. It is likely that a dynamic analysis may be applied to other tendons, leading to an expanded understanding of their pathophysiological failures. For example, dysfunction of the posterior tibial tendon is not an uncommon problem. This condition typically follows severe acute trauma or occurs as a progressive failure, as frequently seen in middle-aged or elderly females.

Normally, there is little motion between the posterior tibial tendon and the posterior surface of the tibia. Although there is asymptomatic subluxation of the peroneal tendons, this has not been observed with the posterior tibial tendon. The presence of atrophic tears of the posterior tibial tendon suggests that there is a component of chronic repetitive trauma. In this situation, kinematic MRI of the ankle would be expected to provide useful information in this group of patients.

During walking and other functional activities, the flexor hallucis longus tendon slides beneath the sustintaculum tali, potentially creating repetitive motion that could be associated with the much less common flexor hallucis longus tendonopathies. Again, kinematic MRI of the ankle would be expected to provide useful information for this condition.

Finally, kinematic MRI of the ankle has been used to assess the Achilles tendon after surgical repair (Figure 7.6). Imaging is typically performed in the sagittal plane, with the ankle in the dorsiflexed position used to apply "stress" to the Achilles tendon.

B. IMPINGEMENT SYNDROMES

In the past, it was thought that impingement syndromes of the ankle were caused primarily by osseous structures, such as an osteophyte on the anterior aspect of the tibia, impacting with the talus during dorsiflexion. However, soft tissue impingement syndromes associated with plantarflexion-inversion injuries of the ankle also have been described.

There are a variety of osseous and soft tissue impingement syndromes encountered about the ankle that result in a loss in range of motion.[19,24-29] These conditions are characterized clinically and are often diagnoses of exclusion. Although MRI correlations exist for these problems, none is specific for impingement. The ability to view the process of impingement syndromes using kinematic MRI offers hope for a better understanding of these clinical entities (Figures 7.7 and 7.8).

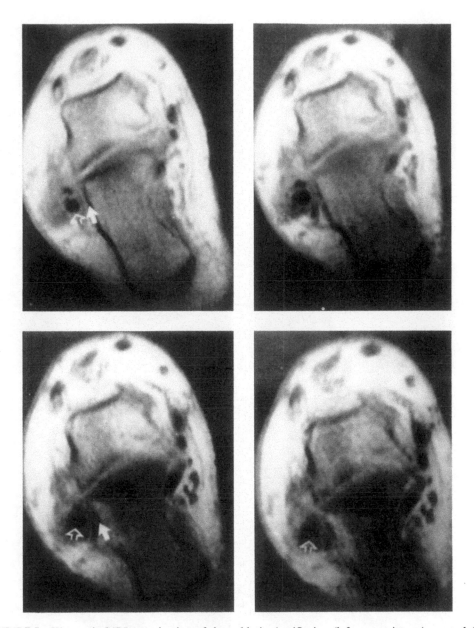

FIGURE 7.5 Kinematic MRI examination of the ankle in dorsiflexion (left, upper image), neutral (right, upper image), partial plantarflexion (left, bottom image), and fully plantarflexion (right, bottom image) positions using incremental, passive positioning technique (axial plane, fast spoiled gradient echo). Lateral subluxation of the abnormally enlarged peroneous longus (open arrow) relative to the lateral border of the calcaneous can be seen on the successive, incremental images. (From Shellock, F. G. et al., *J. Magn. Reson. Imag.*, 7, 451, 1997. With permission.)

Anterolateral impingement syndrome is believed to result from the trapping of thickened synovium in the anterolateral gutter of the ankle. This typically follows an injury to the lateral ankle ligaments, resulting in scarring and capsular hypertrophy. Hypertrophic tissue is believed to become entrapped in the joint when the ankle is moved into a dorsiflexion. Although some investigators have reported fairly specific findings with this syndrome[19] using computerized tomography (CT), Rubin et al.[27] were only able to identify MR findings in the presence of ankle joint

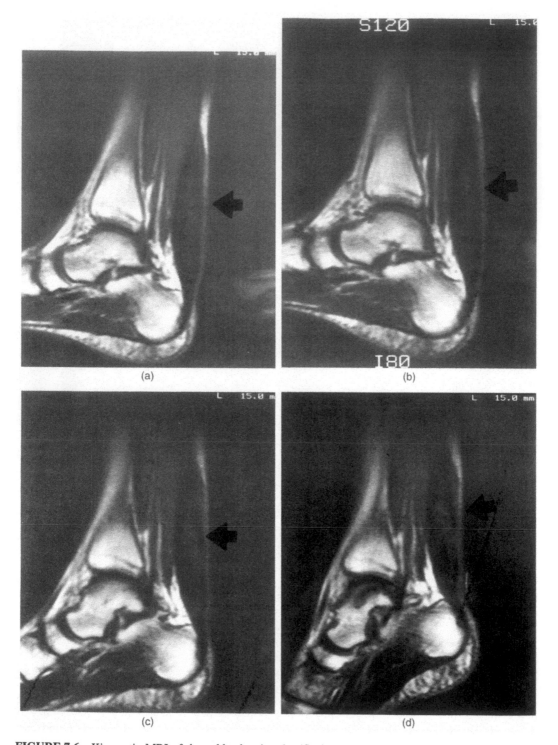

FIGURE 7.6 Kinematic MRI of the ankle showing dorsiflexion (a), neutral (b), partial plantarflexion (c), and full plantarflexion (d) positions (sagittal plane, T1-weighted spin echo). This study was performed to assess the Achilles tendon status post surgical repair. Note the site of the musculotendinous junction where the tendon was repaired (black arrows). (From Shellock, F. G., Kinematic magnetic resonance imaging of the joints, in *Open MRI*, Rothschild, P. A. and Reinking Rothschild, D., Eds., Lippincott, Williams & Wilkins, Philadelphia, 2000, pp. 293–320. With permission.)

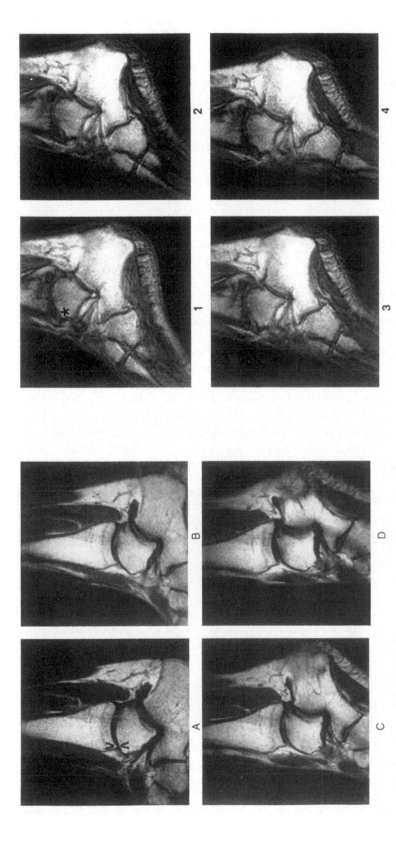

FIGURE 7.7 Example of osseous impingement syndrome. Kinematic MRI examination of the ankle in dorsiflexion (A), neutral (B), partial plantarflexion (C), and full plantarflexion (D) positions (sagittal plane, T1-weighted spin echo). There is an osseous impingement (A, arrow heads) that prevents proper movement into the dorsiflexed position caused by an anterior shift of the talus relative to the tibia. This disorder would go undetected using routine MRI of the ankle because it is position dependent.

FIGURE 7.8 Kinematic MRI examination of the ankle in neutral (1, 2), partial plantarflexion (3), and full plantarflexion (4) positions (sagittal plane, fast gradient echo). There is an osseous impingement resulting from the presence of an osteophyte (1, asterisk) that prevents proper movement into the dorsiflexion position. Similar to the example in Figure 7.7, this disorder would go undetected using routine MRI of the ankle because it is position dependent.

effusion. By comparison, Farooki et al. found MR findings to be quite insensitive.[28] However, it should be noted that this conclusion was reached using static view MRI techniques.

While it is recommended that a dorsiflexed position be used for imaging the ankle to assess anterolateral impingement, this is frequently not done for patient comfort considerations or because of limitations imposed by the RF coil design. The use of kinematic MRI in the evaluation of this syndrome is of considerable value, since it can potentially demonstrate the transient entrapment of thickened scar tissue.

Posterior impingement syndrome typically occurs in individuals whose activities involve repetitive, extreme plantarflexion (e.g., ballet dancers, soccer players, and javelin throwers). The syndrome is associated with several anatomical variants, such as os trigonum and the presence of a posterior intermalleolar ligament.[18,22] However, the os trigonum is a fairly common variant seen in up to 20% of the adult population, as is an enlarged trigonal process. It is evident that the presence of these anatomic abnormalities lack specificity and that assessment with more appropriate imaging is necessary to more completely evaluate the potential causes of this syndrome. Kinematic MRI of the ankle is well suited to this application as this technique is capable of demonstrating the relationships of the anatomical variants to other structures that may become impinged.

C. OSTEOCHONDRAL DEFECTS AND LOOSE BODIES

Osteochondral lesions of the talus are a relatively common problem, occurring in an estimated 6% of severe ankle sprains.[30] These injuries are thought to result from impaction of the talus on the tibia during transient instability of the ankle. This assumption may not be entirely the case, since Hepple et al. found MRI evidence of lateral ligament injury in only 50% of patients with arthroscopically proven osteochondral defects.[30] This raises the possibility that the causative mechanisms may be more complex than previously believed. Kinematic MRI of the ankle in the coronal plane (Figure 7.3) with inversion and eversion positioning may help reveal such mechanisms.

Several classifications exist for osteochondral injuries. Regardless of which is used, the most severe classification is reserved for the situation where a fragment is either loose within the donor site or moves freely within the joint space. This diagnosis can be made using kinematic MRI of the ankle (Figure 7.9).

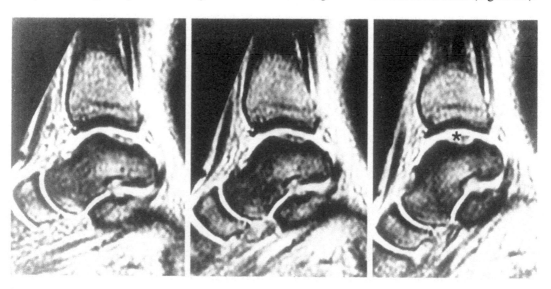

FIGURE 7.9   Kinematic MRI of the ankle obtained using sagittal plane imaging and fast MRI technique with joint in neutral (left), partial plantarflexion (middle), and full plantarflexion positions. This patient was evaluated to identify a possible loose body associated with an osteochondral defect of the talus (right, asterisk). Although free mobility of the loose body is not seen in this example, separation from the talus can be easily detected using this kinematic MRI application. (From Muhle, C. et al., *Acta Radiol.*, 38, 885, 1997. With permission.)

IV. SUMMARY AND CONCLUSIONS

The value of kinematic MRI of the ankle is only now becoming appreciated by those involved in diagnostic imaging. Notably, this imaging procedure is particularly useful for assessment of peroneal tendon subluxation, but also may prove to be beneficial for examination of the posterior tibial and flexor hallicus longus tendons, as well as for evaluation of surgically repaired tendons. Osseous and soft tissue impingement syndromes can be characterized using kinematic MRI procedures, and these procedures can also be used for identification of loose bodies related to osteochondral defects.

REFERENCES

1. Shellock, F. G. and Mandelbaum, B. R., Kinematic MRI of the joints, in *MRI of the Musculoskeletal System: A Teaching File,* Mink, J. H. and Deutsch, A., Eds., Raven Press, New York, 1990, chap. 10.
2. Kneeland, B., Macrandar, S., Middleton, W. D., Cates, J. D., Jesmanowicz, A., and Hyde, J. S., MR imaging of the normal ankle: correlation with anatomic sections, *Am. J. Roentgen.,* 151, 117, 1988.
3. Hajek, P. C., Baker, L. L., Bjorkengren, A., Sartoris, D. J., Neumann, C. H., and Resnick, D., High-resolution magnetic resonance imaging of the ankle: normal anatomy, *Skeletal Radiol.,* 15, 536, 1986.
4. Shellock, F. G., Kinematic MRI of the joints, *Seminars Musculoskeletal Radiol.,* 1, 143, 1997.
5. Shellock, F. G., Kinematic MRI of the joints, in *Magnetic Resonance Imaging in Orthopaedics and Rheumatology,* 2nd edition, Stoller, D. W., Ed., Lippincott-Raven, Philadelphia, 1996, pp. 1023–1058.
6. Hinterman, B. and Nigg, B. M., In vitro kinematics of the axially loaded ankle complex in response to dorsiflexion and plantarflexion, *Foot Ankle Int.,* 16, 514, 1995.
7. Muhle, C., Brinkmann, G., Brossman, J., Wesner, F., and Heller, M., Kinematic MR imaging of the ankle: initial results with ultra-fast imaging, *Acta Radiol.,* 38, 885, 1997.
8. Shellock, F. G., Feske, W., Frey, C., and Terk, M., Peroneal tendons: use of kinematic MR imaging to determine subluxation, *J. Magn. Reson. Imag.,* 7, 451, 1997.
9. Udupa, J. K. et al., Analysis of *in vivo* 3-D internal kinematics of the joints of the foot, *IEEE Trans. Biomed. Eng.,* 45, 1387, 1998.
10. Hirsch, B. E., Udupa, J. K., and Samarasekera, S. S., New method of studying joint kinematics from three-dimensional reconstruction of MRI data, *J. Am. Pod. Med. Assoc.,* 86, 4, 1996.
11. Barnett, C. H., and Napier, J. R., The axis of rotation of the ankle joint in man: its influence upon the form of the talus and the mobility of the fibula, *J. Anat.,* 86, 1, 1952.
12. Singh, A. K. et al., Kinematics of the ankle: a hinge axis model, *Foot Ankle,* 4, 439, 1992.
13. Melchert, U. H. et al., Motion-triggered cine MR imaging of active joint movement, *J, Magn. Reson. Imag.,* 10, 457, 1992.
14. Dumoulin, C. L., Souza, S. P., and Darrow, R. D., Real-time position monitoring of invasive devices using magnetic resonance, *Magn. Reson. Med.,* 29, 411, 1993.
15. Pearle, A. D. et al., Joint motion in an open MR unit using MR tracking, *J. Magn. Reson. Imag.,* 10, 8, 1999.
16. Bruce, W., Christofersen, M. R., and Phillips, D. L., Stenosing tenosynovitis and impingement of the peroneal tendons associated with hypertrophy of the peroneal tubercle, *Foot Ankle Int.,* 20, 464, 1999.
17. Geppert, M. J. et al., Lateral ankle instability as a cause of superior peroneal retinacular laxity: an anatomic and biomechanical study of cadaveric feet, *Foot Ankle,* 14, 330, 1993.
18. Lazarus, M. L., Imaging of the foot and ankle in the injured athlete, *Med. Sci. Sports Exerc.,* 31, S412, 1999.
19. Bencardino, J., Rosenberg, Z. S., and Delfaut, E., MR imaging in sports injuries of the foot and ankle, *MRI Clin. North Am.,* 7, 131, 1999.
20. Monteggia, G. B., *Instituzini Chirurqiche,* Part II, Milan, Italy, pp. 336, 1803.
21. Butler, B. W., Lanthier, J., and Wertheimer, S. J., Subluxing peroneals: a review of the literature and case report, *J. Foot Ankle Surg.,* 32, 134, 1992.
22. Hutchinson, B. L. and Gustafson, L. S., Chronic peroneal tendon subluxation: new surgical technique and retrospective analysis, *J. Am. Pod. Med. Assoc.,* 84, 1994.
23. Yao, L. et al., MR findings in peroneal tendonopathy, *J. Comp. Assist. Tomogr.,* 19, 460, 1995.

24. Steinbach, L. S., Painful syndromes around the ankle and foot: magnetic resonance imaging evaluation, *Topics Magn. Reson. Imag.,* 9, 311, 1998.

25. Hauger, O. et al., Anterolateral compartment of the ankle in the lateral impingement syndrome: appearance on CT arthrography, *Am. J. Roentgen.,* 44, 685, 1999

26. Bassett, F. H., Gates, H. S., Billys, J. B., Morris, H. B., and Nikolaou, P. K., Talar impingement by anteroinferior tibiofibular ligament, *J. Bone Joint Surg.* [*Am.*], 72, 55, 1990.

27. Rubin, D. A. et al., Anterolateral soft-tissue impingement in the ankle: diagnosis using MR imaging, *Am. J. Roentgen.,* 169, 829, 1997.

28. Farooki, S., Yao, L., and Seeger, L. L., Anterolateral impingement of the ankle: effectiveness of MR imaging, *Radiology,* 207, 357, 1998.

29. Fiorella, D., Helms, C. A., and Nunley, J. A., The MR imaging features of the posterior intermalleolar ligament in patients with posterior impingement syndrome of the ankle, *Skeletal Radiol.,* 28, 573, 1999.

30. Hepple, S., Winson, I. G., and Glew, D., Osteochondral lesions of the talus: a revised classification, *Foot Ankle Int.,* 20, 789, 1999.

Part IV

Patellofemoral Joint

8 The Patellofemoral Joint: Functional Anatomy and Kinesiology

Christopher M. Powers

CONTENTS

I. INTRODUCTION

The patellofemoral joint consists of the articulation of the patella and the trochlear surface of the femur and is an integral part of the extensor mechanism. The patellofemoral joint, therefore, plays a key role in normal knee function and lower extremity biomechanics. The ability of this joint to improve mechanical efficiency of the extensor mechanism, and to accept and redirect forces, is dependent on a host of factors, including osseous structure, as well as contributions from various

0-8493-0807-0/01/$0.00+$.50
© 2001 by Frank G. Shellock

soft tissues, such as the quadriceps musculature, quadriceps tendon, patellar tendon, and retinaculum. An understanding of the anatomical structure of this joint is necessary to appreciate both normal and pathological functions. This chapter describes the normal functional anatomy, normal kinesiology, and pathokinesiology of the patellofemoral joint.

II. FUNCTIONAL ANATOMY OF THE PATELLOFEMORAL JOINT

A. OSSEOUS STRUCTURE

1. The Patella

Contained within the quadriceps tendon, the patella has the distinction of being the largest sesmoid bone in the body.[1] Consisting primarily of cancellous bone covered by thin compact lamina, the patella's axial length is approximately 4 to 4.5 cm, while its width is approximately 5 to 5.5 cm. The thickness of the patella varies considerably, attaining a maximum height of 2 to 2.5 cm at its central portion.[2]

The articular surface of the patella is divided into medial and lateral facets by a vertical ridge (median ridge) that roughly bisects the patella (Figure 8.1).[3] Although similar in size, the lateral facet is often slightly larger than the medial.[4] The medial facet is subdivided by a less prominent vertical ridge that separates the medial facet proper and the smaller "odd facet" (Figure 8.1). The articulating surfaces of the patella are covered with aneural hyaline cartilage, which is the thickest cartilage in the body.[5] Maximum cartilage thickness is found at the central portion of the patella (approximately 4 to 5 mm), and decreases from the median ridge to the medial and lateral borders.

The primary function of the patella is to facilitate knee extension by increasing the functional lever arm of the extensor mechanism.[6] In addition to improving the moment arm of the quadriceps muscle, the patella provides protection for the articular cartilage of the trochlea and prevents excessive friction between the quadriceps tendon and the femoral condyles. The patella also acts as a guide for the converging heads of the quadriceps muscle, facilitating transmission of the muscular forces to the patellar tendon.[6]

2. The Trochlear Groove

The femoral condyles form the trochlear groove and the articulating surface of the femur. The lateral anterior femoral condyle is much larger and extends more proximally and anteriorly than

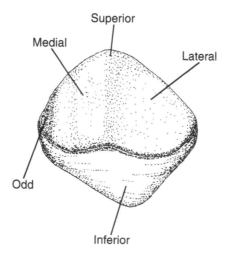

FIGURE 8.1   The articular facets of the patella.

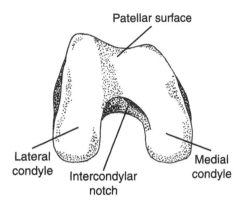

FIGURE 8.2 Inferior aspect of the distal end of the femur.

its medial counterpart, providing an osseous buttress that assists in providing lateral patellar stability (Figure 8.2).[7] In addition, the trochlear groove is shallower proximally than distally, suggesting that osseous stability is compromised as the patella is pulled superiorly during active knee extension.

Similar to the patella, the trochlear surface is covered with aneural hyaline cartilage. However, the cartilage covering the trochlear surface of the femur is much thinner than that of the patella (i.e., 2 to 3 mm).[9]

B. THE SYNOVIUM

The synovial lining of the patellofemoral joint is essentially the synovium of the anterior portion of the knee and consists of three portions: suprapatellar, peripatellar, and infrapatellar. These three portions of the synovium blend imperceptibly with each other, allowing free communication with the knee joint.[8] The peripatellar synovium creates a small synovial fold or fringe less than 1 cm broad that surrounds the patella.[5] Inflammation or scarring of this synovial fold can produce symptoms similar to that of cartilage degeneration and retropatellar pain.[9]

C. VASCULAR SUPPLY

The vascular anatomy of the patellofemoral joint demonstrates relative independence from the knee as it receives its circulation from its own vascular tree.[5] The patellofemoral joint receives its blood supply from a vascular anastomosis with arterial input from the medial superior and inferior genicular arteries, the lateral superior and inferior genicular arteries, and the anterior tibial recurrent artery (Figure 8.3).[10] These vessels are derived from the popliteal artery and form a peripatellar circle that richly supplies the patellar structures.

D. SOFT TISSUE STABILIZERS

The lack of a tightly closed capsule necessitates external assistance in achieving patellar stability within the trochlear groove, which is provided by soft tissue stabilizers. In general, the soft tissue stabilizers of the patellofemoral joint can be described as being either passive or active. Passive stabilizing structures include the medial and lateral retinaculum, while active stabilizing structures consist of the four heads of the quadriceps femoris muscle.

The lateral retinaculum is composed of two distinct portions, a thinner superficial layer and a thicker deep layer. The deep layer is further divided into three fibrous components that connect the patella to the iliotibial band and assist in preventing medial patellar excursion.[11] Because most of the lateral retinaculum originates from the iliotibial band, this structure is drawn posteriorly with knee flexion placing a lateral force on the patella.[12]

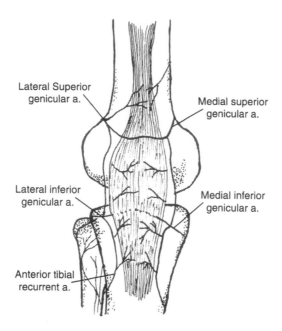

Lateral Superior
genicular a.

Medial superior
genicular a.

Lateral inferior
genicular a.

Medial inferior
genicular a.

Anterior tibial
recurrent a.

FIGURE 8.3   Anatomy of the arterial supply of the patellofemoral joint (a, artery).

The medial retinaculum forms a tough fibrous layer that assists in limiting lateral patellar excursion. The lateral retinaculum is usually thicker than the medial retinaculum and is generally accepted as providing stronger lateral support.[13]

The four heads of the quadriceps femoris muscle (vastus lateralis, vastus medialis, vastus intermedius, and the rectus femoris) insert into the patella and provide dynamic control of the patellofemoral joint. Together, the components of the quadriceps femoris fuse distally to form the quadriceps tendon.

The rectus femoris (RF) inserts into the anterior portion of the superior aspect of the patella with the superficial fibers continuing over the patella and ending in the patellar tendon. The vastus intermedius (VI) inserts posteriorly into the base of the patella but anterior to the joint capsule. Both the vastus lateralis (VL) and vastus medialis (VM) insert into their respective sides of the patella.[14,15]

The lower fibers of the VM insert more distally on the patella and at a greater angle from the vertical compared to the vastus lateralis. In a detailed anatomical analysis, Lieb and Perry[16] determined the angle of insertion of the various heads of the quadriceps muscle with respect to the vertical axis. Thus, the fiber alignment in the frontal plane is as follows: VL, 12 to 15 degrees laterally; RF, 7 to 10 degrees medially; VM (upper fibers), 15 to 18 degrees medially; and the VM (lower fibers), 50 to 55 degrees medially (Figure 8.4). The fibers of the VI lie parallel to the shaft of the femur.

Of note is that the distinct and abrupt change in the fiber orientation between the superior and inferior portions of the vastus medialis led Lieb and Perry[16] to consider each as separate entities. Therefore, the lower fibers are designated as the vastus medialis oblique (VMO) and the upper fibers as the vastus medialis longus (VML). The fiber orientation of the VMO makes this structure particularly effective in providing medial patellar stability.[16]

As a result of the posterior origin of the vasti (linea aspera), any quadriceps muscle contraction (regardless of knee flexion angle) results in compressive forces acting on the patellofemoral joint. Even when the knee is fully extended, substantial joint compression can be present. The posterior angulation of the vastus medialis and vastus lateralis fibers has been reported to be approximately 55 degrees from the vertical (Figure 8.5).[17]

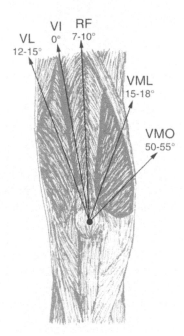

FIGURE 8.4 Frontal plane fiber orientation of the quadriceps musculature in relation to the femur (VL, vastus lateralis; VI, vastus intermedius; RF, rectus femoris; VML, vastus medialis longus; VMO, vastus medialis oblique).

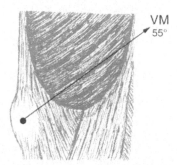

FIGURE 8.5 Two-dimensional representation of the fiber orientation of the vastus medialis (VM; medial view).

III. NORMAL KINESIOLOGY

A. NORMAL PATELLAR KINEMATICS

From a clinical standpoint, the motions of lateral or medial displacement and lateral or medial patellar tilt are most commonly assessed in patients that present with patellofemoral joint pain. However, the inability to directly visualize or determine the relationship between the patella and trochlear groove using physical examination criteria makes assessment of patellar motion an imprecise task. Nonetheless, determination of patellar movement throughout an arc of resisted knee extension can be achieved using kinematic magnetic resonance imaging (MRI) techniques.[18] This diagnostic imaging method has a distinct advantage over static imaging procedures in that the important contribution of the extensor mechanism to patellofemoral joint kinematics can be assessed. Using the *active movement against resistance technique*, Powers et al.[19] quantified patellar tracking patterns in pain-free, healthy adults during non-weight-bearing knee extension against resistance (45 degrees to full extension). The findings of this study are summarized below.

1. Medial and Lateral Movements

The normal position of the patella was found to be one of slight lateral movement throughout the 0 to 45 degree range of motion. The normal kinematic pattern of patellar horizontal motion (frontal plane) was characterized by slight medial movement from 45 to 18 degrees of knee flexion, followed by slight lateral movement at the end range of extension (18 to 0 degrees).[19] This motion pattern has been described previously as the C-curve pattern.[20] The estimated amount of medial and lateral movement was about 3 mm in each direction based on quantitative analysis.[19] Qualitatively, this movement pattern gave an appearance of the patella evenly centered within the femoral trochlear groove throughout this range of motion.[19]

The tendency for the patella to displace medially during knee extension is related to the geometry of the femoral trochlear groove. Because the lateral femoral condyle is typically larger and projects further anteriorly than the medial condyle, the trochlear surface is angled slightly medially when viewed from distal to proximal positions.[21] Additionally, the shift from medial to lateral patellar motions starting at 18 degrees of flexion, can be explained by the screw-home mechanism of the knee. During terminal extension of the non-weight-bearing knee, external rotation of the tibia occurs, as the result of the unequal curvature between the femoral condyles.[22] As demonstrated by van Kampen and Huiskes,[21] patellar motion is highly influenced by rotation of the tibia with external rotation inducing a lateral patellar displacement.

2. Medial and Lateral Tilt

During knee extension from 45 to 0 degrees the patella was found to tilt medially (5 to 7 degrees) from a laterally tilted position.[19] As with medial and lateral patellar displacement, this motion pattern appears to be related to the geometry of the femoral trochlear groove.[19] Again, from a qualitative consideration, this movement pattern gave an appearance of the patella evenly centered within the femoral trochlear groove throughout this range of motion.[19]

3. Influence of Patellar Motion on Patellofemoral Joint Contact Area

As the patella moves from the superior (shallower) portion of the trochlear groove to the inferior (deeper) portion of the trochlear groove during knee flexion, the articulating surface of the patella on the femur varies throughout the range of knee motion.[19] Movement from full extension to 90 degrees of flexion results in a band of contact that moves from the inferior to the superior pole of the patella (Figure 8.6).[23] Between 90 and 135 degrees, the patella rotates laterally with the ridge between the medial and odd facets making contact with the medial condyle. At 135 degrees, the odd facet and the lateral portion of the lateral facet make contact as does the quadriceps tendon.[23]

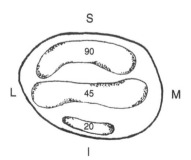

FIGURE 8.6 Patellar contact areas at 20, 45, and 90 degrees of knee flexion. (I, inferior; S, superior; L, lateral; M, medial).

Because the patella enters the deeper portion of the trochlear groove during knee flexion, the area of contact of the patella and the trochlear groove increases. In fact, patellofemoral contact area has been reported to increase threefold from 0.8 cm² at 0 degrees to a maximum of 2.4 cm² at 60 degrees.[17] This increase in contact area with knee flexion functionally serves to distribute joint forces over a greater surface area, thereby minimizing joint stress.

B. MUSCULAR ACTION

1. Role of the Quadriceps Femoris in Knee Extension and Patellar Stabilization

As described above, the various heads of the quadriceps fuse to form a common tendon that envelops the patella and inserts into the tibial tuberosity. As a result, the vasti are powerful extensors of the knee. By virtue of its proximal attachment to the anterior inferior iliac spine, the RF acts to flex the hip and, together with the vasti, assists in knee extension.

It is widely accepted that the vasti work in concert to achieve knee extension. In fact, several studies have confirmed the integrated function of the quadriceps femoris during knee extension, regardless of knee position.[24-27] The visual appearance of medial quadriceps muscle atrophy and the loss of terminal knee extension led early investigators to assign the responsibility for this motion to the VM.[28,29] Unfortunately, this misconception of selective function of the various heads of the quadriceps femoris has erroneously been the basis for many therapeutic exercise programs for the knee.[30]

In a mechanical study using amputated limbs, Lieb and Perry[16] determined that the loss of terminal knee extension was the result of mechanical disadvantage rather than specific muscle action. These authors demonstrated that a 60% increase in quadriceps muscle force was necessary to complete full extension indicating that extensor lag was a function of general quadriceps muscle weakness. In addition, Lieb and Perry[16] noted that the oblique fibers of the VMO could not complete full extension without the assistance of the other vasti. Thus, it was concluded that the only selective function of the VMO would appear to be patellar alignment.[16]

Because the VMO has been widely accepted as being responsible for the prevention of lateral subluxation of the patella, its relationship with respect to the VL has been thoroughly studied. The electromyographic (EMG) activity of the VMO and VL during knee extension while weight bearing was studied by Reynolds et al.[31] to determine the role of these muscles in providing patellar alignment. Both the VMO and VL demonstrated similar levels of activity. Reynolds et al.[31] stated that this is understandable because a balance of forces acting at the patellofemoral joint should be exhibited. Similar results were reported by Mariani and Caruso,[32] who found the EMG activity of the VM and VL in normal individuals to be similar in the last 30 degrees of extension. These studies support the conclusions of Lieb and Perry,[16] who stated that the VMO and VL oppose each other in a critical balance, preventing excessive lateral subluxation of the patella. This controlled balance is essential in preventing pathology of the extensor mechanism and disorders of the patellofemoral joint.

IV. PATHOKINESIOLOGY AND CLINICAL IMPLICATIONS

A. PATELLOFEMORAL PAIN SYNDROME

Patellofemoral pain (PFP) is one of the most common disorders of the knee, with as many as one in four of the general population reporting symptoms.[33] Patellofemoral related problems are prevalent in a wide range of individuals; however, the highest incidence is evident in physically active populations.[34-37] While patellofemoral related problems occur with an incidence of 2 to 1 in females vs. males, men outnumber women (4 to 1) when athletes are studied.[33]

In addition to active individuals, PFP is evident in various other populations. For example, PFP has been reported to be the most common soft tissue syndrome in patients referred for rheumatology consultations[38] and is problematic in children with cerebral palsy.[39] Brick and Scott[40] reported that patellofemoral related problems were the primary reason for total knee arthroplasty revision, while Fulkerson and Hungerford[5] stated that PFP is a common complaint following anterior cruciate ligament or meniscal injury.

B. Pathophysiology of Patellofemoral Pain

Despite the high incidence of PFP in the general population, the pathophysiology of this disorder is not clearly understood. The most commonly accepted hypothesis is related to increased patellofemoral joint stress and subsequent articular cartilage wear.[41-46] Increased shearing and compression associated with abnormal patellar tracking or malalignment is commonly believed to be responsible for articular cartilage degeneration.

Classification of patellofemoral joint disorders based on articular cartilage degeneration has been described in detail.[46-49] Although articular cartilage is aneural and, thus, dismissed as a possible source of pain,[3] it has been proposed that the sub-adjacent endplate is exposed to pressure variations that would normally be absorbed by healthy cartilage.[48] This results in mechanical stress in this pathologic tissue that is believed to stimulate pain receptors in the subchondral bone.[48]

C. Patellar Subluxation

Abnormal patellar tracking that occurs during flexion and extension has been documented as a cause of articular cartilage pain and damage.[43,44] In general, subluxation typically involves increased lateral displacement of the patella;[5] however, medial and lateral-to-medial displacement also can occur.[18,50] Fulkerson and Hungerford[5] have described three types of subluxation: minor recurrent, major recurrent, and permanent lateral subluxation. Minor recurrent subluxation deviated little from the normal patellar course and was not associated with clinically apparent relocation (however, it should be noted that even minor patellar displacements may be associated with significant pain). With major recurrent subluxation, the patella moved across the lateral trochlear facet and returned to the trochlear groove with an audible snap. Permanent lateral subluxation was characterized as a stable lateral displacement where there was no centering of the patella. Other investigators have similarly reported criteria for characterizing abnormal patellofemoral relationships.[18,50,75]

The natural tendency of the patella to track laterally has been described by Fulkerson and Hungerford[5] as the "law of valgus." This is a result of the valgus orientation of the lower extremity. As the quadriceps muscle follows the longitudinal axis of the femur, the quadriceps angle (Q-angle) is formed that creates a lateral force vector acting on the patella (Figure 8.7). This predisposes the patella to lateral tracking forces with quadriceps muscle tension.[51] The Q-angle for women is greater than that of men as a result of a wider pelvis, averaging 15 to 18 degrees. The average for men is approximately 12 degrees.[7] This variation between the sexes may partially explain the greater incidence of PFP in females, as a larger Q-angle would create a larger valgus vector and, therefore, a potentially larger predisposition to lateral tracking.[52]

Medial subluxation of the patella may also occur in patients with PFP. According to Shellock,[18] this abnormal patellar alignment is associated with excessive internal rotation of the lower extremity. However, the precise biomechanical mechanism responsible for this is unknown.

1. Etiology of Patellar Subluxation

As mentioned previously, resistance to the potentially aberrant tracking forces acting on the patella is provided by osseous and soft tissue structures. Disruption of the normal stabilizing forces may lead to patellar malalignment and associated pathology. Possible mechanisms of abnormal patellar tracking include osseous abnormalities, abnormal osseous relationships, and soft tissue imbalance (i.e., imbalance of muscular forces). One or a combination of these factors may be responsible for aberrant patellofemoral relationships.

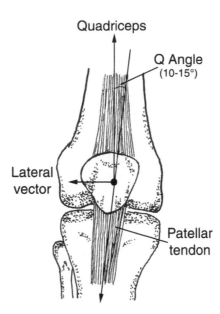

FIGURE 8.7 The angle between the quadriceps tendon and the patellar tendon forms the Q-angle. The Q-angle produces a lateral force on the patella.

2. Osseous Abnormalities

Anatomical variations of the patella and/or distal femur have been shown to contribute to recurrent subluxation.[4,53] Patellar and/or trochlear dysplasias compromise the inherent stability afforded by the interactions between these osseous structures, thus making the patella more susceptible to lateral forces. Other maltracking patterns (e.g., medial and lateral-to-medial displacements) also may occur in association with osseous abnormalities.[18,75]

Apart from the shape of the osseous structure, the position of the patella with respect to the trochlear groove can be a causative factor with respect to abnormal patellar tracking patterns (e.g., patella alta and patella baja). Patella alta, as described by Insall,[51] is evident when the resting position of the patella is above or superior to the femoral groove. The so-called "high riding" patella does not move adequately into the trochlea with knee flexion and, thus, is prone to displacement. Patella alta is usually determined using a lateral radiograph and is considered positive when the patellar tendon is 20% longer than the length of the patella. The excessive length of the patellar tendon is thought to be the primary cause of this condition.[54] Additionally, patella alta may be identified using MRI, whereby successive transaxial section locations obtained through the extended patellofemoral joint show the inferior pole of the patella positioned above the femoral trochlear groove (see Chapter 9).[18]

An excessive inferior position of the patella relative to the femoral trochlear groove (patella baja) also may be responsible for abnormal patellofemoral relationships.[18] Notably, patella baja tends to be caused by iatrogenic mechanisms.

Probably a more influential osseous etiologic factor in patellar subluxation is femoral trochlear dysplasia. As noted previously, the trochlear groove of the femur, especially the larger anterior protrusion of the lateral femoral condyle, provides significant osseous stability for the patella.[55] The normal trochlear facet (sulcus) angle was established by Brattstrom using conventional radiography.[56] Evaluation of 100 normal knees revealed that the values for both sexes were similar, with a mean angle of 143 degrees for males and 142 degrees for females. Higher sulcus angles represented a shallower trochlear groove and were found to been associated with recurrent patellar subluxation.[56,57] According to Hvid et al.,[58] a sulcus angle of greater than 150 degrees is considered representative of trochlear dysplasia.

3. Abnormal Osseous Relationships

Abnormal skeletal alignment has been shown to have a profound effect on the magnitude of the Q-angle and the subsequent laterally directed component of the quadriceps muscle force.[44,59] Huberti and Hayes[59] documented the deleterious effects of an increased Q-angle by measuring patellofemoral contact pressures in 12 fresh cadaver specimens. These authors found that a 10-degree increase in the Q-angle resulted in a 45% increase in peak contact pressure at 20 degrees of knee flexion. In half of the specimens, the area of patella contact shifted laterally, with the peak pressures being evident on the medial portion of the lateral facet.[59] An increased Q-angle is often present when rotational malalignments of the femur and tibia exist. Such abnormalities include femoral anteversion, genu valgum, tibial torsion, and lateral displacement of the tibial tubercle.[33,44,60]

4. Soft Tissue Abnormalities

Both contractile and noncontractile soft tissue structures can contribute to the abnormal forces acting on the patella. As mentioned previously, the lateral retinaculum is capable of exerting a lateral force on the patella, potentially contributing to subluxation. Since the lateral retinaculum has an extensive attachment to the iliotibial band, contraction of the tensor fascia latae may exert a dynamic lateral force through this connection.[55] In some cases, this attachment has been found to be excessive, causing recurrent dislocation of the patella.[61] Evidence exists supporting the concept of a functional anatomic relationship between the patella and the passive lateral structures of the knee. For example, Puniello[12] demonstrated a strong relationship between iliotibial band tightness and decreased passive medial patellar glide in patients with patellofemoral dysfunction. In addition, Hughston and Deese[62] found a high incidence (50%) of medial patellar subluxation following lateral retinacular release, indicating that this structure also plays a role in pulling the patella laterally. Shellock et al.[50] further substantiated this finding using kinematic MRI whereby a high incidence of medial subluxation of the patella was found to be associated with lateral retinacular release.

From a dynamic standpoint, a lack of equilibrium between the VM and VL is widely accepted as a principal cause of patellar subluxation.[7,14,30,31,63] As such, numerous studies have focused on the dynamic factors associated with patellar instability and probable VM insufficiency. For example, VM insufficiency has been associated with muscle atrophy,[24,55] hypoplasia,[55] inhibition due to pain and effusion,[64,65] and impaired motor control.[66]

Documenting imbalances between the VMO and VL in patients with PFP has been of primary interest to clinicians and researchers because conservative treatment of this disorder typically focuses on restoring normal function of the dynamic stabilizers.[60,67] Since an *in vivo* strength assessment of the individual vasti is not possible, EMG has been used to compare the relative recruitment of these muscles with the rationale that decreased activity of the VM relative to the VL is indicative of compromised medial patellar stability. Various investigators have studied the EMG activity of the dynamic patellar stabilizers in subjects with PFP; however, the results of these studies have been equivocal. While some studies reported significant differences in VM and VL activity in patients with PFP,[32,68,69] others did not.[71-73] Direct comparisons of these studies are difficult because of differences in experimental techniques, methods of quantifying the EMGs, and the inherent variability associated with such data.

Since the etiology of PFP is typically considered a dynamic entity, it is logical that a deficiency of the medial stabilizers should result in lateral displacement of the patella. However, it has been documented through radiological examination that less than 50% of patients with PFP demonstrate isolated lateral subluxation.[74,75] This would suggest that lateral patellar tracking is not a universal finding in this disorder and, therefore, such an inference cannot be generalized to all patients.

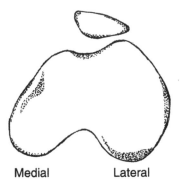

Medial   Lateral

FIGURE 8.8   Increased compression between the lateral patellar facet and femoral condyle as a result of excessive lateral tilting of the patella (axial view).

D. EXCESSIVE LATERAL PRESSURE SYNDROME

The concept of excessive lateral pressure syndrome (ELPS) as a causative factor in patellofemoral articular cartilage pathology was first described in detail by Ficat et al.[76] These authors characterized ELPS as a tilt or compression syndrome where the patella was tilted laterally, thereby increasing compression between the lateral facet and the lateral femoral condyle (Figure 8.8). This position of the patella also unloads the medial facet.

Tilting of the patella can be isolated or associated with lateral patellar subluxation.[18,74] Chronic lateral tilt is determined radiologically and has been shown to have a deleterious effect on the articular cartilage. Increased density of the subchondral bone underlying the lateral facet and a decrease in the medial facet subchondral bone density are signs of the pressure differences (i.e., hyperpressure and hypopressure) exhibited in this syndrome.[5]

Lateral facet overload and deficient medial facet contact can lead to articular cartilage degeneration at both sites. Abnormal articular cartilage loading of the lateral facet may cross the threshold of cartilage resistance leading to the failure.[5] The mechanism of medial facet articular cartilage damage in ELPS appears to be different from lateral facet degeneration, as this area is susceptible to deficient contact. This form of degeneration is likely attributed to impaired nutrition as diminished joint compression would result in decreased flow of synovial fluid.[77] Seedholm et al.[78] has stated that areas of relative contact deficiency develop mild degenerative changes and are most probably asymptomatic. When combined with the shearing of the medial facet associated with lateral patellar subluxation, more extensive medial facet degeneration could occur.[5]

The natural history of ELPS has been described as congenital tilting of the patella followed by adaptive shortening of the lateral retinaculum. Congenital anomalies cited as possible causes of ELPS include genu varum, femoral anteversion, and dysplasia of the hip.[5] The presence of a tight lateral retinaculum produces increased posterolateral tension on this structure with knee flexion. This, in turn, accentuates lateral facet compression. Insall[49] stated that adaptive shortening of the lateral retinaculum was more likely the result of habitual lateral patellar tracking whereby the VM was stretched and the VL contracted. Regardless of the cause of this shortening, excessive tightness of the lateral retinaculum appears to be a secondary adaptive change.

Evidence exists that supports the concept that a shortened retinaculum and insufficient dynamic medial stabilizers contribute to ELPS. For example, Fulkerson and co-workers[79] demonstrated the effectiveness of surgical release of the lateral retinaculum in reducing lateral patellar tilt. Based on pre- and postsurgical evaluations using computerized tomography, these authors reported a mean tilt improvement of 6 degrees at 10 degrees of knee flexion and 15 degrees at 20 degrees of knee flexion. These improvements brought the tilt angles of the patients well within the normal range, as demonstrated in the control group.

Douchette and Goble[80] illustrated the importance of quadriceps muscle weakness and tightness of the lateral structures in contributing to ELPS by demonstrating a decrease in patellar tilt in patients following an eight week quadriceps muscle strengthening and iliotibial band stretching program. In addition, 84% of the previously symptomatic patients were pain free following the conservative exercise program. Thus, results of these studies suggest the contribution of both dynamic and passive factors in the etiology of ELPS.

V. SUMMARY AND CONCLUSIONS

The osseous confines of the trochlea combined with the passive and active soft tissue stabilizers limit patellar excursion, contributing significantly to the stability of the patella. The balance between medial and lateral stability is essential for maintaining appropriate alignment of the extensor mechanism and normal function of the patellofemoral joint. Disruption of the delicate balance of the forces acting on the patella may predispose an individual to altered patellar kinematics and patellofemoral pain syndrome.

REFERENCES

1. Norkin, C. and Levangie, P., *Joint Structure and Function: A Comprehensive Analysis,* 2nd edition, F.A. Davis, Philadelphia, 1983.
2. Reider, B., Marshall, J. L., Koslin, B., Ring, B., and Girgis, F. G., The anterior aspect of the knee joint, *J. Bone Joint Surg.,* 63A, 351–356, 1979.
3. Calliet, R., *Knee Pain and Disability,* 2nd edition, F.A. Davis, Philadelphia, 1990.
4. Wiberg, G., Roentgenographic and anatomic studies on the femoro-patellar joint, *Acta Orthop. Scand.,* 12, 319–410, 1941.
5. Fulkerson, J. P. and Hungerford, D. S., *Disorders of the Patellofemoral Joint,* 2nd edition, Williams & Wilkins, Baltimore, 1990.
6. Kaufer, H., Mechanical function of the patella, *J. Bone Joint Surg.,* 53A, 1551–1560, 1971.
7. Hertling, D. and Kessler, R. M., *Management of Common Musculoskeletal Disorders: Physical Therapy Principles and Methods,* 2nd edition, J.B. Lippincott, Philadelphia, 1990.
8. Romanes, G. J., *Cunningham's Textbook of Anatomy,* 12th edition, Oxford University Press, New York, 1981.
9. Hughston, J. and Andrews, J., The suprapatella plica and internal derangement, *J. Bone Joint Surg.,* 55A, 1318–1319, 1973.
10. Scapinelli, R., Blood supply of the human patella, *J. Bone Joint Surg.,* 49B, 563–570, 1967.
11. Fulkerson, J. P. and Gossling, H. R., Anatomy of the knee joint lateral retinaculum, *Clin. Orthop.,* 153, 183–185, 1993.
12. Puniello, M. S., Iliotibial band tightness and medial patellar glide in patients with patellofemoral dysfunction, *J. Orthop. Sports Phys. Ther.,* 17, 144–148, 1993.
13. Hehne, H. J., Biomechanics of the patellofemoral joint and its clinical relevance, *Clin. Orthop.,* 258, 73–85, 1990.
14. Dye, S. F., Patellofemoral anatomy, in *The Patellofemoral Joint,* Fox, J. M. and Del Pizzo, W., Eds., McGraw-Hill, New York, 1993.
15. Terry, G. C., The anatomy of the extensor mechanism, *Clin. Sports Med.,* 8, 163–177, 1998.
16. Lieb, F. J. and Perry, J., Quadriceps function: an anatomical and mechanical study using amputated limbs, *J. Bone Joint Surg.,* 50A, 1535–1548, 1968.
17. Powers, C. M., Lilly, J. C., and Lee, T. Q., The effects of anatomically based multi-planar loading of the extensor mechanism on patellofemoral joint mechanics, *Clin. Biomech.,* 13, 608–615, 1998.
18. Shellock, F. G., Kinematic MRI of the joints, *Semin. Musculoskeletal Radiol.,* 1, 43–173, 1997.
19. Powers, C. M, Shellock, F. G, and Pfaff, M., Quantification of patellar tracking using MRI, *J. Magn. Reson. Imag.,* 8, 724–732, 1998.
20. Hungerford, D. S. and Barry, M., Biomechanics of the patellofemoral joint, *Clin. Orthop.,* 144, 9–15, 1979.

21. van Kampen, A. and Huiskes, R., The three-dimensional tracking pattern of the human patella, *J. Orthop. Res.,* 8, 372–382, 1990.
22. Soderberg, G. L., *Kinesiology: Application to Pathological Motion,* Williams & Wilkins, Baltimore, 1986.
23. Goodfellow, J., Hungerford, D. S., and Zindel, M., Patello-femoral joint mechanics and pathology: functional anatomy of the patello-femoral joint, *J. Bone Joint Surg.,* 58B, 287–290, 1976.
24. Basmajian, J. V., Harden, T. P., and Regenos, E. M., Integrated actions of the four heads of quadriceps femoris: an electromyographic study, *Anat. Rec.,* 172, 15–20, 1971.
25. Hallen, L. G. and Lindahl, O., Muscle function in knee extension, *Acta Orthop. Scand.,* 38, 434–444, 1967.
26. Jackson, R. T. and Merrifield, H. H., Electromyographic assessment of quadriceps muscle group during knee extension with weighted boot, *Med. Sci. Sports Exercise,* 4, 116–119, 1972.
27. Salzman, A., Torburn, L., and Perry, J., Contribution of rectus femoris and vasti to knee extension: an electromyographic study, *Clin. Orthop.,* 290, 236–243, 1993.
28. DePalma, A. F., *Diseases of the Knee,* J.B. Lippincott, Philadelphia, 1954.
29. Smillie, I. S., *Injuries of the Knee Joint,* 3rd edition, Williams & Wilkins, Baltimore, 1962.
30. Hanten, W. P. and Schulthies, S. S., Exercise effect on electromyographic activity of the vastus medialis oblique and the vastus lateralis muscles, *Phys. Ther.,* 70, 561–565, 1990.
31. Reynolds, L., Levin, T. A., Medeiros, J. M., Adler, N. S., and Hallum, A., EMG activity of the vastus medialis oblique and the vastus lateralis in their role in patellar alignment, *Am. J. Phys. Med.,* 62, 61–70, 1983.
32. Mariani, P. P. and Caruso, I., An electromyographic investigation of subluxation of the patella, *J. Bone Joint Surg.,* 61B, 169–171, 1979.
33. Levine, J., Chondromalacia patellae, *Physician Sportsmed.,* 7, 41–49, 1979.
34. Devereaux, M. and Lachmann, S., Patellofemoral arthralgia in athletes attending a sports injury clinic, *Br. J. Sports Med.,* 18, 18–21, 1984.
35. Renstrom, A. F., Knee pain in tennis players, *Clin. Sports Med.,* 14, 163–175, 1995.
36. Clement, D. B., Tauton, J. E., Smart, G. W., and McNichol, K. L., A survery of overuse running injuries, *Physician Sportsmed.,* 9, 47–58, 1981.
37. Jordan, G. and Schwellnus, M. P., The incidence of overuse injuries in military recruits during basic training, *Military Med.,* 159, 421–426, 1994.
38. Grady, E. P., Carpenter, M. T., Koenig, C. D., Older, S. A., and Battafarano, D. F., Rheumatic findings in Gulf War veterans, *Arch. Intern. Med.,* 158, 367–371, 1998.
39. Samilson, R. L. and Gill, K. W., Patello-femoral problems in cerebral palsy, *Acta Orthop. Belgica,* 50, 191–197, 1984.
40. Brick, G. W. and Scott, R. D., The patellofemoral component of total knee arthroplasty, *Clin. Orthop.,* 231, 163–178, 1998.
41. Fulkerson J. P. and Shea, K. P., Mechanical basis for patellofemoral pain and cartilage breakdown, in *Articular Cartilage and Knee Joint Function: Basic Science and Arthroscopy,* Ewing, J. W., Ed., Raven Press, New York, 1990, 93–101.
42. Grana, W. and Kriegshauser, L., Scientific basis of extensor mechanism disorders, *Clin. Sports Med.,* 4, 247–257, 1985.
43. Heywood, W. B., Recurrent dislocation of the patella, *J. Bone Joint Surg.,* 43B, 508–517, 1961.
44. Insall, J., Falvo, K. A., and Wise, D. W., Chondromalacia patellae: a prospective study, *J. Bone Joint Surg.,* 58A, 1–8, 1976.
45. Moller, B. N., Moller-Larsen, F., and Frich, L. H., Chondromalacia induced by patellar subluxation in the rabbit, *Acta Orthop. Scand.,* 60, 188–191, 1989.
46. Outerbridge, R. E., The etiology of chondromalacia patellae, *J. Bone Joint Surg.,* 43B, 752–757, 1961.
47. Bentley, G. and Dowd, G., Current concepts of etiology and treatment of chondromalacia patellae, *Clin. Orthop.,* 189, 209–228, 1984.
48. Goodfellow, J., Hungerford, D. S., and Woods, C., Patello-femoral joint mechanics and pathology: chondromalacia patellae, *J. Bone Joint Surg.,* 58B, 291–299, 1976.
49. Insall, J., Current concepts review: patellar pain, *J. Bone Joint Surg.,* 64A, 147–152, 1982.
50. Shellock, F. G., Mink, J. H., Deutsch, A., Fox, J. M., and Ferkel, R. D., Evaluation of patients with persistent symptoms after lateral retinacular release by kinematic magnetic resonance imaging of the patellofemoral joint, *Arthroscopy,* 6, 226–234, 1990.

51. Insall, J., Patellar malalignment syndrome, *Orthop. Clin. North Am.*, 10, 117–122, 1979.

52. James, S., *The Injured Adolescent Knee*, Williams & Wilkins, Baltimore, 1979.

53. Rohlederer, O., Atiiologie und symptomatologie der pradeluxio patellae, *Zentralbl. Chir.*, 76, 103–115, 1951.

54. Insall, J. and Salvati, E., Patellar position in the normal knee joint, *Radiology*, 101, 101–109, 1971.

55. Fox, T. A., Dysplasia of the quadriceps mechanism: hypoplasia of the vastus medialis muscle as related to the hypermobile patella syndrome, *Surg. Clin. North Am.*, 55, 199–226, 1975.

56. Brattstrom, H., Shape of the intercondylar groove normally and in recurrent dislocation of the patella, *Acta Orthop. Scand.*, 68, 85–138, 1964.

57. Vainionpaa, S., Laasonen, E., Patiala, H., Rusanen, M., and Rokkannen, P., Acute dislocation of the patella: clinical, radiographic and operative findings in 64 consecutive cases, *Acta Orthop. Scand.*, 57, 331–333, 1986.

58. Hvid, I., Lars, L. I., and Schmidt, H., Patellar height and femoral trochlear development, *Acta Orthop. Scand.*, 54, 91–93, 1983.

59. Huberti, H. H. and Hayes, W. C., Patellofemoral contact pressures: the influence of Q-angle and tendofemoral contact, *J. Bone Joint Surg.*, 66A, 715–724, 1984.

60. Paulos, L., Rusche, K., Johnson, C., and Noyes, F. R., Patellar malalignment: a treatment rationale, *Phys. Ther.*, 60, 1624–1632, 1980.

61. Jeffreys, T. E., Recurrent dislocation of the patella due to abnormal attachment of the ilio-tibial tract, *J. Bone Joint Surg.*, 45B, 740–743, 1963.

62. Hughston, J. C. and Deese, M., Medial subluxation of the patella as a complication of lateral release, *Am. J. Sports Med.*, 16, 383–388, 1988.

63. Outerbridge, R. and Dunlop, J., The problem of chondromalacia patella, *Clin. Orthop.*, 110, 177–196, 1975.

64. Spencer, J. D., Hayes, K. C., and Alexander, I. J. Knee joint effusion and quadriceps reflex inhibition in man, *Arch. Phys. Med. Rehabil.*, 65, 171–177, 1984.

65. Stratford, P., Electromyography of the quadriceps femoris muscles in subjects with normal knees and acutely effused knees, *Phys. Ther.*, 62, 279–283, 1981.

66. Bennett, J. G. and Stauber, W. T., Evaluation and treatment of anterior knee pain using eccentric exercise, *Med. Sci. Sports Exercise*, 18, 526–530, 1986.

67. Papagelopoulus, P. J. and Sim, F. H., Patellofemoral pain syndrome: diagnosis and management, *Orthopedics*, 20, 148–157, 1997.

68. Souza, D. R. and Gross, M. T., Comparison of vastus medialis obliquus: vastus lateralis muscle integrated electromyographic ratios between healthy subjects and patients with patellofemoral pain, *Phys. Ther.*, 71, 310–316, 1991.

69. Wise, H. H., Fiebert, I. M., and Kates, J. L. EMG biofeedback as treatment for patellofemoral pain syndrome, *J. Orthop. Sports Phys. Ther.*, 6, 95–103, 1984.

70. Boucher, J. P., King, M. A., Lefebvre, R., and Pepin, A., Quadriceps femoris muscle activity in patellofemoral pain syndrome, *Am. J. Sports Med.*, 20, 527–532, 1992.

71. MacIntyre, D. L. and Robertson, G. E., Quadriceps muscle activity in women runners with and without patellofemoral pain syndrome, *Arch. Phys. Med. Rehabil.*, 73, 10–14, 1992.

72. Moller, B. N., Krebs, B., Tidemand-Dal, C., and Aaris, K., Isometric contractions in the patellofemoral pain syndrome: an electromyographic study, *Arch. Orthop. Trauma Surg.*, 105, 24–27, 1986.

73. Wild, J. J., Franklin, T. D., and Woods, G. W., Patellar pain and quadriceps rehabilitation: an EMG study, *Am. J. Sports Med.*, 10, 12–15, 1982.

74. Schutzer, S. F., Ramsby, G. R., and Fulkerson, J. P., The evaluation of patellofemoral pain using computerized tomography: a preliminary study, *Clin. Orthop.* 204, 286–293, 1986.

75. Shellock, F. G., Mink, J. H., Deutsch, A. L., and Foo, T. K. F., Kinematic MR imaging of the patellofemoral joint: comparison of passive positioning and active movement techniques, *Radiology*, 184, 574–577, 1992.

76. Ficat, P., Ficat, C., and Bailleux, A., Syndrome d'hyperpression externe de la rotule, *Rev. Chir. Orthop.*, 61, 39–59, 1975.

77. Linn, F. C. and Sokoloff, L., Movement and composition of interstitial fluid of cartilage, *Arthr. Rheum.*, 8, 481–494, 1965.

78. Seedholm, B. B., Takeda, T., Tsubuku, M., and Wright, V., Mechanical factors and patellofemoral osteoarthritis, *Ann. Rheum. Dis.,* 38, 307–316, 1979.
79. Fulkerson, J. P., Schutzer. S. F., Ramsby, G. R., and Bernstein, R. A., Computerized tomography of the patellofemoral joint before and after lateral release or realignment, *Arthroscopy,* 3, 19–24, 1987.
80. Douchette, S. A. and Goble, E. M., The effects of exercise on patellar tracking in lateral patellar compression syndrome, *Am. J. Sports Med.,* 20, 434–440, 1992.

9 Kinematic MRI of the Patellofemoral Joint

Frank G. Shellock and Christopher M. Powers

CONTENTS

I. INTRODUCTION

Abnormalities of the patellofemoral joint are a primary cause of pain and functional instability.[1-7] Imperfect congruence between the patella and femoral trochlear groove is the main causative mechanism responsible for patellofemoral pain (PFP).[1-9] Patellar malalignment and abnormal tracking

0-8493-0807-0/01/$0.00+$.50
© 2001 by Frank G. Shellock

are believed to produce significant shearing forces and excessive contact stress that cause degeneration of the articular cartilage.[1-9] Chronic patellar displacement also may change the load distribution in the patellofemoral joint, producing pain in the absence of a detectable cartilage defect.[1,4,7]

The detection and characterization of patellofemoral joint abnormalities by physical examination is often difficult because the associated symptoms may mimic internal derangement of the knee, and co-existing pathologic conditions are common.[1,4,7,10,11] Patients with persistent symptoms following patellar realignment surgery present a particular challenge.[12] Because identification of abnormal patellofemoral relationships is known to be crucial for proper treatment decisions, diagnostic imaging has played an important role in the evaluation of patients with patellofemoral pain.[1,4,6,7,10-45]

Abnormal patellar alignment and tracking typically exist during the earliest portion of the range of motion (e.g., <20 degrees), as the patella enters and begins to articulate with the femoral trochlear groove.[1,4,5,10] As flexion increases, the patella moves deeper into the femoral trochlear groove. Within this anatomic area, patellar displacement is less likely to occur because the osseous anatomy of the trochlear groove functions to buttress and stabilize the patella.[1,5]

Displacement of the patella is most likely to occur during the initial increments of knee flexion. Therefore, diagnostic imaging techniques that show the patellofemoral joint during the earliest range of motion are best suited for the identification of abnormalities.[1,4,10,12,23,41-45] Imaging the patellofemoral joint at flexion angles of greater than 30 degrees frequently results in clinically important information being overlooked.[1,7,10,23,41,44] In fact, studies have demonstrated that patellar malalignment and abnormal tracking are not reliably or consistently identified by imaging techniques that image the patellofemoral joint at flexion angles greater than 30 degrees (i.e., most conventional radiographic methods).[4,17,21,37,40]

In 1988, a kinematic magnetic resonance imaging (MRI) procedure was developed to provide diagnostic information pertaining to patellar alignment during the initial increments of joint flexion, when subtle position-related abnormalities are most apparent.[16] Since then, many publications have reported that kinematic MRI of the patellofemoral joint is a sensitive and useful technique for identification and characterization of aberrant positions of the patella.[10-12,17-45] Furthermore, this procedure often provides important diagnostic information frequently unappreciated using physical examination criteria.[10]

While conventional and cine computed tomography (CT) also have been used for kinematic examinations,[1,4,44] kinematic MRI has the advantage of showing the soft tissue components (i.e., medial and lateral retinacula, patellar tendon, quadriceps muscles) responsible for static and dynamic stability of the patellofemoral joint. This information is frequently useful because irregularities of one or more of the soft tissue structures may contribute to abnormal patellofemoral relationships.[1-7,12,17,23,41,42,44] Thus, kinematic MRI of the patellofemoral joint is considered to be the diagnostic imaging "technique of choice" for evaluation of the patient with patellofemoral pain.[10,23,41,42,44]

This chapter will describe the various techniques used to perform kinematic MRI of the patellofemoral joint, describe the basic method used to interpret the examination, discuss clinical applications, and present future developments to evaluate patellofemoral relationships.

II. TECHNIQUE

A. THE MAGNETIC RESONANCE SYSTEM

As indicated above, it is important to visualize the earliest increments of the range of motion using kinematic MRI to examine the patellofemoral joint. Fortuitously, this can be accomplished using conventional "tunnel-configured" MR systems (i.e., with the patient in a prone position on a special positioning device that permits unimpaired movement of the patellofemoral articulation; see below).[16,17,23,25,26,29,32-44] While low-field-strength "open" and dedicated-extremity MR systems also may be used to perform the kinematic MRI procedure,[18,21,45] these scanners do not offer any advantages compared with using conventional MR systems for the patellofemoral joint.

B. Positioning Devices and Radiofrequency Coils

Positioning devices are an important requirement for performance of the kinematic MRI procedure. In general, the positioning device is used to maintain the patient's lower extremities in a specific plane of imaging and guide them through a specific range of motion. Additionally, the positioning device must permit flexion and extension of the knee as well as unrestricted rotational movements of the lower extremity to ensure visualization of the inherent biomechanics of the patellofemoral joint.

Positioning devices may incorporate radiofrequency (RF) surface coils to facilitate imaging of the patellofemoral joints and may be used to apply a resistance or stress during the kinematic MRI procedure. There are several commercially available positioning devices that have been developed for the patellofemoral joint in consideration of the above-mentioned factors (Figure 9.1).

In general, high-field-strength MR systems (i.e., >1.0 Tesla) permit imaging with a greater signal-to-noise compared to low- or mid-field-strength MR systems. Therefore, for the kinematic MRI examination of the patellofemoral joint, unilateral or bilateral imaging may be accomplished using the transmit-receive body coil of a high-field-strength MR system, while an RF surface coil is typically required if a low- or mid-field-strength scanner is used.

C. Imaging Parameters and Protocols

Imaging parameters and protocols for the kinematic MRI study of the patellofemoral joint have changed over the years, with a variety of pulse sequences and positioning strategies used for this diagnostic procedure. In general, MR images are acquired through the patellofemoral joint in multiple section locations in the axial plane as the knee moves passively or dynamically from 30 to 40 degrees of flexion to full extension. This procedure best depicts the changing positions of the patella relative to the femoral trochlear groove. Because patellofemoral disorders tend to be bilateral, both joints should be examined using kinematic MRI. The different techniques used for kinematic MRI of the patellofemoral joint can be categorized as follows: (1) incremental, passive positioning; (2) active movement; (3) cine-cyclic; and (4) active movement, against resistance.

1. Incremental, Passive Positioning

The first applications of kinematic MRI of the patellofemoral joint used the incremental, passive positioning technique.[11,12,16-24,27,28,30] This basic technique involves passive movement of the patient's knee from approximately 30 to 40 degrees of flexion to extension in 5 degree increments. The patellofemoral joint is imaged in multiple section locations in the axial plane at each increment of flexion using a T1-weighted, spin echo or spoiled gradient echo (e.g., spoiled GRASS) pulse sequence.

A patient-activated positioning device facilitates performance of the kinematic MRI procedure (Figure 9.1A). Notably, the positioning device must have a cut-out area to permit unimpaired movement of the patellofemoral joint during flexion and extension while the patient is in the prone position. (The kinematics of the patellofemoral joint have been observed to be the same with the patient prone or supine.[23,41,42]) The use of this specific type of device is crucial because direct anterior or lateral pressure that may occur with the patient placed prone (i.e., as a result of the patient's body weight pressing against the table) may be sufficient to displace the patella, resulting in an erroneous diagnosis.[68]

When positioning the patient prone on the device, special care should be taken to maintain the patient's lower extremity alignment (observed while in an upright position). This positioning scheme is unique because it allows rotational movements of lower extremities to occur during flexion and

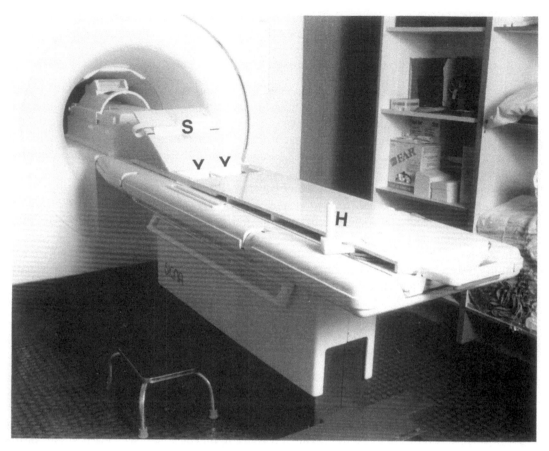

FIGURE 9.1A   Example of a positioning device used for kinematic MRI of the patellofemoral joint. This device is used to perform incremental, passive positioning kinematic MRI of the patellofemoral joint. It has a patient-activated handle (H) that controls a mechanism to move the patellofemoral joints from approximately 30 degrees of flexion to extension in 5 degree increments. A cut-out area (arrow heads) permits uninhibited movements of the patellofemoral joints with the patient placed prone on the positioning device. A Velcro strap (S) is loosely placed around the ankles to maintain the relative alignment of the lower extremities, without impairing rotational movements during joint movements. This positioning device is typically used with the body RF coil for the kinematic MRI examination; however, single or dual RF flex coils also may be used.

extension, which is important because excessive internal or external rotation may be partially responsible for abnormal patellar alignment and tracking.[1,5,7,16,17]

The incremental, passive positioning technique continues to be used in the clinical setting on MR systems that do not have the technical means to achieve the temporal resolution necessary for a dynamic study of the patellofemoral joint (i.e., a temporal resolution of approximately one image per second is required for the use of active movement or active movement, against resistance techniques). Nevertheless, compared to the use of conventional radiographic techniques, this procedure provides an improvement in the diagnostic ability to determine abnormal patellofemoral relationships.[17,21,22,24]

2. Active Movement

The availability of faster MR imaging techniques has enabled kinematic MRI procedures to be accomplished during dynamic movement.[10,29,37,38,41,42,44] The active movement technique uses fast spoiled gradient echo pulse sequences or echo planar imaging to image at the rate of approximately one image per second or faster. The primary advantage of using the active movement technique compared to the incremental, passive positioning method is that the influence of the "activated" quadriceps muscles and associated soft-tissue structures on patellar alignment and tracking can be examined.[10,29,37-39,41,42,44] Additionally, there is no need for a sophisticated positioning device to flex the joint passively and the overall examination time is substantially reduced.[29]

With regard to performing a kinematic MRI examination using the active movement technique, a positioning device is used that has a cut-out area to accommodate the patient in the prone position. Beginning with the knees flexed at approximately 40 to 45 degrees, the patient is instructed to begin moving slowly approximately 1 second after hearing the gradient noise produced by the MR system (indicating that imaging has begun) until reaching full extension. Imaging parameters should be selected to obtain six images at a single section location. In addition, images should be evenly spaced through the range of motion achievable within the bore of the magnet. This procedure should be repeated to acquire three to four different section locations to assess the entire excursion of the patella as it articulates with the femoral trochlear groove. Compared with the incremental, passive positioning technique, a more physiologic examination is obtained, with abnormal patellar tracking being more readily apparent using the active movement technique.[10,23,35,41,42]

a. Axial-loaded, supine

Another technique of performing an active movement kinematic MRI examination of the patellofemoral joint involves the use of the axial-loaded, supine position. This method uses a special positioning device in an attempt to impose weight-bearing forces on the patellofemoral joint (Figure 9.1B). For this kinematic MRI examination, the supine patient presses down on a foot-plate of the device while maintaining the knees at a predetermined angle of flexion (e.g., 20 degrees) using an isometric muscular action.[25] MR images are obtained using a T1-weighted, spin echo or fast spoiled gradient echo pulse sequence. A preliminary report by Shellock et al.[25] indicated that the axial-loaded, supine kinematic MRI procedure is useful for identifying abnormal patellofemoral relationships. However, compared with other active movement techniques, this is technically more difficult to perform and, as such, not used frequently in the clinical setting.

3. Cine-Cyclic

The cine-cyclic method of performing kinematic MRI of the patellofemoral joint (also referred to as "motion-triggered" kinematic MRI) is similar to the gated MRI procedure used to study the heart.[37,44] Using this technique, the knee is flexed and extended repeatedly during acquisition of MR images, which are obtained using an RF surface coil and a T1-weighted, spin echo or gradient echo pulse sequence. Notably, movement of the knee may last from two to several minutes while the MR images are obtained. However, this may be difficult for patients experiencing patellofemoral pain. A special positioning device that incorporates a trigger system to sense the motion of the patella is required to implement this type of kinematic MRI examination.[37,44]

An investigation conducted by Brossmann et al.[37] reported that the cine-cyclic method showed markedly abnormal patellar tracking patterns compared to using an incremental, passive positioning technique, substantiating the importance of using an active movement method to assess patellofemoral relationships. From a clinical MRI consideration, the cine-cyclic technique is rarely used for kinematic MRI of the patellofemoral joint because of the somewhat extensive technical requirements.

4. Active Movement, against Resistance

A major determinant of the function of the patellofemoral joint is the tolerance displayed in reaction to the external forces encountered during activity or weight bearing.[1,5,46,47] As the quadriceps muscle force increases in response to an external load, so does the reaction force imposed upon the patellofemoral joint.[5,7,46,47] Notably, patients with patellofemoral disorders usually experience pain or increased symptoms during activity or stress of the joint.[1,5,7,46,47] Therefore, in consideration of

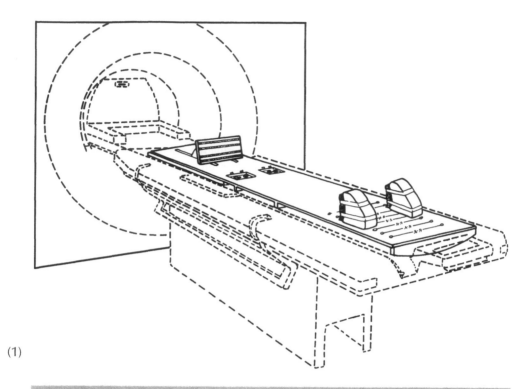

(1)

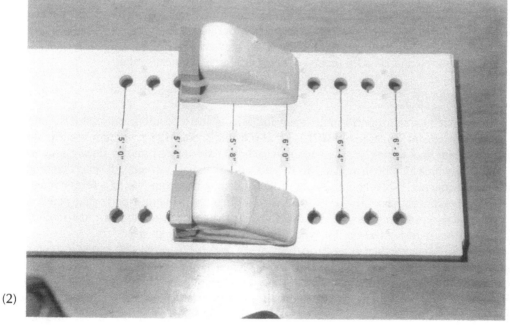

(2)

FIGURE 9.1B Schematic drawing of a positioning device designed for axial-loaded, supine kinematic MRI examination of the patellofemoral joint (1). This device has shoulder supports that may be adjusted to accommodate the height of the patient (2). A series of valves (V) are turned "on" or "off" to control the axial load (range 50–220 lbs). For the kinematic MRI examination, the patient is placed supine on the device and presses down on the foot-plate (FP), while maintaining the patellofemoral joints at a predetermined angle of flexion (e.g., 20 degrees) using isometric muscle action (3, 4). MR images are obtained using a T1-weighted or fast spoiled gradient echo pulse sequence. This example of axial loading of the patellofemoral joint shows a patient with lateral subluxation of the patella (5).

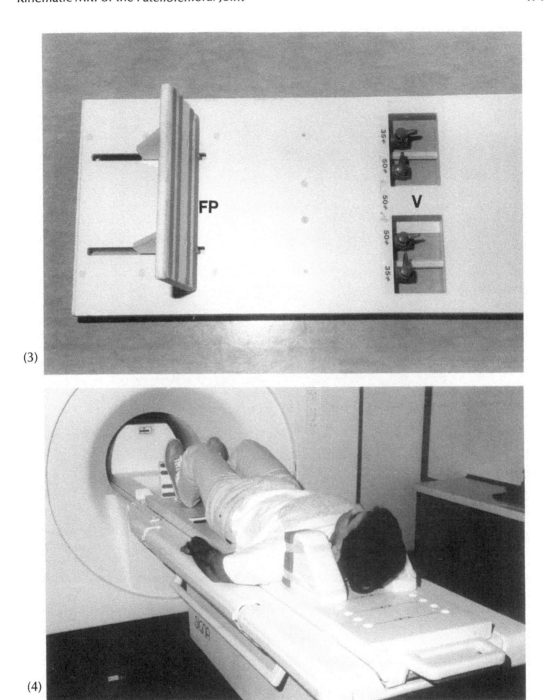

(3)

(4)

FIGURE 9.1B   (continued).

these biomechanic principals and in an effort to improve the diagnostic yield of the kinematic MRI examination, a technique was developed to assess the patellofemoral joint during "active movement, against resistance."[36] Conceptually, this procedure was designed to stress the quadriceps and associated soft tissue structures, thereby permitting identification of abnormal patellofemoral relationships in the presence of unbalanced or disruptive forces.[36]

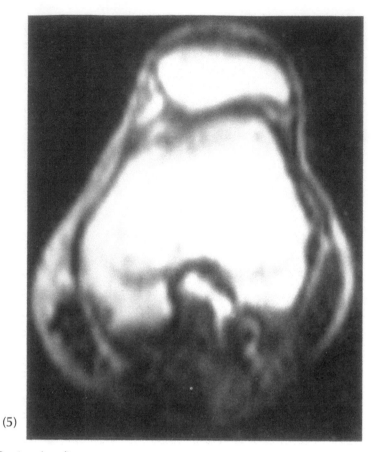

(5)

FIGURE 9.1B   (continued).

Clinical use of the active movement, against resistance technique has shown that the application of an external load to the patellofemoral joint elicits aberrant positions of the patellar and tracking deviations that may not be observed during "unloaded" examinations.[10,36,41,42,44] Therefore, this kinematic MRI technique offers an improved diagnostic method for identifying abnormal patellofemoral relationships.[10,36,41,42,44]

The active movement against resistance technique is performed using a positioning device that incorporates a mechanism with an adjustable resistance (Figures 9.1C to 9.1E). Various manufacturers make such a device (e.g., General Electric Medical Systems, Milwaukee, WI; CHAMCO, Cocoa, FL). The design of the typical positioning device used for this kinematic MRI procedure is such that a bilateral or unilateral examination may be used to assess the patellofemoral joints during movement from approximately 40 to 45 degrees of flexion to full extension.[36] With the patient prone, the positioning device primarily imposes a load during this open-chain activity.[36,41,42] Of note is that the "loaded" condition of the active movement, against resistance technique is imposed during the earliest increments of flexion when the required muscle force is substantial. The associated patellofemoral joint reaction forces are the greatest during this time.[36,46,47]

Similar to other active movement techniques, imaging parameters should be selected to achieve a temporal resolution of approximately one image per second or faster. The basic protocol requires acquisition of five to six images at three to four different section locations to properly assess patellofemoral relationships.[36,41,43]

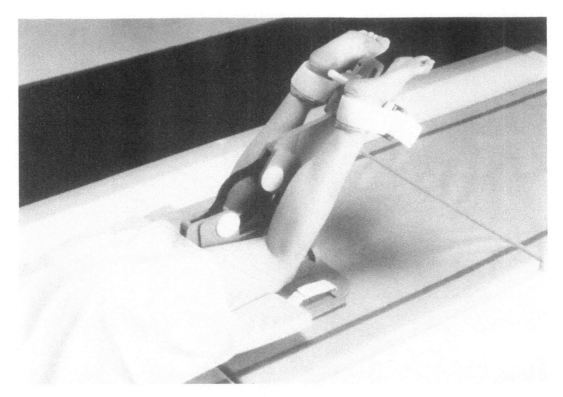

FIGURE 9.1C Positioning device used for kinematic MRI of the patellofemoral joints using the active movement, against resistance technique (General Electric Medical Systems, Milwaukee, WI). The patient is placed prone on this device. The patellofemoral joints are suspended above the MR system table to allow unrestricted movements. Velcro straps are placed around the ankles to hold them within small cradles that swivel 360 degrees. Thus, there is no limitation of lower extremity rotation. This positioning device is designed for use with a body RF coil, single- or dual-circumferential surface RF coils, or single- or dual-flex RF coils.

D. INTERPRETATION OF THE KINEMATIC MRI EXAMINATION

1. Anatomic Considerations

Careful review of the MR images obtained from the kinematic MRI examination frequently provides diagnostic information related to anatomy known to predispose to abnormal patellofemoral relationships.[41,42,48,49] For example, because the patella articulates with the femoral trochlear groove during knee flexion, congruent shapes of these structures are crucial for proper function of the patellofemoral joint.[1-9,46,47,50] Dysplastic osseous anatomy is commonly observed in conjunction with patellofemoral instability;[1,6,7,50] therefore, inspection of the shapes of the patella and femoral trochlear groove may provide evidence of a patellofemoral abnormality (however, the existence of dysplastic osseous morphology does not always preclude normal patellar alignment and tracking).[1-7,9] Furthermore, it is important to determine the position of the patella (i.e., with the knee extended) relative to the femoral trochlear groove, or patellar height, because an excessively "high-" or "low-riding" patella (i.e., patella alta or patella baja) is frequently associated with an abnormal patellofemoral relationship.[1,7,51-53]

When performing the kinematic MRI examination of the patellofemoral joint, evaluation of the anatomic features of the patella and femoral trochlear groove is easily accomplished using images acquired in multiple section locations in the axial plane with the joint extended (i.e., these MR images are obtained to determine the position of the patella relative to the femoral trochlear groove to prescribe section locations for the subsequent "flexion-to-extension" portion of the kinematic

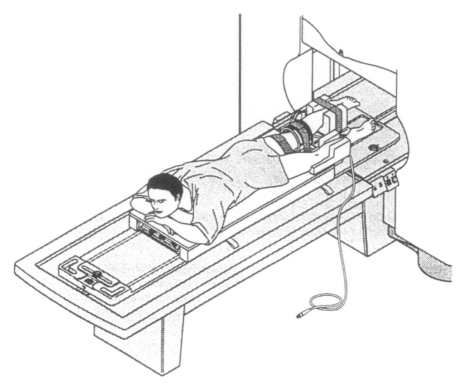

FIGURE 9.1D Positioning device used for kinematic MRI of the patellofemoral joint using the active movement, against resistance technique (CHAMCO, Inc., Cocoa, FL). The patient is placed prone on this device. It is designed for a unilateral examination of the patellofemoral joint using the body RF coil, a circumferential surface RF coil, or single flex RF coil.

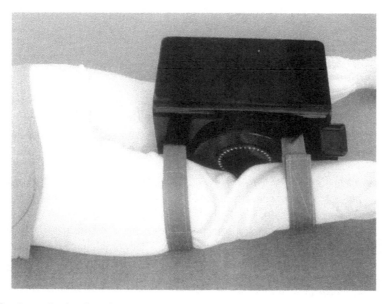

FIGURE 9.1E A newly developed positioning device designed for kinematic MRI of the patellofemoral joint using the active movement, against resistance technique (CHAMCO, Inc., Cocoa, FL). The patient is placed prone on this device. It is designed for a unilateral examination of the patellofemoral joint using the body RF coil, a circumferential surface RF coil, or single flex RF coil.

MRI study). Additionally, these MR images are useful for determining the position of the inferior pole of the patella relative to the femoral trochlear groove to assess patellar height.[41,42,48,53]

a. The patella

Dysplastic shapes of the patella are commonly observed in conjunction with patellofemoral arthrosis, chondromalacia, recurrent dislocation, and instability.[1-3,13-15,42,43,48,49] While various descriptions of patellar shape have been published over the years, these were based on the use of conventional radiographs (i.e., plain film x-rays) that showed the configuration of the subchondral bone of the patella on a tangential projection.[1,7,13-15] Studies using the tomographic capabilities of CT and MR imaging have reported that the shape of the patella appears to change from one section location to another, a finding that casts suspicion on the value of the previously published classification systems for patellar shapes that relied on x-rays.[1,48-50] Nevertheless, consideration of the shape of the patella and how it corresponds with the shape of the femoral trochlear groove (see below) is diagnostically useful for evaluation of the patellofemoral joint.

b. The femoral trochlear groove

The femoral trochlear groove provides a mechanical restraint that helps stabilize and guide the patella during flexion of the knee.[1,5,7,46,47,50] The normal shape of the femoral trochlear groove has been described to have a "deep" sulcus with well-defined medial and lateral facets that are either equal in size or with a slightly larger lateral facet.[1,5,7,46,47,50] Most importantly, the shape of the groove should conform to the shape of the patella for proper articulation. Abnormal shapes of the femoral trochlear groove are variable insofar as the medial or lateral aspects may be hypoplastic or dysplastic (Figure 9.2). A shallow, flattened, or convex femoral trochlear groove has been reported to be associated with patellofemoral joint instability.[1,5,7,41,42,46,47,50]

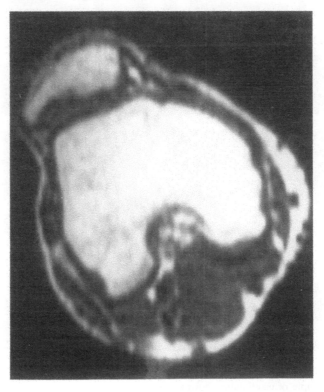

FIGURE 9.2   Axial plane MR image of the right patellofemoral joint showing dysplastic (i.e., flattened) femoral trochlear groove (T1-weighted, spin echo). This geometric osseous abnormality tends to be associated with patellofemoral instability.

c. Patellar height

As previously mentioned, proper position of the patella relative to the femoral trochlear groove is important for normal function of the patellofemoral joint.[5,46,47,51-53] Contact points between the cartilaginous surfaces of the patella and femoral trochlear groove during flexion are drastically altered if the patella is positioned too high or too low, potentially leading to pain and instability. Additionally, abnormal patellar height may be partially responsible for patellar malalignment and abnormal tracking.[1,7,51-53]

Using MRI, axial plane section locations obtained with the patellofemoral joint extended will show a normal patellar height when the inferior pole of the patella is positioned in the superior aspect of the femoral trochlear groove.[41,42,53] Patella alta, an abnormally high position of the patella, is associated with various patellofemoral problems, including patellofemoral joint instability, patellar dislocation, and chondromalacia patella,[51,52] and is found more often in women than men. On sequential, axial plane MR images, patella alta is present when the inferior pole of the patella is positioned above the superior aspect of the femoral trochlear groove[53] (Figure 9.3A).

Patella baja (sometimes called "patella infera"), an abnormally low position of the patella, is often seen in conjunction with Osgood-Schlatter disease, a traumatic disturbance in the development

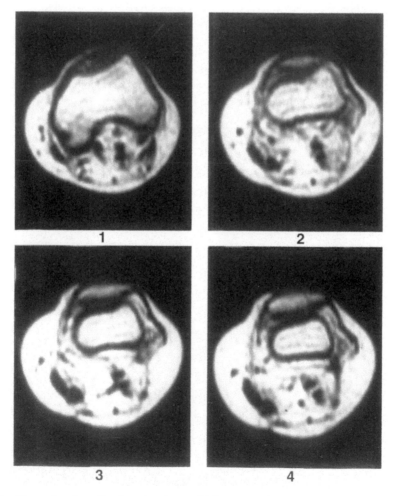

FIGURE 9.3A   Example of patella alta, showing multiple, sequential axial plane images obtained through the left patellofemoral joint (T1-weighted, spin echo). The inferior pole of the patella is positioned well above the femoral trochlear groove (2). In addition, the patella has a dysplastic shape (4, mid-patellar section location), and the medial aspect of the femoral trochlear groove (1) is hypoplastic.

of the tibial tuberosity in adolescents.[1,7,51] Patella baja may also be found after patellar realignment surgery that involves repositioning or shortening of the patellar tendon or ligament.[51] On sequential, axial plane MR images, patella baja is present when the entire patella is positioned in or below the femoral trochlear groove with the knee joint extended.

2. Use of Qualitative Criteria

Kinematic MRI examinations may be interpreted using either quantitative or qualitative criteria.[10,11,12,16-44] Notably, the qualitative method tends to be used most often in the clinical setting because of the known limitations of using quantification schemes to analyze kinematic MRI studies.[10,12,17,41,42,50,56] These limitations include the following:

1. The majority of the quantitative techniques were designed for use with plain film radiographs obtained at a single increment of joint flexion, usually greater than 30 degrees. The use of these measurement techniques is not practical for analyzing kinematic MRI examinations, because multiple images are obtained during the earliest increments of joint flexion. Furthermore, the validity of applying techniques developed for projection views to assess tomographic images is unknown.
2. Abnormal patellofemoral joints often have associated anatomic irregularities (e.g., dysplastic patellae, dysplastic bony anatomy, patella alta, patella baja). These conditions preclude an accurate assessment of patellar positions using quantification schemes that rely on specific and consistent landmarks for characterization of patellofemoral relationships. For example, in the case of patella alta, there is no acceptable means to determine the relationship of the patella relative to the femoral trochlear groove (i.e., the osseous landmarks are not present on the section location that shows the patella) (Figure 9.3B).
3. There is no general agreement on the usefulness of any quantification technique for evaluation of patellofemoral relationships.
4. There is a poor correlation between quantified indices and clinical findings.[7,10,41,42]
5. A recent investigation by Staubli et al.[50] reported that indices developed to describe osseous contours of the patellofemoral joint using conventional radiography and computed tomography do not provide the specific relationships of the surface geometry of the articulating cartilaginous surfaces, as visualized on MR images.
6. Importantly, orthopedic surgeons and clinicians rarely use the quantitative information to guide the use of surgical or rehabilitation treatments.

In consideration of these issues, most studies using kinematic MRI techniques have reported that it is more appropriate and practical to use qualitative criteria to describe patellofemoral relationships viewed on kinematic MRI examinations.[10-12,16,17,19,20,23,25-29,32,34-36,41,42,45,56] Thus, the qualitative technique is the predominant method used to interpret kinematic MRI examinations in the clinical setting.

a. Normal patellar alignment and tracking

Using qualitative criteria to analyze kinematic MRI examinations, normal patellar alignment and tracking are displayed when the median ridge of the patella is positioned in the center of the femoral trochlear groove and this orientation is maintained throughout the range of motion (Figure 9.4). Additionally, the patella maintains a horizontal orientation relative to the femoral trochlear groove (i.e., there is no "tilt" present). Abnormalities of patellar alignment and tracking are apparent on the kinematic MRI examination when there is any deviation of this normal pattern of patellar movement exhibited on one or more section locations at approximately five degrees of joint flexion or greater.[12,17,41,42] This is typically seen as some form of transverse displacement of the patella relative to the femoral trochlear groove and/or change in position from horizontal to a vertical orientation (i.e., tilt).

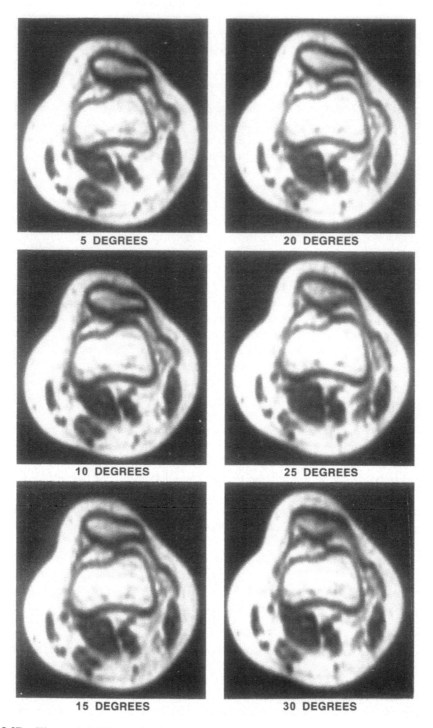

FIGURE 9.3B   Kinematic MRI examination performed using the incremental, passive positioning technique (axial plane; T1-weighted, spin echo) showing lateral subluxation, lateral tilt, and marked patella alta. Note that the patella is articulating well above the femoral trochlear groove.

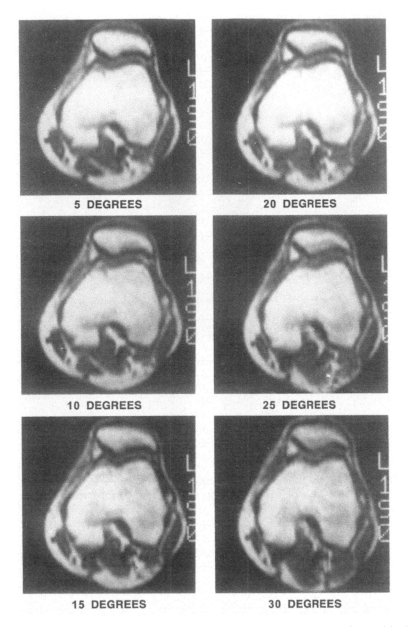

5 DEGREES   20 DEGREES

10 DEGREES   25 DEGREES

15 DEGREES   30 DEGREES

FIGURE 9.4A   Kinematic MRI examination performed using the incremental, passive positioning technique (axial plane; T1-weighted, spin echo) showing normal patellar alignment and tracking.

b. Lateral subluxation

Lateral subluxation of the patella is a form of patellar malalignment where the median ridge of the patella is laterally displaced relative to the femoral trochlear groove or the centermost part of the femoral trochlea. Typically, the lateral facet of the patella is seen to overlap or extend beyond the lateral aspect of the femoral trochlea.

c. Excessive lateral pressure syndrome and lateral tilt

Excessive lateral pressure syndrome (ELPS) and lateral tilt are exhibited by a change in the patella from a horizontal to a slight vertical orientation relative to the femoral trochlear groove (as viewed

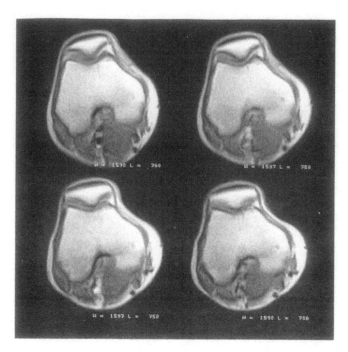

FIGURE 9.4B   Kinematic MRI examination performed using the active movement, against resistance technique (axial plane; fast spoiled GRASS) showing normal patellar alignment and tracking. Note that each example shows the median ridge of the patella positioned in the center of the femoral trochlear groove.

on images obtained in the axial plane). On the kinematic MRI examination, this abnormal patellofemoral relationship often gives the appearance of a gap between the articulating surfaces of the median ridge of the patellar and the trochlear groove. There may be slight lateralization of the patella associated with the higher increments of joint flexion. It should be noted that tilting of the patella onto the lateral aspect of the femoral trochlear groove may shift the medial facet of the patella medially.

d. Medial subluxation of the patella

Medial subluxation of the patella is distinguished by medial displacement of the patellar median ridge relative to the femoral trochlear groove or the centermost part of the femoral trochlea. Typically, impaction between the median ridge and medial aspect of the femoral trochlea may occur.

e. Medial-to-lateral subluxation

Medial-to-lateral subluxation of the patella is a pattern of abnormal patellar alignment and tracking whereby the patella is positioned medially in the higher increments of flexion, moves into and across the femoral trochlear groove, and then displaces laterally during terminal extension.

f. Display of the kinematic MR images

To optimally assess patellar alignment and tracking using kinematic MRI, three to four different section locations, obtained through the femoral trochlear groove or femoral trochlea (depending on the position of the patella) during the initial increments of the range of motion, should be evaluated. The MR images can be analyzed individually or, more effectively, displayed as a "cine-loop."[12,17,41,42] The cine-loop is created using software available on virtually all MR systems, to "page-through" the multiple images obtained at a given section location (i.e., the images should be ordered from beginning to end to beginning). This display technique facilitates review of the multiple images and best shows subtle patellar alignment and tracking abnormalities.[10,12,17,41,42]

The severity of disordered patellofemoral relationships may be characterized by determining the various positional changes of the patella as the joint moves from flexion to extension.[41,42] For example, for minor abnormalities, patellar subluxation is transient, with the patella tending to be displaced less in association with the greater increments of joint flexion (however, as indicated previously, even a subtle patellar displacement can alter the load distribution on the patellofemoral joint, creating pain in the absence of a detectable cartilage lesion).[1,3,7] If the abnormality is more severe, the patella is either maintained in its displaced position or is further displaced (i.e., progressive subluxation) in association with greater increments of joint flexion.

III. CLINICAL APPLICATIONS

A. LATERAL SUBLUXATION

Lateral subluxation of the patella is the most common form of patellar malalignment and abnormal tracking encountered in patients with patellofemoral pain.[1-10,12-24,30,37-42] This aberrant patellofemoral relationship occurs with varying degrees of severity (Figures 9.5 to 9.7). Imbalanced or insufficient forces from lateral soft tissues, sometimes combined with insufficient counterbalancing forces from medial soft tissues, are typically the cause of lateral subluxation of the patella. Additional findings often associated with this condition include dysplastic osseous anatomy and patella alta (Figure 9.3B).

The presence of a lax or redundant lateral retinaculum is sometimes observed in cases of lateral subluxation of the patella (Figure 9.8). This is an especially important finding that may be identified using kinematic MRI, indicating that patellar displacement is not caused by excessive force from the lateral retinaculum. Therefore, surgical release of the lateral retinaculum (i.e., a procedure frequently performed in an attempt to realign a laterally subluxated patella) may not be appropriate for such patients.

Lateral subluxation of the patella also may occur secondary to substantial joint effusions (Figure 9.9). Increased join pressure from the effusion is believed to be responsible for, or contribute to, patellar displacement. Removal of joint fluid will tend to reduce the degree of lateral subluxation.[69]

B. EXCESSIVE LATERAL PRESSURE SYNDROME AND LATERAL TILT

Excessive lateral pressure syndrome (ELPS) is a form of patellar malalignment that is a clinico-radiologic entity, characterized clinically by anterior knee pain and radiologically by tilting of the patella with patellar lateralization. The lateral tilt of the patella usually occurs onto a dominant lateral facet.[1] A small amount of lateral displacement of the patella may or may not be present during joint flexion, as increasing tension from one or more overly taut soft tissue structures tilt the patella, displacing it vertically (as viewed on an axial plane image) (Figure 9.10). Studies suggest that the main pathologic component responsible for this abnormality is excessive force from the lateral retinaculum.[1,4]

Because the patellar tilt that occurs with ELPS may be either transient (i.e., centralization or correction of the patellar malalignment occurs during joint flexion) or progressive (i.e., there is additional tilting with increasing increments of joint flexion), kinematic MRI techniques used to study the patellofemoral joint are particularly useful for identifying and characterizing this abnormality.[41,42]

Notably, the underlying hyperpressure found in ELPS can produce significant destruction of the articular cartilage.[1,4] Lateral joint line narrowing (i.e., seen on conventional radiographs) is often present as a result of a decrease in cartilage thickness or due to gross cartilage degeneration along the median ridge and lateral facet of the patella.[1,4] A dysplastic patella and/or femoral trochlear groove is commonly encountered with ELPS, particularly if this abnormality is present during growth and development of the patellofemoral joint (i.e., the final shapes of the patella and femoral trochlea are typically modified by use). Therefore, the presence of ELPS is likely to be involved in modification of the associated bone anatomy.[1]

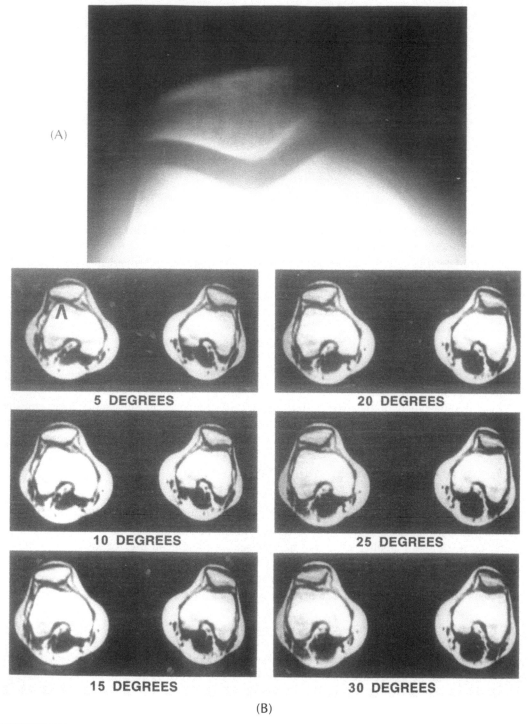

FIGURE 9.5 (A) Sky-line view (approximately 40 degrees of flexion) of the right patellofemoral joint showing normal patella alignment. (B) Kinematic MRI examination performed using the incremental, passive positioning technique (axial plane; T1-weighted, spin echo) showing severe (right joint, arrow head) lateral displacement of the patella (in the same patient as shown in [A]). Note that the patella moves into a more centralized position during the higher increments of flexion (e.g., 30 degrees). This example illustrates the failure of conventional radiography to identify abnormal patellofemoral relationships.

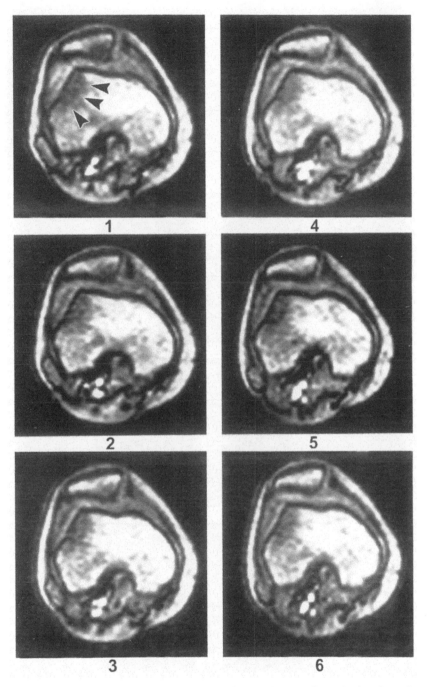

FIGURE 9.6 Kinematic MRI examination of the patellofemoral joint performed using the active movement, against resistance technique (axial plane; fast spoiled GRASS). This patient has lateral subluxation of the patella. Additionally, there are areas of decreased signal intensity in the lateral femoral condyle (1, arrow heads) and median ridge of the patella indicative of bone contusions. These findings suggest that the patient had a previous traumatic lateral dislocation of the patella.

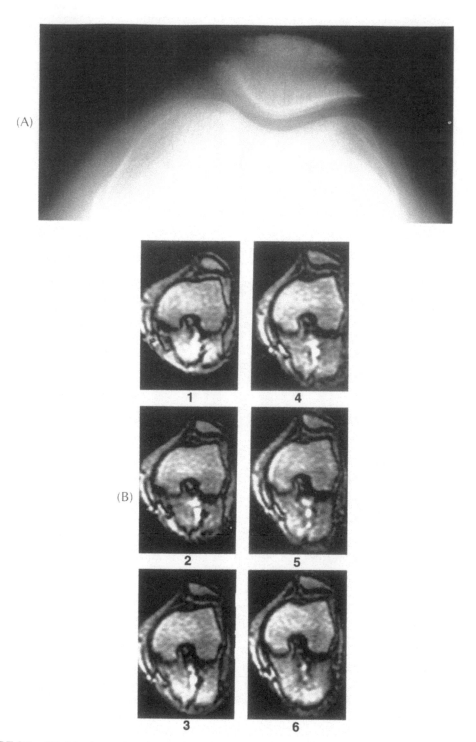

FIGURE 9.7 (A) Merchant view (approximately 45 degrees of flexion) of the left patellofemoral joint showing normal patella alignment. (B) Kinematic MRI examination of the left patellofemoral joint performed using the active movement, against resistance technique (axial plane; fast spoiled GRASS). This study shows lateral subluxation and lateral tilt of the patella (in the same patient as shown in [A]). Additionally, the Merchant view did not show the abnormal patellar displacement which mostly exists during the initial increments of range of motion (i.e., views 1, 2, 3, 4).

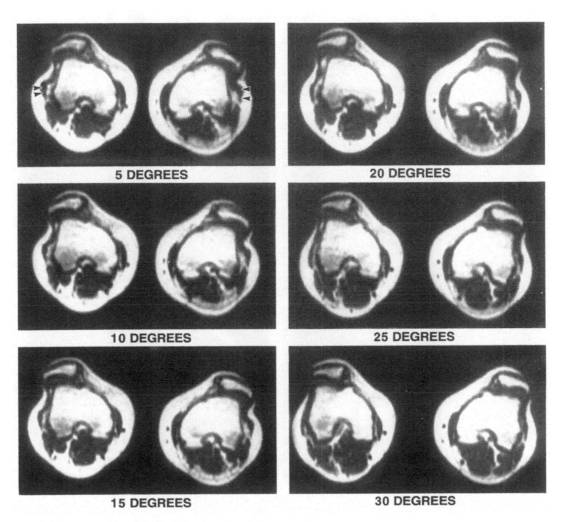

FIGURE 9.8 Kinematic MRI examination of bilateral patellofemoral joints obtained using the incremental, passive positioning technique (axial plane; T1-weighted, spin echo). This patient has bilateral lateral subluxation of the patellae. Notably, there is also laxity of the lateral retinacular structures seen on both joints (5 degrees, arrow heads), suggesting that a lateral release may not be appropriate surgical treatment for this patient.

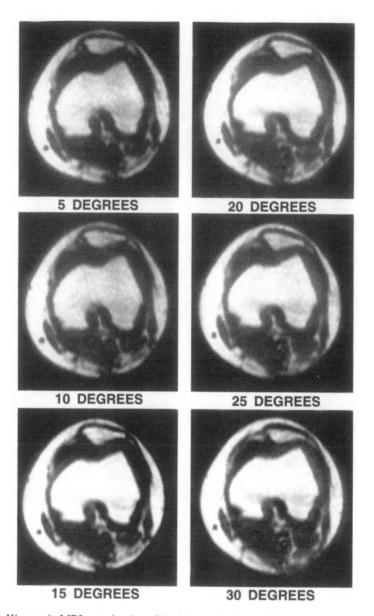

FIGURE 9.9A   Kinematic MRI examination of the left patellofemoral joint obtained using the incremental, passive positioning technique (axial plane; T1-weighted, spin echo). There is a large joint effusion likely to be partially responsible for the mild lateral displacement of the patella.

ELPS is usually treated effectively by surgical release of the lateral retinaculum.[1] It should be noted that using the above criteria, substantial lateral forces acting on the patella may shift the patellar median ridge medially, producing an appearance of medial subluxation (Figure 9.11).

C. Medial Subluxation (Patella Addentro)

Medial subluxation of the patella (or patella addentro) is predominantly shown by medial displacement of the patellar median ridge relative to the femoral trochlear groove (Figure 9.12). This abnormal patellofemoral relationship has been studied extensively using clinical and diagnostic imaging techniques.[7,12,17,27,32,41,42,54,55]

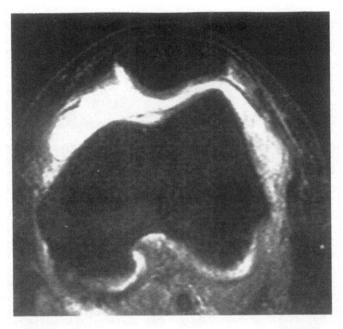

FIGURE 9.9B   MR image showing large joint effusion (axial plane, short tau inversion recovery or STIR pulse sequence) and mild lateral subluxation.

Medial subluxation of the patella is found frequently in patients after surgical patellar realignment procedures in which there has been overcompensation of the lateral tethering or stabilizing mechanisms of the patellofemoral joint (Figure 9.13).[12,27,32,54,55] For example, the lateral soft tissue structures of the patellofemoral joint may be cut excessively during a lateral retinacular release procedure, causing a patella that was laterally subluxated to become medially displaced. Medial subluxation may also be observed in patients without previous patellar realignment surgery[12,27,32,54] (Figures 9.14 and 9.15).

Various factors, existing either separately or in combination, may be responsible for producing this type of aberrant patellar alignment and tracking, including an excessively tight medial retinaculum, insufficient lateral retinaculum, abnormal patellofemoral anatomy, and imbalances of the quadriceps. Extreme internal rotation of the lower extremities and atrophy of the vastus lateralis are common clinical findings in patients with medial subluxation[1,27,54] (Figure 9.16). Identifying this abnormal patellofemoral relationship and distinguishing it from lateral subluxation are diagnostically crucial for selection of the proper rehabilitative or surgical intervention.

Currently, it is unknown whether the appearance of medial subluxtion of the patella on kinematic MRI examinations is the result of a true transverse displacement or due to some element of patellar rotation in the coronal plane (i.e., causing the inferior pole to impact with the medial aspect of the trochlear during flexion or extension). Regardless, abnormal patellar displacement is present and may be a contributing factor to pain and patellofemoral dysfunction.

D. Medial-to-Lateral Subluxation

Medial-to-lateral subluxation of the patella is a patellofemoral abnormality whereby the patella moves slightly lateral during the initial increments of joint flexion (i.e., 5 to 10 degrees), moves into and across the femoral trochlear groove (or femoral trochlea) as flexion increases, and displaces medially during the higher increments of flexion. This relatively uncommon abnormality is typically found in association with patella alta and/or dysplastic bony anatomy because of the inherent lack

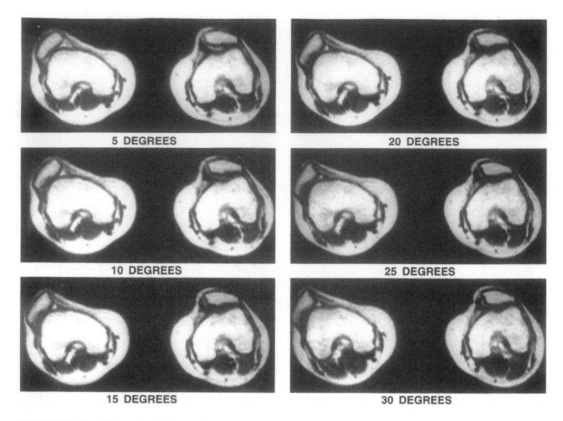

FIGURE 9.10   Kinematic MRI examination of bilateral patellofemoral joints obtained using the incremental, passive positioning technique (axial plane; T1-weighted, spin echo). This study shows excessive lateral pressure syndrome (ELPS), lateral tilt of the left patellofemoral joint. Note the appearance of a "gap" between the median ridge of the patella and femoral trochlear groove. There is severe lateral dislocation of the patella on the right patellofemoral joint.

of stabilization provided by the articulating surfaces.[35,38] In addition, medial-to-lateral subluxation may occur iatrogenically secondary to failed surgery.

The actual biomechanic factors responsible for medial-to-lateral subluxation of the patella are obviously quite complicated. Apparently, various disordered or uncoordinated forces that act on the patella during joint flexion cause this pattern of abnormal patellar alignment and tracking.[41,42] Similar to other types of dysfunctional patellofemoral relationships, the kinematic MRI examination is particularly suited to identify medial-to-lateral subluxation because it shows the movements of the patella during the earliest increments of the range of joint motion.[17,41,42]

E. EVALUATION OF TREATMENT

Many different physical rehabilitation and surgical protocols have been used to manage patients with patellofemoral pain.[1,7,54,57-60] Understandably, the results of these treatments are varied and no one therapeutic technique has been found to be useful for every patient. Non-operative regimens that include the use of physical rehabilitation, bracing, and/or taping are recommended typically for the initial treatment of patellofemoral pain, reserving surgical interventions for the most severe or difficult cases.[26-39]

Besides being used in the initial diagnostic evaluation of the patellofemoral joint, kinematic MRI has been applied to assess the effect of conservative treatments and surgical interventions on patellofemoral relationships.[12,24,30,31,33,39,40,56,61-66] Additionally, for patients with persistent

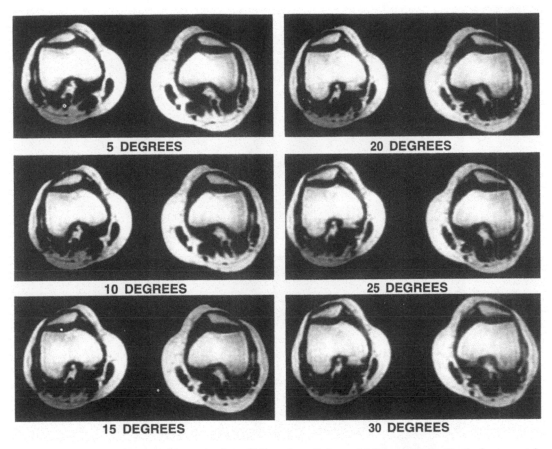

FIGURE 9.11A Kinematic MRI examination of bilateral patellofemoral joints obtained using the incremental, passive positioning technique (axial plane; T1-weighted, spin echo) showing medial subluxation of the patellae.

symptoms following surgery, this diagnostic imaging technique has been reported to be beneficial for assessment of problematic cases.[12] For example, symptomatic patients following lateral retinacular release were found to have unresolved patellar malalignment as demonstrated by kinematic MRI.[12]

When a conservative treatment such as bracing or taping is used, it is advantageous to immediately determine if there has been improvement in patellar displacement.[39,56,61-67] Otherwise, valuable time may be wasted or, more importantly, unwanted cartilage contact stress may be induced that creates another problem for the patient (e.g., if bracing or taping moves the patella in an unacceptable manner).

Theoretically, the function of bracing is to reduce the displaced patella, with secondary functions that include providing warmth to the tissues, changing tension of soft tissue structures, and reducing sensations of joint instability.[58,59] Various investigations have used kinematic MRI to examine the effect of bracing on patellofemoral relationships.[39,56,61-67] Using the incremental, passive positioning technique, Koskinen and Kujala[30] were the first investigators to apply this diagnostic procedure to study the influence of bracing on the displaced patella. Later, Worrell et al.[61,62,64-66] reported that bracing was capable of changing the position of the patella in certain cases, based on findings from kinematic MRI. Using a dedicated extremity MR system, Shellock et al.[63] found that bracing could improve or correct abnormal patellar positions as shown on kinematic MRI examinations analyzed using qualitative criteria.

Studies of bracing also have been conducted using the active movement against resistance technique. In investigations involving two different patellar realignment braces, Shellock et al.[39,63]

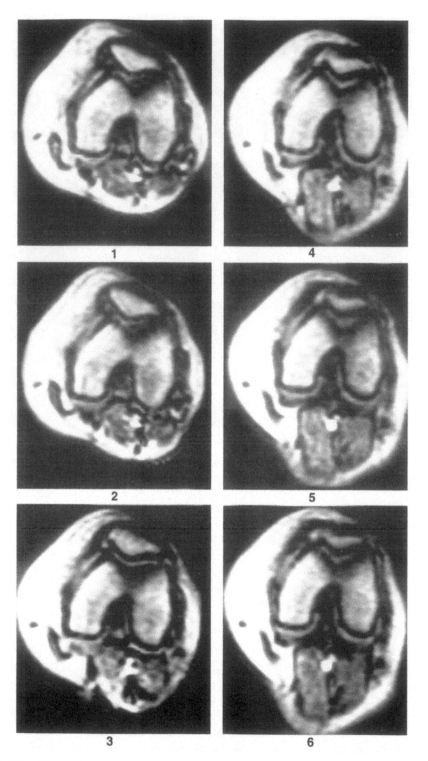

FIGURE 9.11B   Kinematic MRI examination of the left patellofemoral joint performed using the active movement, against resistance technique (axial plane; fast spoiled GRASS). Using qualitative criteria, these examples (9.11A and 9.11B) appear to exhibit medial subluxation of the patella. However, it is possible that substantial lateral forces acting on the patella displace the median ridge of the patella onto the medial aspect of the femoral trochlear groove.

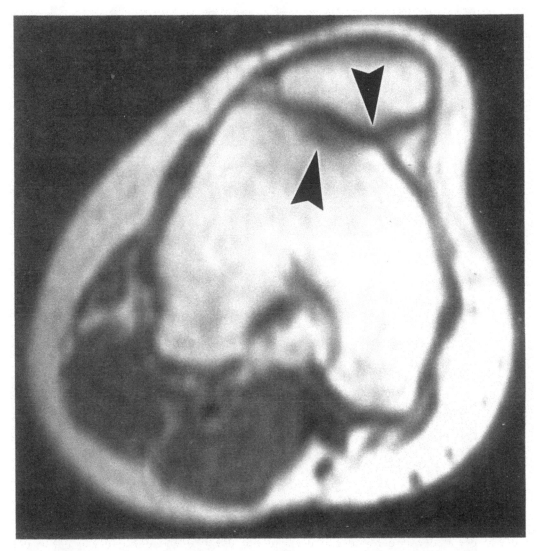

FIGURE 9.12 MR image acquired during kinematic MRI examination using the incremental, passive positioning technique (axial plane; T1-weighted, spin echo) showing example of medial subluxation of the patella. Note the substantial medial displacement of the patellar median ridge relative to the femoral trochlear groove (arrow heads).

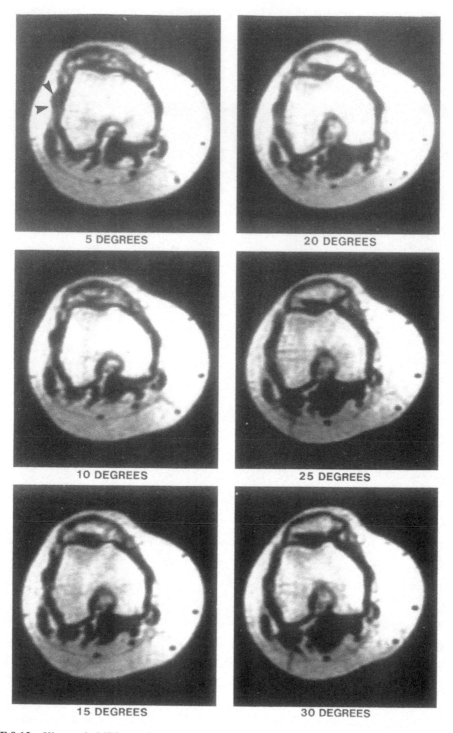

FIGURE 9.13   Kinematic MRI examination of the right patellofemoral joint obtained using the incremental, passive positioning technique (axial plane; T1-weighted spin echo). This patient has severe medial subluxation of the patella. A thickened lateral retinaculum (5 degrees, arrow heads) is noted secondary to two prior lateral retinacular release surgeries.

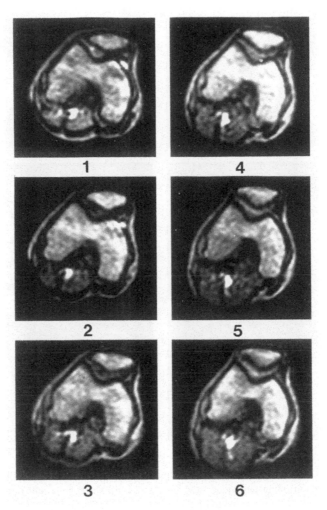

FIGURE 9.14 Kinematic MRI examination of the right patellofemoral joint obtained using the active movement against resistance technique (axial plane; fast spoiled gradient echo) showing medial subluxation of the patella. Notably, this patient did not undergo prior patellar realignment surgery.

found that bracing improved or corrected patellar malalignment for most patients (Figures 9.17 to 9.19). Conversely, Powers et al.[66] and Muhle et al.[67] reported that bracing had no substantial effect with regard to altering patellofemoral relationships. These latter studies used quantitative criteria to interpret the kinematic MRI examinations, while data obtained by Shellock et al.[39,63] were assessed using qualitative criteria.

While findings from kinematic MRI investigations generally support the use of bracing, there are cases where this conservative treatment fails to improve or correct patellar malalignment. This typically occurs in association with patella alta and/or dysplastic osseous anatomy.[39,56,63] Additionally, bracing may not be able to alter the position of the patella in overweight patients (i.e., those with excessive subcutaneous fat).[56] Externally applied force produced by the functional components of the brace is unlikely to work if the anatomy does not permit repositioning of the patella (e.g., in patella alta or dysplastic osseous anatomy) or if the brace is unable to properly interact with the patella (e.g., by "gripping" it).[56] Kinematic MRI may be used effectively in a timely manner to obtain objective findings regarding whether bracing is successful in treating subluxation of the patella.

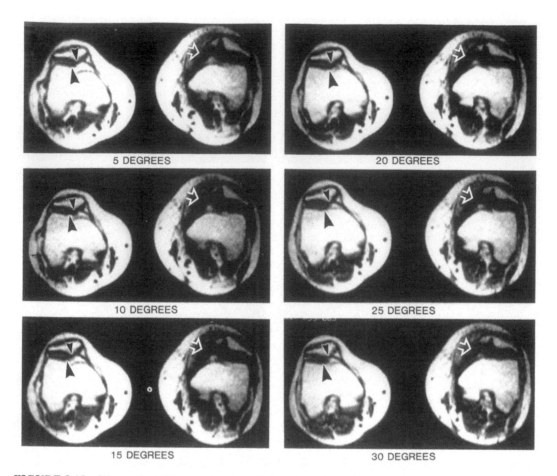

FIGURE 9.15   Kinematic MRI examination of the bilateral patellofemoral joints obtained using the incremental, passive positioning technique (axial plane; T1-weighted spin echo). This patient has medial subluxation on the left (black arrow heads) patellofemoral joint. The left patellofemoral joint has a large effusion probably responsible for the apparent lateral tilting of the patella (open white arrows) of the patella. A thickened lateral retinaculum (5 degrees, arrow heads) is noted secondary to two prior lateral retinacular release surgeries.

Recently, our group has been involved in an investigation designed to assess the patellofemoral joint during open-chain (i.e., with the foot off the ground, the tibia moving "freely") and closed-chain (i.e., with the foot on the ground, the tibia "fixed" during weight-bearing movement) activities. To accomplish this, we used a vertically opened MR system (0.5 Tesla, Signa SP, General Electric Medical Systems, Milwaukee, WI) that permits the patient to undergo dynamic MR imaging (i.e., using a fast spoiled GRASS pulse sequence) in upright and seated positions (Figure 9.20A). To our knowledge, this is the first time that patellofemoral relationships have been visualized with the patient in a weight-bearing position. Additionally, the goal of this research was to evaluate the effects of two different braces on patellofemoral relationships with the patient performing open- and closed-chain movements (Figures 9.20B to 9.20E). Preliminary results have indicated that patellar tracking is qualitatively different comparing open- and closed-chain activity, while bracing may or may not improve the abnormal position of the patella, depending on the underlying anatomy and severity of patellofemoral dysfunction for a given patient.

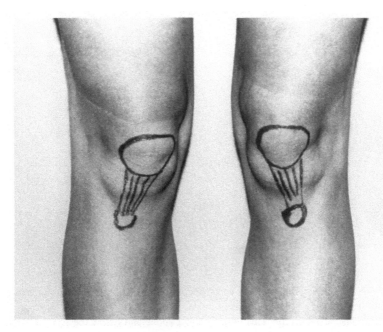

FIGURE 9.16   Bilateral internal rotation of the lower extremities. Medial subluxation of the patella has been reported to occur in association with excessive internal rotation.

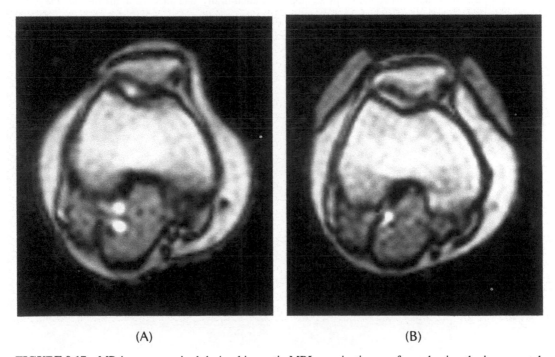

(A)   (B)

FIGURE 9.17   MR images acquired during kinematic MRI examinations performed using the incremental, passive positioning technique (axial plane; T1-weighted, spin echo) to illustrate the effect of conservative treatment. (A) MR image shows severe medial subluxation of the patella. (B) MR image obtained with application of a patellar realignment brace (P3, Baurfeind, Kennesaw, GA). Note that the brace moved the patella into a more centralized position relative to the femoral trochlear groove.

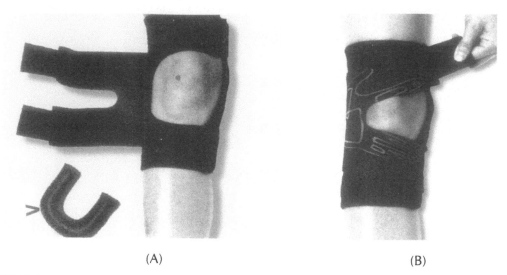

(A)   (B)

FIGURE 9.18   The Shields Patellar Stabilizing Brace used for conservative treatment of patellar subluxation. (A) This brace consists of a neoprene cuff with a posterior cut-out, a U-shaped buttress (arrow), and two Neoprene straps. The cuff is placed around the knee and fastened above and below the patellofemoral joint via Velcro components. Care is taken to ensure that the patella is centrally located within the brace. The patella is palpated and the U-shaped buttress is placed directly against the lateral side of the patella. (B) Next, the buttress is pushed medially while the straps are applied, pulled firmly, and attached to the medial side of the brace, creating a counter force acting on a laterally subluxated patella.

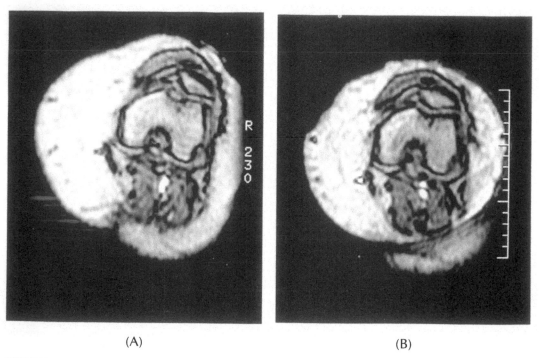

(A)   (B)

FIGURE 9.19   MR images acquired during kinematic MRI examinations performed using the active movement against resistance technique (axial plane; fast spoiled gradient echo) to illustrate the effect of conservative treatment. (A) MR image shows lateral subluxation of the patella. (B) MR image obtained after application of the Shields Patellar Stabilizing Brace. Note that the brace moved the patella into a more centralized position relative to the femoral trochlear groove.

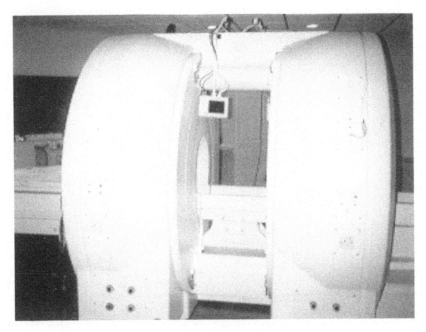

FIGURE 9.20A Vertically opened MR system (0.5 Tesla, Signa SP, General Electric Medical Systems, Milwaukee, WI) used for upright, loaded kinematic MRI examination.

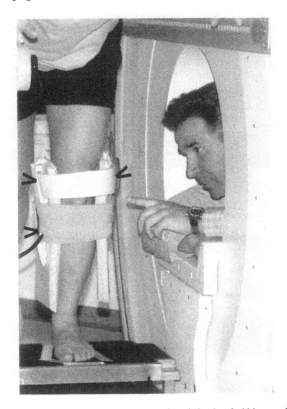

FIGURE 9.20B Preparation of patient for performance of upright, loaded kinematic MRI examination. Note the investigator inside the bore of the magnet, positioned to monitor the degree of joint flexion. Also shown is the flexible transmit-receive RF coil used for this procedure (arrow heads).

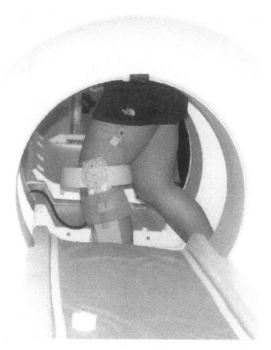

FIGURE 9.20C   Side view of patient performing upright, loaded movement of the patellofemoral joint.

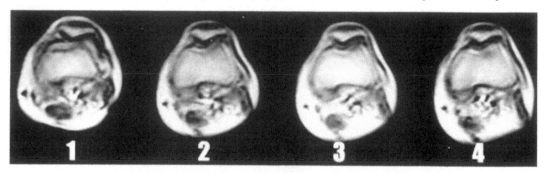

FIGURE 9.20D   Kinematic MRI examination of the left patellofemoral joint obtained using the upright, loaded technique (axial plane; fast spoiled gradient echo) showing lateral subluxation of the patella during the early increments of knee flexion (1, 2). Note the centralization of the patella at the higher increments of knee flexion (3, 4).

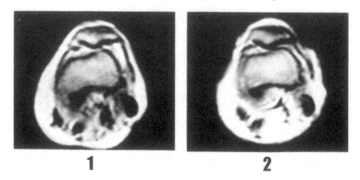

FIGURE 9.20E   MR images acquired during kinematic MRI examinations performed using the upright, loaded technique (axial plane; fast spoiled gradient echo) to illustrate the effect of conservative treatment (1, no brace; 2, brace applied). (1) Without the brace, there is substantial lateral subluxation of the patella and patella alta. (2) Application of the brace improves the position of the patella, moving it into a more central position.

IV. SUMMARY AND CONCLUSIONS

Proper identification and classification of abnormal patellar alignment and tracking is crucial for an optimal decision to be made concerning appropriate treatment. While the use of clinical criteria to document and characterize patellofemoral disorders is often challenging, objective functional information can be obtained for patellar alignment and tracking using kinematic MRI. Therefore, the use of this imaging procedure should be considered when evaluating the patient with patellofemoral pain.

REFERENCES

1. Fulkerson, J. P. and Hungerford, D. S., *Disorders of the Patellofemoral Joint,* 2nd edition, Williams & Wilkins, Baltimore, 1990.
2. Insall, J., Falvo, K. A., and Wise, D. W., Patellar pain and incongruence. II. Clinical application, *Clin. Orthop.,* 176, 225, 1983.
3. Moller, B. N., Krebs, B., and Jurik, A. G., Patellofemoral incongruence in chondromalacia and instability of the patella, *Acta Orthop. Scand.,* 57, 232, 1986.
4. Schutzer, S. F., Ramsby, G. R., and Fulkerson, J. P., Computed tomographic classification of patellofemoral joint pain patients, *Orthop. Clin. North Am.,* 17, 235, 1986.
5. Amis, A. A. and Faramand, F., Biomechanics of the knee extensor mechanism, *Knee,* 3, 73, 1996.
6. Pfirrmann, C. W. A., Zanetti, M., Romero, J., and Hodler, J., Femoral trochlear dysplasia: MR findings, *Radiology,* 216, 858, 2000.
7. Fox, J. and Del Pizzo, W., *The Patellofemoral Joint,* McGraw-Hill, New York, 1993.
8. Moller, B. N., Moller-Larsen, F., and Frich, L. H., Chondromalacia induced by patellar subluxation in the rabbit, *Acta Orthop. Scand.,* 60, 188, 1989.
9. Insall, J., Chondromalacia patellae: patellar malalignment syndrome, *Orthop. Clin. North Am.,* 10, 117, 1979.
10. Brown, S. M. and Bradley, W. G., Kinematic magnetic resonance imaging of the knee, *MRI Clin. North Am.,* 2, 441, 1994.
11. Shellock, F. G., Deutsch, A., and Mink, J. M., MR imaging assessment of internal derangement of the knee and patellar tracking abnormalities: high incidence of combined abnormalities, *Radiology,* 201(P), 170, 1996.
12. Shellock, F. G., Mink, J. H., Deutsch, A. L., Fox, J. M., and Ferkel R. D., Evaluation of patients with persistent symptoms after lateral retinacular release by kinematic magnetic resonance imaging of the patellofemoral joint, *Arthroscopy,* 6, 226, 1990.
13. Merchant, A. C., Mercer, R. L., Jacobsen, R. H., and Cool, C. R., Roentgenographic analysis of patellofemoral congruence, *J. Bone Joint Surg.,* 56A, 1391, 1974.
14. Laurin, C. A., Dussault, R., and Levesque, H. P., The tangential X-ray investigation of the patellofemoral joint: X-ray technique, diagnostic criteria and their interpretation, *Clin. Orthop.,* 144, 16–26, 1979.
15. Carson, W. G., James, S. L., Larson, R. L., Singer, K. M., and Winternitz, W. W., Patellofemoral disorders: physical and radiographic evaluation. II. Radiographic examination, *Clin. Orthop. Relat. Res.,* 185, 178–186, 1984.
16. Shellock, F. G., Mink, J. H., and Fox, J. M., Patellofemoral joint: kinematic MRI to assess tracking abnormalities, *Radiology,* 168, 551, 1988.
17. Shellock, F. G., Mink, J. H., Deutsch, A. L., and Fox, J. M., Evaluation of patellar tracking abnormalities using kinematic MRI: clinical experience in 130 patients, *Radiology,* 172, 799, 1989.
18. Kujala, U. M., Osterman, K., Kormano, M., Komu, M., and Schlenzka, D., Patellar motion analyzed by magnetic resonance imaging, *Acta Orthop. Scand.,* 60, 13, 1989.
19. Shellock, F. G., Mink, J. H., Deutsch, A. L., and Fox, J. M., Kinematic magnetic resonance imaging for evaluation of patellar tracking, *Physician Sports Med.,* 17, 99, 1989.
20. Shellock, F. G., Mink, J., Deutsch, A., and Fox, J., High incidence of medial subluxation of the patella identified by kinematic MR imaging, *Med. Sci. Sports Exercise,* 21, S90, 1989.
21. Kujala, U. M., Osterman, K., Kormano, M., Nelimarkka, O., Hurme, M., and Taimela, S., Patellofemoral relationships in recurrent patellar dislocation, *J. Bone Joint Surg. [Br.],* 71B, 788–792, 1989.

22. Kujala, U. M., Osterman, K., Kormano, M., Komu, M., and Schlenzka, D., Patellar motion analyzed by magnetic resonance imaging. *Acta Orthop. Scand.*, 60, 13–16, 1989.

23. Shellock, F. G. and Mandelbaum, B., Kinematic MRI of the joints, in *MRI of the Musculoskeletal System: A Teaching File*, Mink, J. H. and Deutsch, A., Eds., Raven Press, New York, 1990.

24. Koskinen, S. K., Hurme, M., Kujala, U. M., and Kormano, M., Effect of lateral release on patellar motion in chondromalacia: an MRI study of 11 knees, *Acta Orthop. Scand.*, 61, 311–312, 1990.

25. Shellock, F. G., Mink, J. H., Deutsch, A., Meeks, T., Fox, J., and Molnar, T., Axial loaded stress views and kinematic MRI evaluation of patellar alignment and tracking: results in 98 patellofemoral joints, *Radiology*, 177(P), 263, 1990.

26. Shellock, F. G., Cohen, M. S., Brady, T., Mink, J. H., and Pfaff, J. M., Evaluation of patellar alignment and tracking: comparison between kinematic MRI and "true" dynamic imaging by hyperscan MRI, *J. Magn. Reson. Imag.*, 1, 148, 1991.

27. Shellock, F. G., Fox, J. M., Deutsch, A., and Mink, J. H., Medial subluxation of the patella: Radiologic and physical findings, *Radiology*, 181(P), 179, 1991.

28. Shellock, F. G., Mink, J. H., and Fox, J. M., Identification of medial subluxation of the patella in a dancer using kinematic MRI of the patellofemoral joint: a case report, *Kinesiol. Med. Dance*, 13, 1–9, 1991.

29. Shellock, F. G., Foo, T. K. F., Deutsch, A., and Mink, J. H., Patellofemoral joint: evaluation during active flexion with ultrafast spoiled GRASS MR imaging, *Radiology* 180, 581–585, 1991.

30. Koskinen, S. K. and Kujala, U. M., Effect of patellar brace on patellofemoral relationships, *Scand. J. Med. Sci. Sports*, 1, 119–122, 1991.

31. Koskinen, S. K., Hurme, M., and Kujala, U. M., Restoration of patellofemoral congruity by combined lateral release and tibial tuberosity transposition as assessed by MRI analysis, *Int. Orthop.*, 15, 363–366, 1991.

32. Powers, C. M., Pfaff, M., and Shellock, F. G., Active movement, loaded kinematic MRI of the patellofemoral joint: reliability of quantitative measurements, *J. Magn. Reson. Imag.*, 8, 724–732, 1998.

33. Koskinen, S. K. and Kujala, U. M., Patellofemoral relationships and distal insertion of the vastus medialis muscle: a magnetic resonance imaging study in nonsymptomatic subjects and in patients with patellar dislocation, *Arthroscopy*, 8, 865–868, 1992.

34. Shellock, F. G., Mink, J. H., Deutsch, D. L., and Molnar, T., Effect of a newly-designed patellar realignment brace on patellofemoral relationships: a case report, *Med. Sci. Sports Exercise*, 27, 469, 1995.

35. Shellock, F. G., Mink, J. H., Deutsch, A. L., and Foo, T. K. F., Kinematic MR imaging of the patellofemoral joint: comparison between passive positioning and active movement techniques, *Radiology*, 84, 574–577, 1992.

36. Shellock, F. G., Mink, J. H., Deutsch, A. L., Foo, T. K. F., and Sullenberger, P., Patellofemoral joint: identification of abnormalities using active movement, "unloaded" vs "loaded" kinematic MR imaging techniques, *Radiology*, 88, 575–578, 1993.

37. Brossmann, J., Muhle, C., Schroder, C., Melchert, U. H., Spielmann, R. P., and Heller, M., Motion-triggered cine MR imaging: evaluation of patellar tracking patterns during active and passive knee extension, *Radiology*, 187, 205–212, 1993.

38. Brossmann, J., Muhle, C., Bull, C. C., Schroder, C., Melchert, U. H., Ziplies, J., Spielmann, R. P., and Heller, M., Evaluation of patellar tracking in patients with suspected patellar malalignment: cine MR imaging vs. arthroscopy, *Am. J. Roentgen.*, 162, 361–367, 1993.

39. Shellock, F. G., Mink, J. H., Deutsch, A. L., Fox, J., Molnar, T., and Kvitne, R., Effect of a patellar realignment brace on patellofemoral relationships: evaluation using kinematic MR imaging, *J. Magn. Reson. Imag.*, 4, 590–594, 1994.

40. Brossmann, J., Muhle, C., Bull, C. C., Zieplies, J., Melchert, U. H. et al., Cine MR imaging before and after realignment surgery for patellar tracking: comparison with axial radiographs, *Skeletal Radiol.*, 24, 191–196, 1995.

41. Shellock, F. G., Kinematic MRI of the joints, in *Magnetic Resonance Imaging in Orthopaedics and Rheumatology*, 2nd edition, Stoller, D. W., Ed., Lippincott-Raven, Philadelphia, 1996.

42. Shellock, F. G., Kinematic MRI of the joints, *Semin. Musculoskeletal Radiol. MR Imag. Sports Med.*, 1, 143, 1997.

43. Witonski, D. and Goraj, B., Pateller motion analyzed by kinematic and dynamic axial magnetic resonance imaging in patients with anterior knee pain syndrome, *Arch. Orthop. Trauma Surg.,* 119, 46–49, 1999.

44. Muhle, C., Brossmann, J., and Heller, M., Kinematic CT and MR imaging of the patellofemoral joint, *Eur. Radiol.,* 9, 508–518, 1999.

45. Shellock, F. G., Stone, K. R., Crues, J. V., Development and clinical application of kinematic MRI of the patellofemoral joint using an extremity MR system, *Med. Sci. Sports Exercise,* 31, 788–791, 1999.

46. Otis, J. C. and Gould, J. D., The effect of external load on torque production by knee extensors, *J. Bone Joint Surg.,* 68A, 65–70, 1986.

47. Nordin, M. and Frankel, V. H., *Basic Biomechanics of the Musculoskeletal System,* 2nd edition, Lea & Febiger, Philadelphia, 1989.

48. Deutsch, A. D., Shellock, F. G., and Mink, J. H., Imaging of the patellofemoral joint: emphasis on advanced techniques, in *The Patellofemoral Joint,* Fox, J. and Del Pizzo, W., Eds., McGraw-Hill, New York, 1993.

49. Conway, W. F., Hayes, C. W., Loughran, T., Totty, W. G., Griffeth, L. K., El-Khoury, G. Y., and Shellock, F. G., Cross-sectional imaging of the patellofemoral joint and surrounding structures, *RadioGraphics,* 11, 195–211, 1991.

50. Staubli, H. U., Durrenmatt, U., Porcellini, B., and Rauschning, W., Anatomy and surface geometry of the patellofemoral joint in the axial plane, *J. Bone Joint Surg. [Br.],* 81B, 452–458, 1999.

51. Lancourt, J. E. and Cristini, J. A., Patella alta and patella infera. Their etiological role in patellar dislocation, chondromalacia, and apophysitis of the tibial tubercle, *J. Bone Joint Surg.,* 57A, 1112, 1975.

52. Marks, K. E. and Bentley, G., Patella alta and chondromalacia, *J. Bone Joint Surg.,* 60B, 71, 1978.

53. Shellock, F. G., Kim, S., Mink, J., Deutsch, A., and Fox, J., "Functional" patella alta determined by axial plane imaging of the patellofemoral joint: association with abnormal patellar alignment and tracking, *J. Magn. Reson. Imag.,* 2(P), 93, 1992.

54. Eppley, R. A., Medial patellar subluxation, in *The Patellofemoral Joint,* Fox, J. and Del Pizzo, W., Eds., McGraw-Hill, New York, 1993, chap. 9.

55. Hughston, J. C. and Deese, M., Medial subluxation of the patella as a complication of lateral release, *Am. J. Sports Med.,* 16, 383, 1988.

56. Shellock, F. G., The effect of a patellar stabilizing brace on lateral subluxation of the patella: assessment using kinematic MRI, *Am. J. Knee Surg.,* 13, 137, 2000.

57. Arroll, B., Ellis-Pegler, E., Edwards, A., Sutcliffe, G., Patellofemoral pain syndrome. A critical review of the clinical trials on nonoperative therapy, *Am. J. Sports Med.,* 25, 207–212, 1997.

58. Henry, J. H., Conservative treatment of patellofemoral subluxation, in *Clinics in Sports Medicine: Patellofemoral Problems,* Henry, J. H., Ed., Saunders, Philadelphia, 1990, 261–278.

59. Molnar, T. J., Patellar rehabilitation, in *The Patellofemoral Joint,* Fox, J. and Del Pizzo, W., Eds., McGraw-Hill, New York, 1993, chap 24.

60. McConnell, J. S., The management of chondromalacia patellae, *Aust. J. Phys.,* 31, 215, 1986.

61. Worrell, T., Ingersoll, C. D., Brockrath-Pugliese, K., and Minis, P., Effect of patellar taping and bracing on patellar position as determined by MRI in patients with patellofemoral pain, *J. Athletic Training,* 33, 16–20, 1998.

62. Worrell, T. W., Ingersoll, C. D., and Farr, J., Effect of patellar taping and bracing on patellar position. An MRI study, *J. Sports Rehabil.,* 3, 146–153, 1994.

63. Shellock, F. G., Mullen, M., Stone, K., Coleman, M., and Crues, J. V., Kinematic MRI evaluation of the effect of bracing on patellar positions: qualitative assessment using an extremity MR system, *J. Athletic Training,* 35, 44–49, 2000.

64. Worrell, T., Ingersoll, C. D., Bockrath-Pugliese, K., and Minis, P., Effect of patellar taping and bracing on patellar position as determined by MRI in patients with patellofemoral pain, *J. Athletic Training,* 33, 16–20, 1998.

65. Worrell, T. W., Ingersoll, C. D., and Farr, J., Effect of patellar taping and bracing on patellar position: an MRI case study, *J. Sports Rehabil.,* 3, 146–153, 1994.

66. Powers, C. M., Shellock, F. G., Beering, T. V., Garrido, D. E., Goldbach, R. M., and Molnar, T., Effect of bracing on patellar kinematics in patients with patellofemoral joint pain, *Med. Sci. Sports Exercise,* 31, 1714–1720, 1999.
67. Muhle, C., Brinkmann, G., Skaf, A., Heller, M., and Resnick, D., Effect of a patellar realignment brace on patients with patellar subluxation and dislocation. Evaluation with kinematic magnetic resonance imaging, *Am. J. Sports Med.,* 27, 350, 1999.
68. Shellock, F. G., Unpublished observations, 1987.
69. Shellock, F. G., Unpublished observations, 1990.

Part V

Shoulder

10 The Shoulder: Functional Anatomy and Kinesiology

Gretchen B. Salsich and Samuel R. Ward

CONTENTS

0-8493-0807-0/01/$0.00+$.50
© 2001 by Frank G. Shellock

I. INTRODUCTION

The glenohumeral joint allows for a high degree of upper limb mobility, which is necessary to move the hand through space. However, the configuration of the shoulder articulation sacrifices stability.[1] As a result, the shoulder requires substantial muscle activity and ligamentous support to maintain its integrity and move against resistance.[1] This combination of a high degree of mobility, limited bony stability, and high muscular demand places the shoulder at risk for various injuries and subsequent development of joint pathology. This chapter will present the functional anatomy, normal kinesiology, and pathokinesiology of the shoulder.

II. FUNCTIONAL ANATOMY

A. OSSEOUS ANATOMY AND ARTICULATING SURFACES

1. The Humerus and Glenoid Fossa

The convex head of the humerus and the concave glenoid fossa of the scapula form the articulating surfaces of the glenohumeral joint (Figure 10.1). The surface of the glenoid is shallow and is approximately one third the size of the humeral head,[2] resulting in poor bony congruency. The orientation of the humeral head is such that its articulating surface faces superiorly, medially, and posteriorly,[2] forming angles between the humeral head and the humeral shaft of approximately 130 to 150 degrees in the frontal plane and 20 to 30 degrees in the transverse plane (posterior).[3] The shape of the glenoid fossa has been described as an inverted comma,[4] narrow at the superior margin and broad inferiorly.

In the transverse plane, the orientation of the articulating surface is variable. Saha reported that, in normal subjects, the fossa is oriented posteriorly, while subjects with recurrent anterior dislocation have an anteriorly oriented fossa.[2] In the frontal plane, the orientation of the glenoid is described as being inferior.[2,4-6]

2. The Acromion

The acromion process of the scapula is located superior and posterior to the glenoid fossa and plays an important role in both normal and pathologic shoulder mechanics (Figure 10.1). Forming

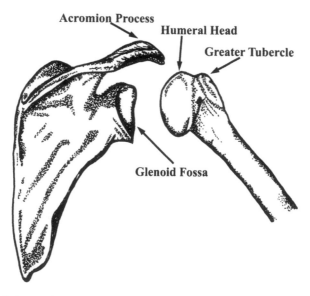

FIGURE 10.1   Articulating surfaces of the glenohumeral joint.

the postero-superior aspect of the coracoacromial arch, the acromion provides protection for the rotator cuff tendons.[1] However, the acromium may also contribute to irritation of subacromial structures due to its proximity to the humeral head. Weiner and Macnab reported acromio-humeral distances of 7 to 14 mm in subjects without shoulder pathology, suggesting that individuals with intervals less than 5 mm may be at risk for rotator cuff injuries.[7]

3. The Coracoid Process

The coracoid process arises from the neck of the scapula and is anterior and inferior to the acromion process. Structurally, the coracoid is an important site for ligamentous and muscular attachment. It forms the anterior portion of the coracoacromial arch.[1] By partially covering the humeral head, the coracoacromial arch adds protection, anteriorly.[4]

B. EXTRACAPSULAR STRUCTURES

1. The Capsule and Ligaments

The shoulder capsule is a multilayered structure composed of collagen fiber bundles.[8] It surrounds the glenohumeral joint and is approximately twice the volume of the humeral head, allowing for a high degree of mobility[4] (Figure 10.2). Although the configuration of the capsule varies among individuals, it generally arises from the glenoid labrum and surrounding bone, inserting distally on the upper portion of the anatomic neck of the humerus.[4]

The inside of the capsule is covered by a synovial membrane that extends distally to line the bicipital groove.[4] When the arm is abducted and externally rotated, the joint capsule twists upon itself and becomes taut, making abduction and external rotation the close-packed position of the glenohumeral joint.[9]

As a result of the orientation of the fibers and the amount of collagen fibers present, the regions of the joint capsule vary in strength. Gohlke et al. reported that the anteroinferior portion of the

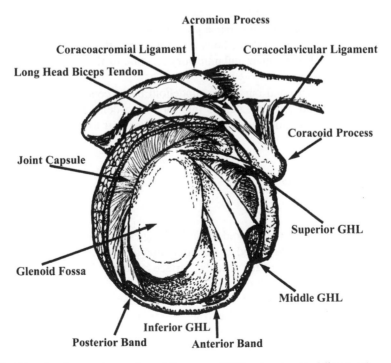

FIGURE 10.2 The glenohumeral capsule and ligaments (GHL, glenohumeral ligament).

capsule is thickest and strongest.[8] Anteriorly, the capsule thickens to form three glenohumeral ligaments (superior, middle, and inferior) that enhance the stability of the glenohumeral joint by preventing anterior subluxation of the humeral head[10-13] (Figure 10.2).

The superior glenohumeral ligament arises from the antero-superior labrum and inserts superior to the lesser tuberosity of the humerus[10] (Figure 10.2). The middle glenohumeral ligament originates from the glenoid labrum, just inferior to the superior glenohumeral ligament, and inserts on the lesser tuberosity with the tendon of the subscapularis.[10,14] The middle glenohumeral ligament is important for anterior stability in the midrange of arm elevation. The inferior glenohumeral ligament originates from the antero-inferior labrum and inserts on the medial border of the lesser tuberosity of the humerus (Figure 10.2).

O'Brien and co-workers describe three portions of the inferior glenohumeral ligament: (1) the anterior band, (2) the posterior band, and (3) the axillary pouch.[12] The inferior gleno-humeral ligament is important for inferior stability at higher ranges of arm elevation, but more importantly, for anterior inferior stability with the arm in abduction and external rotation (similar to a throwing motion). Posteriorly, the glenohumeral joint capsule is thinnest and has no distinct ligaments.[15]

In addition to the glenohumeral ligaments, the coracoacromial and coracohumeral ligaments have important anatomical and functional significance for the shoulder. The coracohumeral ligament arises from the base of the coracoid process and inserts on the greater and lesser tuberosities of the humerus,[10] adding anterior support to the capsular structures. The coracoac-romial ligament, extending from the superior surface of the coracoid process to the anterior surface of the acromion, forms the antero-superior portion of the coracoacromial arch[4] (Figure 10.2). The coracoacromial arch provides protection for the humeral head and rotator cuff tendons. Notably, the coracoacromial arch is frequently the site of impingement for subacromial structures during elevation of the arm.[4]

2. Bursae

The subacromial bursa is a fluid-filled sac situated between the supraspinatus and deltoid muscles in the subacromial space. Normally, this bursa provides for smooth gliding between the coracoac-romial arch and the rotator cuff tendons; however, it may be affected by calcification or tears of the tendonous structures. The resultant inflammatory reaction of the bursa may promote impinge-ment of subacromial structures.[4]

In addition to the subacromial bursa, the subdeltoid bursa contributes to the smooth gliding characteristics of the shoulder joint. Located inferior to the deltoid muscle and superior to the rotator cuff tendons, the subdeltoid bursa permits the rotator cuff to glide beneath the deltoid and acromion as the arm is elevated.[16]

C. Intracapsular Structures

1. The Glenoid Labrum

Surrounding the outer edge of the glenoid fossa is the glenoid labrum, a band of dense fibrous connective tissue that has been described as a continuation of the joint capsule[11] (Figure 10.3). The labrum increases the contact area of the articular surface by deepening the glenoid fossa,[11,17,18] and provides an attachment site for the long head of the biceps.

The functional significance of the labrum remains unclear. It appears to offer little structural support,[11,19] as it provides minimal resistance to anterior translation of the humeral head.[20] However, Pagnani et al. reported mild to moderate increases in glenohumeral translations after inducing superior labral lesions by detaching the biceps tendon.[21]

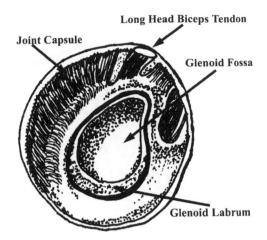

FIGURE 10.3 The glenoid fossa and labrum.

III. NORMAL KINEMATICS

A. OSTEOKINEMATICS

Osteokinematic movements of the glenohumeral joint are generally described relative to the sagittal, frontal, and transverse planes[22] (Figure 10.4). The large degree of motion available in each plane allows the upper extremity to move through space and position the hand for optimal function. In addition, the scapula provides a stable base for the humerus and contributes to shoulder motion by upwardly rotating as the arm is moved away from the body.

1. Humeral Elevation

Elevation is the general term used to describe movement of the humerus away from the thorax (e.g., in front or to the side of the body). Abduction is elevation of the humerus in the frontal plane, and most authors report maximal humeral abduction values of approximately 120° with the scapula fixed.[16,23] If the scapula is free to rotate in an upward direction, approximately 180° of shoulder abduction can be achieved.[22,23]

Sagittal plane elevation (flexion) has maximal humeral and scapular range values that are similar to those of abduction.[16,23] In addition to frontal and sagittal plane elevation, elevation of the humerus

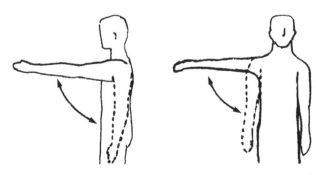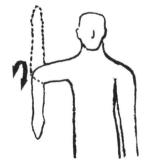

Flexion/Extension   Abduction/Adduction   Internal/External Rotation

FIGURE 10.4 Osteokinematic motions of the glenohumeral joint: (A) flexion and extension, (B) abduction and adduction, (C) internal and external rotation.

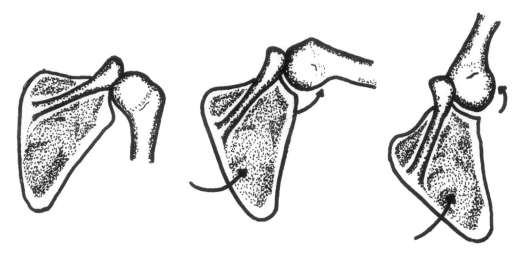

FIGURE 10.5   Humeral elevation with associated scapular rotation.

has been described relative to the plane of the scapula, located approximately 30 degrees anterior to the frontal plane.[5,24] In this position, the shoulder capsule is relatively untwisted, and the humerus and scapula are oriented in the same plane allowing more "pure" humeral elevation.[24] Maximum elevation in the scapular plane is similar to that of flexion and abduction.[25]

While researchers generally agree that upward rotation of the scapula is necessary to achieve full shoulder elevation, there are inconsistencies regarding the ratio of humeral to scapular movement. Inman et al.[23] described a 2:1 relationship during shoulder abduction from 30° to 170°, in that for every two degrees of humeral abduction, there is 1° of upward rotation of the scapula.

When shoulder elevation in the plane of the scapula was assessed, Freedman and Munro observed a 3:2 ratio over the full range of elevation,[5] while Poppen and Walker reported a 5:4 ratio beyond 30° of humeral elevation.[6] While the relative contributions of the scapula and humerus to shoulder elevation remain unclear, it is widely accepted that upward scapular rotation is a necessary component of full shoulder elevation (Figure 10.5).

2. Humeral Rotation

Rotation of the humerus in the transverse plane is another functionally important shoulder motion. With internal rotation, the humerus rotates toward the midline of the body, whereas with external rotation the humerus rotates away from the body's center. Maximum range values for internal and external rotation vary considerably, depending on the degree of humeral elevation. In general, approximately 90° of both internal and external rotation can be achieved, for a total range of 180°.[22,26]

3. Coupled Motions (Rotation with Elevation)

In addition to providing greater degrees of freedom for the hand to function in space, glenohumeral rotation is a necessary component of maximal humeral elevation. However, there is some controversy regarding the direction of rotation that occurs with elevation.

In general, with humeral elevation greater than 90°, the configuration of the glenohumeral articulating surfaces produces external rotation,[16,23,27] which allows the greater tuberosity to clear the acromion process. Findings to the contrary have been observed by Blakely and Palmer,[28] who reported internal humeral rotation with active elevation in the sagittal plane (flexion). Regardless of the direction of rotation or the plane of elevation, full humeral elevation cannot be achieved without the coupling motion of rotation.

B. ARTHROKINEMATICS

1. Humeral Elevation

To achieve maximal joint motion with minimal joint stress during shoulder movements, subtle humeral head motion occurs at the glenohumeral articulating surface. Three types of surface motion (arthrokinematics) have been described — rotation, rolling, and translation (gliding). These motions may occur in any given plane.[22]

During rotation, the contact point on the glenoid remains constant, while the contact point on the humeral head changes (Figure 10.6). This rotation permits the humeral head to remain in contact with the glenoid as it rotates. During rolling, both contact surfaces change by an equal amount, the consequence of which would be humeral dislocation if left unopposed (Figure 10.6). During translation, the contact area on the humerus remains constant while the contact area on the glenoid changes, resulting in a gliding motion of the humerus on the glenoid[22] (Figure 10.6).

During humeral elevation in individuals without shoulder pathology, the primary arthrokinematic motion of the glenohumeral joint is rotation, but some translation and rolling may occur.

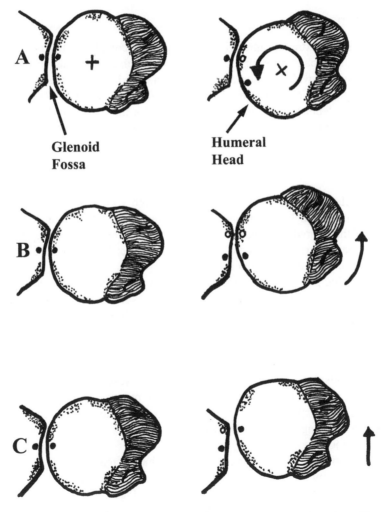

FIGURE 10.6 Arthrokinematic motions of the glenohumeral joint: (A) rotation, (B) rolling, (C) translation (gliding). (Adapted from Nordin, M. and Frankel, V. H., *Basic Biomechanics of the Musculoskeletal System*, 2nd edition, Lea & Febiger, Philadelphia, 1989, 231. With permission.)

Poppen and Walker reported that the average upward movement of the humeral head in the glenoid (an indication of translation or rolling) was 3 mm during humeral elevation from 0° to approximately 60°.[6] After 60° of elevation, superior humeral movement was approximately 1 mm.[6] Similar findings regarding humeral head movement during abduction in healthy subjects have been reported by Beaulieu et al.[29] (notably, Bealieu et al. characterized these movements using kinematic MRI of the shoulder; see Chapter 11 in this text). These investigators stated that the average humeral head displacement throughout the entire range of abduction was less than 3 mm.[29]

2. Humeral Rotation

In addition to assisting humeral elevation, arthrokinematic motions assist internal and external rotation of the humerus. As in elevation, the primary arthrokinematic motion during internal and external rotation is rotation, indicating that the humeral head remains fairly well stabilized within the glenoid. Beaulieu et al.[29] report humeral head translations in the anterior/posterior direction of less than 4 mm throughout the range of internal and external rotation, while Rhoad et al.[30] report average humeral head translations of 2.1 mm.

C. Muscular Action

Movement of the upper extremity through space requires a complex pattern of muscle activity. In general, elevation of the humerus requires muscle force to raise the arm against gravity, to stabilize the humeral head and provide a stable axis of rotation,[23] and to rotate the scapula on the thorax. Based on these functional requirements, the muscles acting at the shoulder can be grouped into three categories: (1) glenohumeral (muscles responsible for movement of the humerus); (2) rotator cuff (muscles responsible for stabilizing the humeral head within the glenoid); and (3) scapulothoracic (muscles responsible for stabilizing and moving the scapula on the thorax).

1. Abduction

The primary muscles responsible for humeral abduction (prime movers) are the deltoid and supraspinatus muscles, which act throughout the entire range of motion[23,31] (Figure 10.7). The middle portion of the deltoid, originating from the acromion process and inserting on the deltoid tubercle of the humerus, provides the strongest abduction force;[32] however, the supraspinatus muscle also adds a significant abduction component.[32]

In addition to being prime movers, stabilizing muscles must be active to achieve full abduction. The rotator cuff muscles (supraspinatus, infraspinatus, teres minor, and subscapularis) stabilize the humeral head in the glenoid fossa and provide a relatively fixed axis of rotation. Without rotator cuff muscle activity, full humeral elevation would not be possible.[23,32]

The supraspinatus arises from the supraspinous fossa and inserts on the superior aspect of the greater tuberosity, between the infraspinatus and subscapularis tendons (Figure 10.8).[32] The infraspinatus originates from the infraspinous fossa of the scapula, and the teres minor from the lateral border of the scapula. Both muscles insert into the posterior aspect of the greater tuberosity (Figure 10.8).[32] The subscapularis originates on the costal surface of the scapula and inserts into the lesser tuberosity. Fusing with the shoulder capsule, the rotator cuff tendons add reinforcement to the glenohumeral joint.[1]

The fiber orientation of the supraspinatus is such that it creates a superior shear force acting on the glenohumeral joint,[3,32] which is counteracted by the inferior shear force components of the infraspinatus, teres minor, and subscapularis muscles[3,32] (Figure 10.8). Furthermore, the anterior force component of the subscapularis is counteracted by the posterior force component of the infraspinatus and teres minor, which minimizes horizontal humeral displacement.[2] The end result is that with shoulder abduction, almost pure rotation occurs about the glenohumeral joint axis.

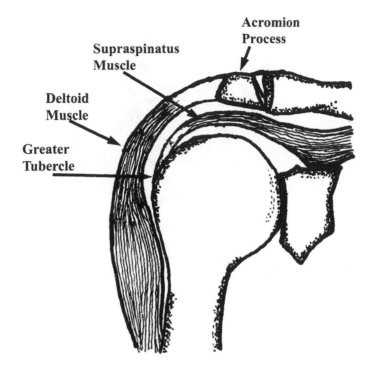

FIGURE 10.7   Prime movers for humeral abduction (deltoid and supraspinatus muscles).

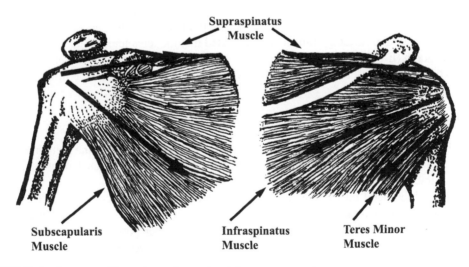

FIGURE 10.8   Rotator cuff muscles and associated force components.

2. Flexion

There are many biomechanical similarities between shoulder flexion and abduction, but slight differences in muscle requirements exist. The activity of the rotator cuff muscles in stabilizing the humeral head is essentially the same in flexion as it is in abduction;[23] however, prime mover activity is somewhat different. The clavicular head of the pectoralis major and the anterior portion of the deltoid are the major muscles of flexion,[4,23,33] while the biceps muscle (both long and short heads) contributes to a lesser extent.[31]

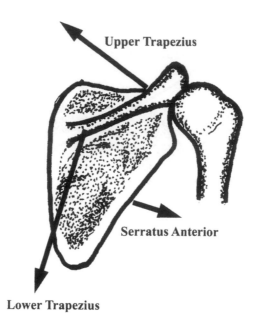

FIGURE 10.9   Muscular force couple of the scapula.

3. Humeral Rotation

Internal humeral rotation is achieved primarily through activation of the pectoralis major and latissimus dorsi muscles;[1] however, the subscapularis and anterior deltoid also contribute.[34] The teres major, while anatomically oriented to contribute to internal rotation, appears to be most active in maintaining static positions.[23] Inman et al. reported that the teres major muscle had the greatest electromyograph (EMG) activity at 90° abduction and that muscle activity increased with increasing loads.[23] The primary muscles responsible for external humeral rotation are the infraspinatus, teres minor, and posterior deltoid.[35]

4. Scapular Rotation

Although the muscles responsible for scapular rotation do not act directly at the glenohumeral joint, they make an important contribution to glenohumeral mechanics. As stated previously, upward rotation of the scapula is necessary for full humeral elevation.

The scapulohumeral muscles responsible for creating this rotation comprise a "force couple" in that their opposing translatory force components offset each other, resulting in almost pure rotation of the scapula. For example, the upper trapezius, upper portion of the serratus anterior, and levator scapula elevate the scapula via their superior force vectors (Figure 10.9). The lower trapezius and lower portion of the serratus anterior move the scapula inferiorly, and the middle trapezius acts to fix the scapula against the thorax.[23] The net result of simultaneous activity of these scapular muscles during humeral elevation is upward rotation of the scapula,[16,23] which permits full humeral elevation.

IV. PATHOKINESIOLOGY: CLINICAL IMPLICATIONS AND RELEVANCE

Shoulder movement is complex, requiring the synchronized motion of multiple articulations. The complexity of this motion leaves a variety of tissues at risk for pathology. Common pathologies include impingement syndrome and glenohumeral instability. Both of these conditions involve a variety of contributing factors. This section will define some of the subcategories of impingement syndrome and instability, as well as explain various contributing factors for these common clinical entities.

A. IMPINGEMENT SYNDROME

Impingement syndrome is defined as pathologic compression of the subacromial soft tissues between the proximal humerus and the acromion process of the scapula. This disorder spans a continuum of severities, ranging from simple edema to tendinitis to frank tendon tears.

The clinical presentation of impingement syndrome varies with the severity of the injury. Neer originally described impingement syndrome as mechanical impingement of the subacromial bursa, supraspinatus tendon, or long head of the biceps tendon under the acromial arch.[36] He proposed a classification system (stages I to III), based on a patient's clinical presentation, that describes the extent to which structures are affected.[36]

Stage I is the mildest form of impingement and is usually found in younger patients. It involves edema and hemorrhage of the subacromial soft tissues; however, patients appear strong on clinical examination.[36] Stage I usually manifests itself as pain when elevating the arm in an arc from 60° to 120° of abduction, or as point tenderness at the supraspinatus tendon.

Stage II is a moderate form of impingement, usually found in patients from 25 to 40 years of age. It involves tendinitis of the supraspinatus and/or long head of the biceps tendon and bursitis. Patients with stage II impingement syndrome may have limitations in range of motion in addition to pain.

Finally, stage III is the most severe form of impingement, usually affecting patients over 40 years of age. Clinically, stage III is characterized by weakness in shoulder abduction and external rotation.[36] These patients often have bone spur formation on the acromion and tendon disruption of either the supraspinatus or long head of the biceps tendon.[36]

1. Etiology

Although a variety of factors may contribute to impingement syndrome, only the most common will be discussed here. It is important to note that this condition is multifactorial in nature, meaning a variety of factors may contribute to impingement in any one patient.

a. Acromial architecture

Morrison and Bigliani proposed abnormal subacromial architecture may predispose tissues beneath the acromion to abnormal levels of compression.[37] These investigators described three shapes of the inferior surface of the acromion: type I, flat; type II, curved; type III, hooked[37] (Figure 10.10).

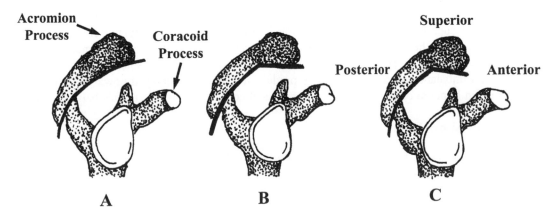

FIGURE 10.10   Acromial architecture: (A) type I (flat); (B) type II (curved); (C) type III (hooked).

From a functional standpoint, curved or hooked acromions would decrease the suprahumeral space and predispose tissues to abnormal compression. Dissection of 140 cadaver shoulders revealed a 34% incidence of full thickness rotator cuff tendon tears. Within this group 70% had type II or type III acromions.[37] The results of this study indicated that the relationship between narrowing of the suprahumeral space and impingement should be appreciated.

b. Vascular contributions to rotator cuff pathology

The region of greatest subacromial compression on the supraspinatus tendon is called the "critical zone." This region lies approximately 5 to 10 mm proximal to the insertion of this muscle onto the humeral tuberosity. The blood supply to the supraspinatus tendon is composed of the anastomoses of the arcuate artery (a branch of the anterior humeral circumflex artery that perfuses the humeral head), the suprascapular artery, and the posterior humeral circumflex artery. The orientation of these arteries was thought to leave the "critical zone" relatively hypovascular, predisposing this region to degeneration. However, recent *in vivo* studies suggest that this region becomes hypervascular in symptomatic cases of impingement.[38] Additionally, one group of investigators found subacromial pressures to exceed capillary refill pressures during forward shoulder flexion with a 1 kg weight in the hand.[39] The significance of these findings is that relatively small loads may impair circulation to this region. Therefore, hypovascularity may not cause symptomatic lesions in the "critical zone," but instead, repeated compression with high stress overhead activities may impair circulation, thereby contributing to lesion formation.

c. Biomechanical contributions to pathology

The second set of conditions contributing to impingement syndrome is biomechanical in nature. For example, poor dynamic control of shoulder elevation (particularly abduction) has been implicated as a cause of abnormal subacromial compression. As mentioned previously, contraction of the deltoid causes the humerus to elevate and the humeral head to slide vertically up the face of the glenoid (upward shear). If unrestrained, this shear effect would cause a significant amount of soft tissue compression between the humerus and the acromial arch.

The lower three rotator cuff muscles (subscapularis, infraspinatus, and teres minor) help to minimize subacromial compression by creating downward shear and compressive forces between the humeral head and the face of the glenoid. The infraspinatus and teres minor muscles also externally rotate the humerus during abduction to move the greater tubercle laterally, away from the acromion. Failure of the rotator cuff muscles to restrain upward shear of the humeral head and/or create enough external rotation to clear the humeral tuberosity from the acromion are potential causes of subacromial impingement.[40]

Abnormal scapular motion also has been implicated in subacromial impingement. During arm elevation, the scapula upwardly rotates which provides continued congruency between the glenoid and the humeral head, assures the length tension relationship of the rotator cuff muscles, and maintains the suprahumeral space. As previously mentioned, the primary muscles that control upward rotation of the scapula are the upper and lower portions of the trapezius muscle and the serratus anterior muscle. The balance of these muscular forces creates a smooth upward rotation; however, an imbalance in these forces may produce inadequate or delayed upward rotation. This may result in humeral contact with the acromion and compression of the tissues between them.[41]

B. GLENOHUMERAL INSTABILITY

As with impingement syndrome, the clinical presentation of a patient with instability varies with the severity of the injury. Mild instability may produce symptoms similar to impingement, while severe instability may present as a frank dislocation. Failure of the static stabilizers to maintain proper bony alignment can manifest itself as pain, clicking, and/or joint subluxation. The relationship between joint laxity, impingement, and subluxation will be discussed in the following sections.

1. Anterior Instability and Glenoid Labral Tears

Ninety-eight percent of all cases of shoulder instability are anterior in nature.[42] Stretching or tearing of the anterior-inferior glenohumeral ligaments causes anterior instability. Shoulder abduction and external rotation produce tension in the anterior and inferior glenohumeral ligaments as well as the anterior-inferior glenoid labrum. Activities that impart high loads to the arm in abduction and external rotation place the glenohumeral joint at risk for anterior instability.

The dynamic stabilizers located on the anterior and inferior surfaces of the joint (subscapularis and teres major) help to unload to static stabilizers in this area. Weakness of these muscles makes the joint even more susceptible to injury. For example, the combination of poor muscular support and high forces across the anterior-inferior joint during the throwing motion makes the inferior glenohumeral ligament, capsule, and labrum susceptible to permanent stretching (plastic deformation) or tearing. The exact mechanism by which capsulo-ligamentous stretching and/or labral tearing occurs is poorly understood, but the shoulder position at the time of injury is typically the same.

Permanent stretching of the anterior capsule and its associated ligaments is recognized clinically as hypermobility when the joint is stressed anteriorly. In extreme cases there may be a tear in the subscapularis tendon or a capsular–periosteal separation at the anterior-inferior glenoid (i.e., Bankart lesion).[43] Lesions to the labrum not only make the joint unstable but have been attributed to reduction in rotator cuff strength of up to 40%.[44]

2. Relationship between Anterior Ligamentous Laxity and Impingement

Another consideration in persons with anterior instability is the risk of secondary impingement syndrome. As anterior capsulolabral structures prevent excessive anterior translation of the humeral head across the glenoid face, instability may allow the humeral tuberosity to slide forward, approximating it with the anterior-inferior edge of the acromion process. Therefore, repeated anterior subluxation may contribute to supraspinatus pathology.

A staging system that reflects the relationship between impingement and anterior instability has been proposed by Jobe and Glousman.[45] Stage I is pure mechanical impingement and diagnosed with positive impingement signs in the absence of instability. Stage II is anterior instability and associated impingement, diagnosed with positive impingement and instability tests. Stage III is anterior instability and associated impingement, diagnosed with the same positive tests as stage II but also associated with generalized joint hyperelasticity. Stage IV is pure anterior instability, diagnosed with positive instability tests only.[45]

3. Posterior and Multidirectional Instability

Posterior glenohumeral dislocation and instability are much less common than anterior instability, accounting for only 2 to 4% of all cases.[42] Stretching or tearing of the posterior-inferior joint capsule, posterior band of the inferior glenohumeral ligament, and posterior labrum causes posterior instability. Biomechanically, activities that require internal rotation and horizontal adduction of the shoulder (i.e., deceleration phase of pitching) produce tension in these structures and can cause deformation. Traumatic events, such as falling on an outstretched arm, which force the humeral head posteriorly on the glenoid surface, also can damage the posterior capsule.

Multidirectional instability is more common than posterior instability but less common than anterior instability. Although the etiology of multidirectional instability is poorly understood, over 50% of these patients show signs of generalized ligamentous laxity.[42] These patients usually show signs of increased joint volume associated with laxity in the joint capsule and surrounding ligaments.[42]

Multidirectional instability is typically classified as follows: type I, global instability with dislocation of the humeral head in the inferior, posterior, and anterior directions; type II, instability that is characterized as dislocation in the anterior and inferior directions and subluxation in the posterior direction; type III, dislocation in the posterior and inferior directions and mild instability in the anterior-inferior direction; and type IV, instability in the anterior and posterior directions and no abnormal inferior translation.[42]

V. SUMMARY AND CONCLUSIONS

Shoulder movement is complex, requiring the synchronized motion of multiple articulations. The complexity of this motion, a result of muscle contraction and passive restraint, leaves a variety of tissues at risk for pathology. Common pathologies include impingement syndrome, glenohumeral instability, and glenoid labral tears. Accurate diagnosis and effective treatment of these conditions requires a thorough understanding of shoulder anatomy and biomechanics.

REFERENCES

1. Norkin, C. C. and Levangie, P. K., *Joint Structure and Function — A Comprehensive Analysis,* 2nd edition, F. Davis, Philadelphia, 1992, 207.
2. Saha, A. K., Dynamic stability of the glenohumeral joint, *Acta Orthop. Scand.,* 42, 491, 1971.
3. Sarrafian, S. K., Gross and functional anatomy of the shoulder, *Clin. Orthop. Relat. Res.,* 173, 11, 1983.
4. Rothman, R. H., Marvel, J. P. J., and Heppenstall, R. B., Anatomic considerations in glenohumeral joint, *Orthop. Clin. North Am.,* 6, 341, 1975.
5. Freedman, L. and Munro, R. R., Abduction of the arm in the scapular plane: scapular and glenohumeral movements. A roentgenographic study, *J. Bone Joint Surg. [Am.],* 48, 1503, 1966.
6. Poppen, N. K. and Walker, P. S., Normal and abnormal motion of the shoulder, *J. Bone Joint Surg. [Am.],* 58, 195, 1976.
7. Weiner, D. S. and Macnab, I., Superior migration of the humeral head. A radiological aid in the diagnosis of tears of the rotator cuff, *J. Bone Joint Surg. [Br.],* 52, 524, 1970.
8. Gohlke, F., Essigkrug, B., and Schmitz, F., The pattern of the collagen fiber bundles of the capsule of the glenohumeral joint, *J. Shoulder Elbow Surg.,* 3, 111, 1994.
9. MacConnail, M. A. and Basmajian, J. V., *Muscles and Movement: A Basis for Human Kinesiology,* Williams & Wilkins, Baltimore, 1969.
10. DePalma, A. F., Callery, G., and Bennett, G. A., Shoulder joint. I. Variational anatomy and degenerative lesions of the shoulder joint, Instructional Course Lectures, *American Academy of Orthopaedic Surgeons,* 6, 255, 1949.
11. Moseley, H. F. and Overgaard, B., The anterior capsular mechanism in recurrent anterior dislocation of the shoulder, *J. Bone Joint Surg. [Br.],* 44, 913, 1962.
12. O'Brien, S. J., Neves, M. C., Arnoczky, S. P., Rozbruck, S. R., Dicarlo, E. F., Warren, R. F., Schwartz, R., and Wickiewicz, T. L., The anatomy and histology of the inferior glenohumeral ligament complex of the shoulder, *Am. J. Sports Med.,* 18, 449, 1990.
13. Turkel, S. J., Panio, M. W., Marshall, J. L., and Girgis, F. G., Stabilizing mechanisms preventing anterior dislocation of the glenohumeral joint, *J. Bone Joint Surg. [Am.],* 63, 1208, 1981.
14. Ferrari, D. A., Capsular ligaments of the shoulder. Anatomical and functional study of the anterior superior capsule, *Am. J. Sports Med.,* 18, 20, 1990.
15. Moore, K. L., *Clinically Oriented Anatomy,* third edition, Williams & Wilkins, Baltimore, 1992.
16. Lucas, D. B., Biomechanics of the shoulder joint, *Arch. Surg.,* 107, 425, 1973.
17. Bowen, M. K. and Warren, R. F., Ligamentous control of shoulder stability based on selective cutting and static translation experiments, *Clin. Sports Med.,* 10, 757, 1991.
18. Howell, S. M. and Galinat, B. J., The glenoid-labral socket. A constrained articular surface, *Clin. Orthop. Relat. Res.,* 243, 122, 1989.
19. Reeves, B., Experiments on the tensile strength of the anterior capsular structures of the shoulder in man, *J. Bone Joint Surg. [Br.],* 50, 858, 1968.
20. Townley, C. O., The capsular mechanism in recurrent dislocation of the shoulder, *J. Bone Joint Surg. [Am.],* 32, 370, 1950.

21. Pagnani, M. J., Deng, X. H., Warren, R. F., Torzilli, P. A., and Altchek, D. W., Effect of lesions of the superior portion of the glenoid labrum on glenohumeral translation, *J. Bone Joint Surg. [Am.],* 77, 1003, 1995.

22. Zuckerman, J. D. and Matsen, F. A., *Basic Biomechanics of the Musculoskeletal System,* 2nd edition, Nordin, M. and Frankel, V. H., Eds., Lea & Febiger, Philadelphia, 1989, p. 225.

23. Inman, V. T., Saunders, J. B., and Abbott, L. C., Observations on the function of the shoulder joint, *J. Bone Joint Surg. [Am.],* 26, 1, 1944.

24. Johnston, T. B., The movements of the shoulder joint; a plea for the use of the 'plane of the scapula' as the plane of reference for movements occurring at the humero-scapular joint, *Br. J. Surg.,* 25, 252, 1937.

25. Browne, A. O., Hoffmeyer, P., Tanaka, S., An, K. N., and Morrey, B. F., Glenohumeral elevation studied in three dimensions, *J. Bone Joint Surg. [Br.],* 72, 843, 1990.

26. Bechtol, C. O., Biomechanics of the shoulder, *Clin. Orthop. Relat. Res.,* 37, 67, 1980.

27. An, K. N., Browne, A. O., Korinek, S., Tanaka, S., and Morrey, B. F., Three-dimensional kinematics of glenohumeral elevation, *J. Orthop. Res.,* 9, 143, 1991.

28. Blakely, R. L. and Palmer, M. L., Analysis of rotation accompanying shoulder flexion, *Phys. Ther.,* 64, 1214, 1984.

29. Beaulieu, C. F., Hodge, D. K., Bergman, A. G., Butts, K., Daniel, B. L., Napper, C. L., Darrow, R. D., Dumoulin, C. L., and Herfkens, R. J., Glenohumeral relationships during physiologic shoulder motion and stress testing: initial experience with open MR imaging and active imaging-plane registration, *Radiology,* 212, 699, 1999.

30. Rhoad, R. C., Klimkiewicz, J. J., Williams, G. R., Kesmodel, S. B., Udupa, J. K., Kneeland, J. B., and Iannotti, J. P., A new *in vivo* technique for three-dimensional shoulder kinematics analysis, *Skeletal Radiol.,* 27, 92, 1998.

31. Basmajian, J. V., The surgical anatomy and function of the arm-trunk mechanism, *Surg. Clin. North Am.,* 43, 1471, 1963.

32. Rosse, C. and Gaddum-Rosse, P., *Hollinshead's Textbook of Anatomy,* Lippincott-Raven, Philadelphia, 1997.

33. Basmajian, J. V. and Latif, A., Integrated actions and functions of the chief flexors of the elbow, *J. Bone Joint Surg. [Am.],* 39, 1106, 1957.

34. Schenkman, M. and Rugo De Cartaya, V., Kinesiology of the shoulder complex, *J. Orthop. Sports Phys. Ther.,* 8, 438, 1987.

35. Kendall, F. P., McCreary, E. K., and Provance, P. G., *Muscles, Testing and Function,* Williams & Wilkins, Baltimore, 1993.

36. Neer, C. S., Impingement lesions, *Clin. Orthop. Relat. Res.,* 173, 70, 1983.

37. Morrison, D. S. and Bigliani, L. U., The clinical significance of variations in acromial morphology, *Orthop. Trans.,* 11, 43, 1987.

38. Chansky, H. A. and Iannotti, J. P., The vascularity of the rotator cuff, *Clin. Sports Med.,* 10, 807, 1991.

39. Sigholm, C., Styf, J., Korner, S. et al., Pressure recording in the subacromial bursa, *J. Orthop. Res.,* 6, 123, 1988.

40. Magee, D. J., *Shoulder, Orthopedic Physical Assessment,* Magee, D. J., Ed., W.B. Saunders, Philadelphia, 1992, p. 90.

41. Paine, R. M. and Voight, M., The role of the scapula, *J. Orthop. Sports Phys. Ther.,* 18, 386, 1993.

42. Pagani, M. J. and Warren, R. F., Instability of the shoulder, in *The Upper Extremity in Sports Medicine,* Vol. 2, Nicholas, J. A. and Hershman, E. B., Eds., Mosby, St. Louis, 1995, p. 173.

43. Mattalino, A. J., Instabilities, in *Physical Therapy of the Shoulder,* Vol. 3, Donatelli, R. A., Ed., Churchill Livingstone, New York, 1997, 435.

44. Thein, L. A. and Greenfield, B. H., Impingement syndrome and impingement related instability, in *Physical Therapy of the Shoulder,* Donatelli, R. A., Ed., Churchill Livingstone, New York, 1997, chap. 3.

45. Jobe, F. W. and Glousman, R. E., Rotator cuff dysfunction and associated glenohumeral instability in the throwing athlete, in *Operative Techniques in Shoulder Surgery,* Paulos, L. E. and Tibone, J. E., Eds., Aspen Publishers, Gaithersburg, MD, 1991, 85.

11 Kinematic MRI of the Shoulder: Stress Testing and MR-Guided Physical Examination

Christopher F. Beaulieu and Garry E. Gold

CONTENTS

I. INTRODUCTION

The shoulder or glenohumeral (GH) joint is unique in that there exists a fine balance between mobility and stability. A certain amount of laxity (defined as asymptomatic passive translation of the humeral head on the glenoid) is required for maximal rotational mobility. Instability is a pathologic condition defined by pain or discomfort in association with excessive glenohumeral translation during active shoulder motion.[1,2]

Bankart[3] and Perthes[4] originally described detachment of the labrum and its closely associated anterior inferior glenohumeral ligament complex from the glenoid rim and scapular neck as the "essential lesion" leading to recurrent anterior dislocation. With subsequent clinical experience and biomechanical studies clarifying the roles of various glenohumeral components,[5-8] it is now generally recognized that recurrent anterior dislocation probably requires an additional component besides the Bankart lesion, such as stretching or plastic deformation of the capsule and/or tearing of the glenohumeral ligaments.[9,10]

Bankart, or "labral-ligamentous," lesions are often detectable using static, unenhanced magnetic resonance (MR) imaging[11,12] or MR arthrography.[12-16] When diagnosed, a variety of open and arthroscopic surgical methods exist for repair of the Bankart lesion. However, attempts using conventional, static view MRI to understand capsular contributions to GH joint stability have largely

0-8493-0807-0/01/$0.00+$.50
© 2001 by Frank G. Shellock

failed.[14,16] As such, the first task in operative GH joint stabilization is mainly a diagnostic one in which examination under anesthesia and diagnostic arthroscopy are used to correct or refine the preoperative diagnosis.[17] Obviously, this is not ideal for the patient or the orthopedist, neither of whom knows preoperatively whether open surgery or an entirely arthroscopic approach will be required to effectively treat the condition.

Based on emerging concepts from evaluation of GH joint instability using a specially designed, vertically opened MR system (0.5 Tesla Signa SP; General Electric Medical Systems, Milwaukee, WI), we believe that performance of a kinematic MRI examination involving joint motion and physical examination can provide a unique functional assessment of the capsular components of GH joint stability. If combined with high-quality, static MR imaging of anatomic components, a comprehensive diagnostic imaging evaluation of instability may become practical in the clinical setting.

In this chapter, we first discuss techniques for kinematic MRI of the shoulder using a vertically opened MR system, followed by a description of normal glenohumeral motion patterns and observations from other investigators using kinematic MRI techniques to evaluate the shoulder. Next, we describe findings obtained using kinematic MRI of the shoulder in patients with instability and early observations on mechanical impingement. Finally, needs for future research and validation will be addressed.

II. TECHNICAL ASPECTS

A. THE MAGNETIC RESONANCE SYSTEM AND PATIENT POSITIONING

Using a vertically opened MR system (0.5 Tesla, Signa SP; General Electric Medical Systems, Milwaukee, WI), basic techniques were developed to perform a kinematic MRI examination of the shoulder during active joint motion and physical examination. In addition, measurement tools were created for the quantification of glenohumeral motion patterns.[18,19]

Figure 11.1 shows an example of how the subject is positioned in the vertically opened MR system. Note that in this MR system, the subject can be positioned in either a sitting or lying position, and has a wide range of available physiologic motion of the shoulder. The vertically opened MR system configuration allows an examiner to approach the patient during the examination. While somewhat similar patient motions are possible in MR systems that are horizontally opened, this configuration is less amenable to an examiner working directly with the patient during a kinematic MRI procedure. Additionally, the vertically opened MR system is useful not only for motion imaging of the joint, but for static assessments of joint derangement in positions of function or stress, such as the apprehension position or in abduction and external rotation (ABER).[20,21] Facilitation of this type of kinematic MRI examination of the shoulder is augmented by the presence of a monitor (liquid crystal display or LCD screen) that permits viewing of the acquired MR images during the procedure (Figure 11.1).

B. KINEMATIC MRI: TYPES OF TECHNIQUES

As shown in other chapters of this book and in the literature,[22,23] a number of studies have illustrated the benefits of imaging joints undergoing their native motions. In this context, it is important to distinguish the various types of kinematic MRI techniques: *incremental passive positioning*, *active movement*, and *active movement, against resistance*.

For the incremental passive positioning technique, a series of images is obtained at different positions through a specific range of motion of the joint. For the active movement technique, the patient freely moves the joint limb and a rapid MR imaging technique is used to acquire images for the kinematic MRI examination. Finally, for the active movement, against resistance technique, stress is applied to load or resist the joint while the patient freely moves the joint and/or limb and a rapid imaging technique is used to acquire MR images. Obviously, the distinction between passive and active kinematic MRI techniques is important because joint alignment in a state of muscle relaxation may differ from alignment when under the influence of active muscle contraction.[24,25]

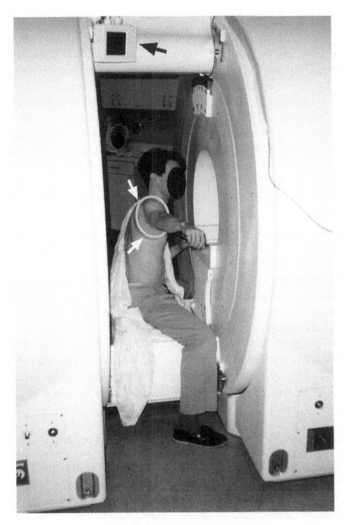

FIGURE 11.1 Positioning of the subject for shoulder abduction in the vertically opened MR system. The subject straddles the connector bar between the two magnet rings of the MR system. A circular transmit-receive RF coil is placed around the shoulder (white arrows). In this example, the subject's arm is abducted to approximately 80°. Note that MR images may be viewed on a monitor (LCD screen, black arrow) during examination of the patient.

Using each of the above techniques, MR images are typically acquired at different section locations. The resulting series is replayed and viewed as a "cine-loop" that simulates joint motion.

C. IMAGING PARAMETERS AND PROTOCOL

Using the vertically opened MR system, the general MR imaging parameters and protocol that would allow examination of the shoulder in an "interactive" time frame were determined. Basically, the parameters studied were patient positioning, pulse sequences, repetition time (TR), echo time (TE), flip angle, field of view (FOV), section thickness, and number of excitations (NEX).

MR images were acquired using a fast spin echo (FSE) pulse sequence, as follows: TR, 200 msec; TE, 16 msec; echo train length (ETL), 8; matrix size, 256 × 128 to 256 × 192; NEX, 1 to 2; FOV, 16 to 36 cm; and section thickness, 5 to 20 mm. The minimum acquisition time for a single section, FSE, T1-weighted image was approximately 4 seconds.

MR imaging using a fast gradient echo (GRE) was performed, as follows: TR, 19.8 msec; TE, 7.2 to 20 msec; flip angle, 10 to 110°; matrix size, 256 × 128 to 256 × 256; bandwidth, 16 to 32 kHz; NEX, 1 to 2; FOV, 16 to 36 cm; and section thickness, 5 to 20 mm. Kinematic MRI of the shoulder is performed without and with MR tracking (see below) during the use of the fast GRE pulse sequences. The minimum acquisition time for a single section, fast GRE pulse image was 2 to 2.5 seconds. Both FSE and fast GRE pulse sequences yielded images of acceptable quality for evaluation of gross anatomy in relatively rapid image acquisition times (2 to 4 sec/image).

MR Tracking is specialized hardware and software that enables active scan plane registration. This system was developed by Dumoulin et al.[26] Our group adapted MR tracking for use in the musculoskeletal system,[26,27] and have found the system extremely valuable for capturing anatomy of interest over a wide range of joint motion.

In brief, MR Tracking incorporates a miniature radiofrequency (RF) coil surrounding a sample containing gadolinium solution. RF pulses that sample signal from the small tracker coil are interleaved with imaging sequences. The image plane location is determined by the spatial location of the tracker RF coil. By interactively adjusting the location of the tracker coil on the patient, the scan location is also modified.

Notably, in the absence of MR tracking, images tend to be highly variable in their depiction of anatomy. Specifically, without direct control over the section location relative to the patient, it may be impossible to keep structures of interest, such as the glenoid, labrum, and the humeral head, within a constant scan plane.

From within the range of imaging parameters coupled to the existing MR tracking system, the following imaging parameters are used for an interactive, kinematic MRI study of the shoulder, with emphasis on the glenohumeral joint: patient sitting perpendicular to the magnet bore; fast GRE sequence; TR, 19.8 msec; TE, 7.2 msec; flip angle, 30 to 40°; matrix size, 256 × 128; FOV, 18 to 24 cm; section thickness, 7 mm; and NEX, 1.

D. Physical Examination of the Shoulder Using Kinematic MRI

A fundamental difference exists between physical examination of a patient with instability and current diagnostic imaging methods. Whereas the physical examination is dynamic and interactive between patient and physician, static MR imaging is usually performed on a subject deep within the bore of a magnet, and whose muscles are in a state of relaxation. Thus, it is not surprising that despite the use of high image quality, static MR imaging and MR arthrography provide only limited insight into the cause of a specific patient's shoulder dysfunction. Through the use of a vertically opened MR system and the development and implementation of the necessary tools for efficient kinematic MRI of the shoulder, the gap between physical examination and diagnostic imaging can be closed or at least narrowed.

Initially, the concepts of an MR-guided, physical examination of the shoulder have been applied to volunteer subjects and patients by performing stress testing during the MRI procedure. In this procedure, an examiner either applies direct force to the humeral head or uses the arm as a lever to apply stress to the joint. Figure 11.2 illustrates this examination technique and Figure 11.3 shows MR images that demonstrate moderate translation of the shoulder joint.

In the group of asymptomatic volunteer subjects, the kinematic MRI of the shoulder stress testing procedure resulted in as much as 6 mm of anterior translation and 13 mm of posterior translation.[19] While in its infancy, this type of interactive imaging appears to be extremely promising.

III. NORMAL GLENOHUMERAL MOTION PATTERNS

Until the development of MRI techniques that incorporated fast image acquisition methods, assessment of dynamic glenohumeral motion was limited to x-ray-based methods. Mostly because of the risks associated with the use of ionizing radiation, very little research has been done on normal motion patterns.

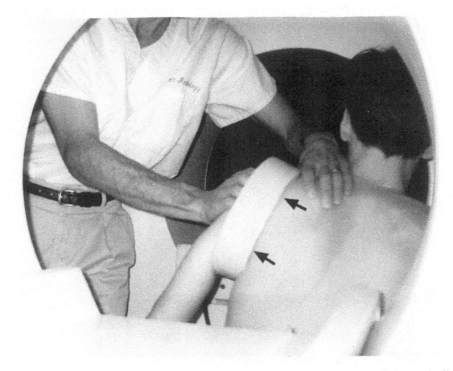

FIGURE 11.2   Kinematic MRI of the shoulder: stress testing. View from the end of the vertically opened MR system showing a seated subject with a circular transmit-receive RF coil placed on the left shoulder (black arrows). A physician examiner stabilizes the shoulder girdle with his left hand and applies a direct force to the humeral head with the right hand. The subject is positioned so that the shoulder is maintained as closely as possible within the center of the magnet to facilitate imaging.

Using static radiographs obtained at different arm positions, Poppen and Walker[29] studied the motion of the glenohumeral joint in the plane of the scapula. Beginning with the arm in adduction, these researchers found that the humeral head of normal volunteers remained centered in the glenoid between 30° and maximum abduction. Between 0° and 30°, the humeral translated superiorly about 3 mm. Thereafter its position remained constant, moving only 1 mm or at most 2 mm superiorly to inferiorly with successive abduction increments.

Conventional "tunnel-shaped" and open MR systems have subsequently been used to evaluate glenohumeral alignment in normal subjects using kinematic MRI techniques (Figure 11.4). Typically, this type of kinematic MRI examination is performed using standard or "fast" gradient echo pulse sequences with the subject's arm placed in maximal internal and external rotated positions.

Using the vertically opened MR system, we studied ten normal subjects with no prior shoulder problems or abnormal conditions to determine motion patterns during abduction/adduction and internal/external rotation.[18,19] Kinematic MRI of the shoulder using the stress testing technique as described above was performed. Figure 11.5 shows examples of MR images taken from the kinematic MRI examinations obtained during abduction. Figure 11.6 displays a graphic depiction of normal GH joint positioning as a function of the glenohumeral abduction angle.

In these initial studies, consistent superior translation of the humeral head on the glenoid during the early phases of abduction was not observed, such as was described by Poppen and Walker.[29] This may be due to the small number of subjects who have been evaluated or to the accuracy and precision of the respective measurement techniques. However, it should be noted that an advantage of tomographic methods, such as MRI, is that projection-related errors, inherent to plain film radiographic techniques, are eliminated. Instead, one has to contend with errors that might arise because successive sections evaluate different portions of the bony anatomy. To address the problem

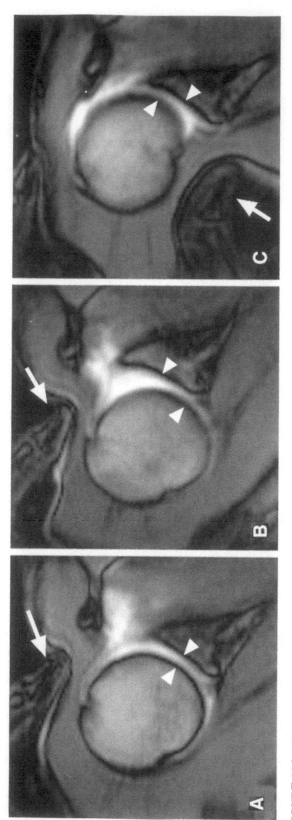

FIGURE 11.3 Kinematic MRI of the shoulder: MR images acquired during stress testing. In (A), the axial plane MR image shows that the humeral head remains well centered on the glenoid, as illustrated by alignment of the arrowheads. Note the appearance of the examiner's fingers in the images (white arrows). With anterior-posterior force (B), the humeral head shifted by approximately half its diameter on the glenoid. In (C), posterior-anterior force is applied. In this direction, the humeral head only shifted by approximately 25% of its diameter on the glenoid.

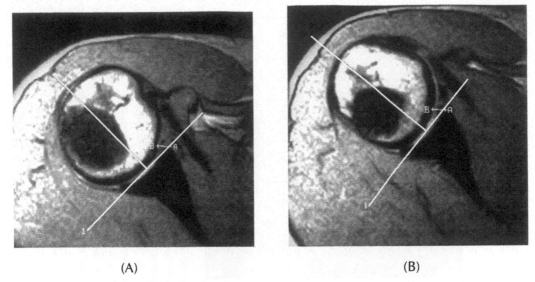

(A)   (B)

FIGURE 11.4 Normal glenohumeral alignment shown on kinematic MRI examination of the shoulder. Axial plane, kinematic MRI series demonstrating glenohumeral congruence in maximal internal (A) and external (B) rotation positions. Note that the humeral head remains centered on the glenoid, without anterior or posterior translation and that no abnormal widening of the anterior aspect of the joint occurs during external rotation (figure provided courtesy of John D. Reeder, M.D., Chief, Musculoskeletal Imaging Division, ProScan International, Cincinnati, OH).

of complex anatomy more effectively, Graichen and colleagues[25,30] have applied three-dimensional rendering techniques to MR imaging data, with the shoulder in different positions. Early results from this group are quite compelling.

In measuring glenohumeral relationships during internal and external rotation of the humerus, we found that the humeral head remained precisely centered in the glenoid over the full range of physiologic motion.[18,19] Figure 11.7 shows an example of the spatial relationships we have characterized using kinematic MRI of the shoulder.

In a static, plain film, radiographic study of glenohumeral motion in the horizontal (or axial plane), Howell et al.[31] studied 20 normal subjects and demonstrated precise positioning of the humeral head within the glenoid in all positions except maximum extension and external rotation. In this position, normal subjects experienced approximately 4 mm of posterior translation of the humeral head on the glenoid.

By comparison, our studies of internal and external rotation differed in arm position from those of Howell et al.,[31] in that our subjects were evaluated with the arm in adduction. In this position, we found no evidence of significant translation of the humeral head on the glenoid between maximum internal rotation and maximum external rotation.

Using conventional "tunnel-shaped" MR systems, kinematic MRI of the shoulder has been reported for normal subjects. Sans et al.[32] performed kinematic MRI procedures on 39 shoulders. This group characterized the shape and signal intensity of the glenoid labrum as well as labral position. They found that the anterior labrum showed changes in shape and signal intensity with internal rotation in over half the subjects, whereas the posterior labrum remained motionless in 97% of the subjects. These studies were performed with a mechanical positioning device, to which the patient's arm was strapped, and motion was restricted to internal and external rotation in an adducted position. Imaging time was approximately 32 sec per position (an incremental passive positioning kinematic MRI technique was used). No quantitative analysis of humeral head position on the glenoid was reported. Similar qualitative features were reported by Cardinal

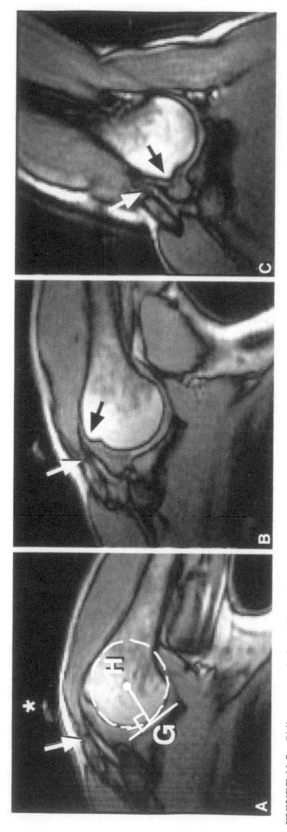

FIGURE 11.5 Oblique coronal plane, kinematic MRI (TR 19.8, TE 7.2; flip angle 30°) examination of the glenohumeral joint during abduction in an asymptomatic 26-year-old man. This kinematic MRI study was performed using an active movement technique. In (A), the asterisk marks the location of the MR tracking coil. MR images show successive degrees of abduction: (A) 40°; (B) 68°; (C) 127° of abduction. Measurement techniques are illustrated in (A) in which a circle is prescribed along the articular surface of the humeral head (H) to determine its geometric center (white dot). A line between the superior and inferior margins of the glenoid (G) is used to define its center point. A perpendicular line from the humeral head center to the glenoid line allows measurement of translation in humeral position relative to the glenoid center point. The degree of glenoid (scapular) and humeral elevation relative to the fully adducted position is determined by measuring and following the angles of the glenoid and a line prescribed along the humeral shaft (not shown) relative to the vertical axis of the image. Note that with abduction, the relationship of the humeral head, in particular the greater tuberosity (black arrow), can be evaluated relative to the acromion (white arrow) for assessment of mechanical impingement.

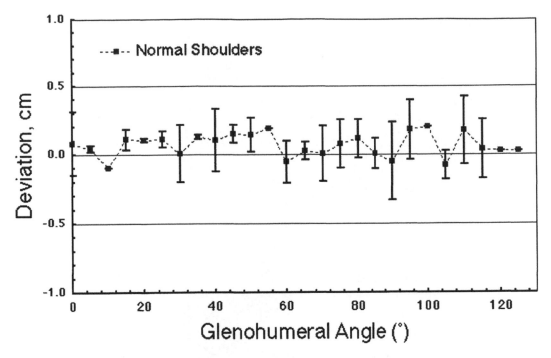

FIGURE 11.6   Normal glenohumeral alignment during abduction. Measurements of humeral head position relative to the glenoid center were made on serial oblique coronal plane kinematic MRI examinations during abduction/adduction in ten asymptomatic shoulders. The glenoid center point is represented by 0 cm on the Y axis. The humeral head remained well centered on the glenoid, with fluctuations in position on the same order of magnitude as standard deviations of the measurements.

et al.[33] These latter investigators also pointed out the value of kinematic MRI in assessment of the shoulder capsule.

In an earlier study by Bonutti et al.,[34] a positioning device was used in a 0.6 Tesla MR system to evaluation internal/external rotation in 24 asymptomatic subjects. MR image acquisition time was 2.2 min per position (again, incremental passive positioning kinematic MRI). These authors reported that glenohumeral alignment was well depicted by kinematic MRI of the shoulder using a positioning device (Figures 11.8 and 11.9). However, using noncontrast MR imaging, it was difficult to clearly evaluate for labral motion due to its location immediately adjacent to the anterior capsule and subscapularis tendon.[34]

In summary, the total number of normal subjects studied to date using kinematic MRI techniques to assess the shoulder is relatively small, but early results suggest that this type of specialized MRI examination can provide unique functional insight into the biomechanics of this complex articulation.

IV. CLINICAL APPLICATIONS

A. GLENOHUMERAL INSTABILITY

Whereas there is considerable literature on the appearance of the glenohumeral joint with static view MR imaging and MR arthrography,[11,12,14-16,33,34] there are no systematic reports of kinematic MRI of the shoulder in patients with instability. In our initial studies, we have found that pathological motion patterns and anatomic derangements can be identified in many patients with instability, using kinematic MRI of the shoulder.[19,35,36]

In a study of patients with unilateral instability, we found a correlation between GH joint motion patterns, findings on clinical examination, and examinations under anesthesia (EUA).[38] We studied

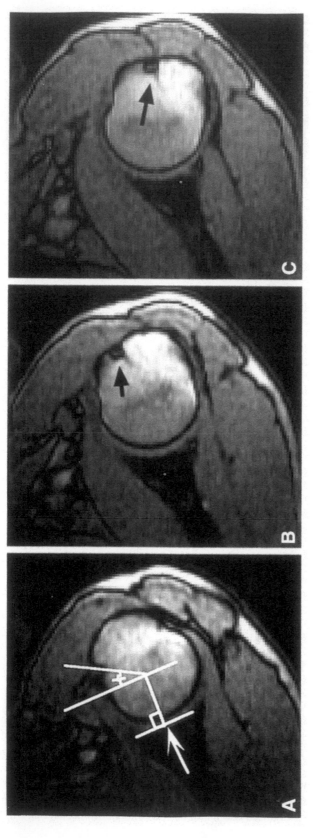

FIGURE 11.7 Axial plane, kinematic MRI (TR 19.8, TE 7.2; flip angle 30°) examination of the shoulder with images obtained through the center of the glenohumeral joint during (A) 24°, (B) 61°, and (C) 99° of external rotation. Measurement techniques are illustrated in (A), in which a line defined by the anterior and posterior margins of the glenoid determine its center point (white arrow); a line perpendicular to the glenoid line through the humeral head center defines the position of the humeral head on the glenoid. By using a line from the humeral head center through the bicipital groove (black arrows in [B] and [C]), the rotation angle is determined relative to a line parallel to the glenoid face. As with abduction/adduction, the normal humeral head remains well centered in the glenoid throughout a full range of physiologic internal and external rotation.

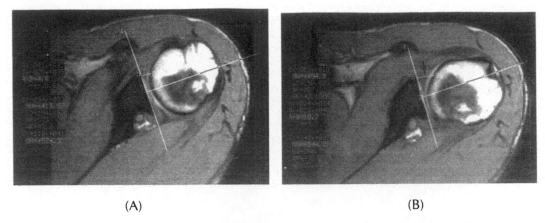

(A)   (B)

FIGURE 11.8   Glenohumeral instability demonstrated by kinematic MRI of the shoulder. This study was performed using a conventional open MR system. Axial plane MR images were obtained for this kinematic MRI series in a patient with symptomatic glenohumeral instability, revealing normal glenohumeral alignment in internal rotation (A) but posterior translation of the humeral head relative to the glenoid in external rotation (B). Also, note that the width of the anterior aspect of the joint doubles (arrow) as the shoulder progresses from internal to external rotation, indicative of capsular laxity. (Figure provided courtesy of John D. Reeder, M.D., Chief, Musculoskeletal Imaging Division, ProScan International, Cincinnati, OH.)

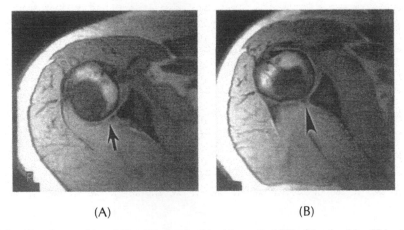

(A)   (B)

FIGURE 11.9   Glenohumeral instability demonstrated by kinematic MRI of the shoulder. This study was done using a conventional open MR system. Axial plane MR images were obtained for this kinematic MRI performed in a patient who demonstrated posterior subluxation (arrow) of the humeral head relative to the glenoid in internal rotation (A) with reduction of the malalignment (arrowhead) occurring during external rotation (B). By placing rotational demands on the capsular mechanism of the shoulder, the use of the kinematic MRI technique improves the sensitivity of MRI in the detection of glenohumeral instability. (Figure provided courtesy of John D. Reeder, M.D., Chief, Musculoskeletal Imaging Division, ProScan International, Cincinnati, OH.)

symptomatic shoulders in eleven subjects and compared them to the subject's contralateral asymptomatic shoulder. Each shoulder was studied through a range of abduction/adduction and internal/external rotation to quantify translation of the humeral head in relation to the glenoid. Additionally, an examiner performed kinematic MRI stress testing on each shoulder.

   Each shoulder was assigned an instability grade from the kinematic MRI stress test and this was correlated with: (1) clinical instability grade assigned during preoperative assessment by an orthopedic surgeon, and (2) intraoperative instability grade determined by EUA immediately preceding shoulder arthroscopy.

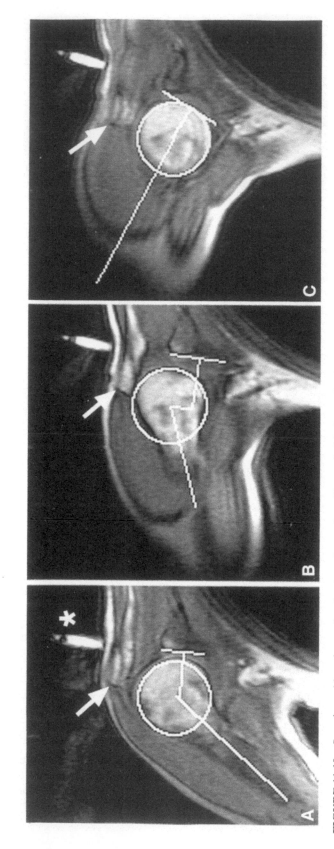

FIGURE 11.10 Superior subluxation and reduction observed on kinematic MRI examination of the shoulder. Successive oblique coronal plane MR images were acquired in this kinematic MRI series. This patient was a 26-year-old woman who complained that her humeral head dislocated inferiorly with abduction. The position of the MR tracking coil is marked with an asterisk and is represented by the bright cylinder in the images. The acromion is shown by the white arrows. The humeral head is described by a circle along its articular surface with the center of the circle representing the geometric center of the humeral head. Note that when progressing from an adducted position (A), to approximately 75° of abduction (B), the humeral head subluxes superiorly. With further abduction to approximately 110° (C), the humeral head reduces into the glenoid fossa.

During patient-initiated motions, the humeral head typically remained well centered on the glenoid, in both symptomatic and asymptomatic GH joints. However, in two individuals, dramatic examples of subluxation were directly observed. MR images obtained from one of the kinematic MRI studies on these individuals are shown in Figure 11.10. The interesting observation in this patient was that both she and her orthopedist thought that the shoulder "clunk" she experienced was due to inferior subluxation with abduction. In actuality, the clunk was due to relocation of the humeral head in the glenoid from an unusual position of superior subluxation. In another patient, we observed anterior-inferior subluxation only when the shoulder was placed in a position of extreme abduction and external rotation, known clinically as the apprehension position (illustrated in Figure 11.11).

The MR grading or characterization of GH joint instability agreed with clinical instability grade in 7 of 10 cases, whereas three subjects were given lower MR instability grades than clinical grades. By comparison, MR grading of instability tended to underestimate the degree of laxity observed during EUA.

The relatively good correlation between kinematic MRI stress testing and clinical instability grades provides encouragement that relevant information is being derived from this maneuver. The fact that kinematic MRI stress testing underestimated instability compared with EUA suggests that muscle tone, even in relaxed subjects, provides some constraint to GH joint translation. Additional clinical experience will be required to draw conclusions regarding the overall value of the kinematic MRI stress test procedure.

Over the past three years, we have increasingly applied our interactive kinematic MRI techniques to examine the GH joint in patients with shoulder pain and symptoms of clicking, grinding, or instability. Notably, we have performed comprehensive static and kinematic MRI examinations on over 60 patients using the vertically opened MR system and have reported preliminary findings.[37] These patients were most often referred to confirm the presence and primary direction of instability (anterior or posterior) or to determine whether multidirectional laxity was present. Many of the patients had undergone static-view MRI examinations of the shoulder that did not fully explain their clinical picture.

In the study group, there were 43 subjects (28 males, 15 females), with an average age of 30 years (range 16 to 72 years). GH joint motion was primarily evaluated using kinematic MRI with the patient in a seated position using a flexible, transmit-receive circular RF coil and MR tracking. Kinematic MRI stress testing was performed by the examining radiologist or during maneuvers in which the patient could evoke pain, clicking, or instability.

To improve the image contrast during the kinematic MRI examination, 18 patients underwent MR arthrography using MR-guided GH joint injection of 15 to 20 cc dilute Gd-DTPA (1:200 with sterile normal saline). (Notably, MR-guided injection of the GH joint is straightforward, and perhaps technically easier than the x-ray fluoroscopy approach, as the trajectory of an MR-compatible 20 gauge spinal needle can be tracked on cross-sectional images.[39]) In our experience, GH joint injection was successful in all attempts, in agreement with previous reports of excellent success both in horizontal[40] and vertically opened MR systems.[41] GH joint alignment was assessed both subjectively and with quantitative methods, as described by Beaulieu et al.[19] The minimum GH joint shift required to classify a shoulder as "unstable" was translation of the humeral head on the glenoid by at least 25% of the humeral head diameter. In most of the cases in the instability categories, the shift was 25 to 50% of the humeral head diameter.

Table 11.1 summarizes results from kinematic MRI stress testing studies or patient-provoked instability maneuvers in the 43 patients. Fifteen shoulders showed no significant humeral head translation. Eleven showed patterns of anterior or anteroinferior instability. In these cases, assessment of the GH joint relationship was frequently most revealing in a position of extreme abduction and external rotation (apprehension), using an oblique coronal imaging plane (Figure 11.11). Ten shoulders showed posterior instability, best assessed on axial plane section locations. Multidirec-

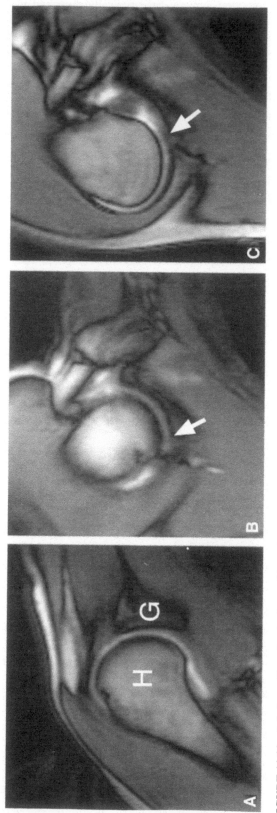

FIGURE 11.11 Inferior subluxation in the position of apprehension, shown using kinematic MRI of the shoulder. In (A), the shoulder is adducted and the humeral head is well centered in the glenoid. With abduction to approximately 120°, the humeral head (H) remained centered in the glenoid (G) as shown in (B). With further abduction and external rotation (C), the humeral head shifted inferiorly such that over half the humeral head diameter was beyond the inferior margin of the glenoid. Bright signal within the joint space is a result of MR-guided injection of intra-articular contrast at the beginning of the study.

TABLE 11.1
Instability Patterns Observed on Kinematic MRI
Examinations of the Shoulder

No Instability	Anterior/Inferior	Posterior	Multidirectional
15 (35%)	11 (26%)	10 (23%)	7 (16%)

Note: Total number and percentage of patients in each category (43 total). Categories for anterior and inferior instability were combined as the motion direction was typically a combination of the two. Three patients in this category had isolated inferior instability.

tional instability was assigned when abnormal motion was observed in at least two directions, usually anterior and posterior.

In addition to the kinematic MRI information regarding GH joint translation, static view MR images demonstrated anecdotal examples of labral tears, detachment, and labral deformation. Figure 11.12 shows an example of a posterior labral tear of the shoulder, apparent only when the GH joint was placed in a position of external rotation.

While overall patient numbers remain small, results obtained to date for kinematic MRI examinations of the shoulder are encouraging. Broader support for the concept of performing MR imaging during joint motions or at least in various joint positions is also beginning to accrue in the radiological and orthopedic communities, as indicated by the studies described herein and in the list of references for this chapter.

In another relatively recent study, Allmann et al.[42] studied the GH joint in 20 patients, performing kinematic MRI examinations in both the axial and oblique coronal planes. A positioning device was used to standardize the shoulder movements. This investigation reported that kinematic MRI of the shoulder was useful for visualizing the capsular-ligament complex of the shoulder in instability, both pre- and postoperatively.

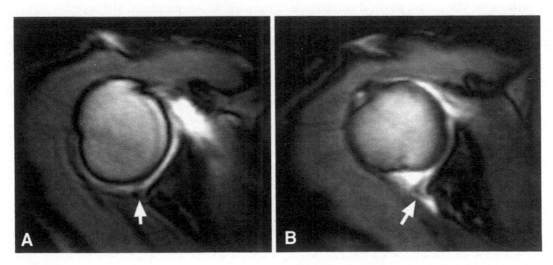

FIGURE 11.12   Demonstration of labral tear with external rotation seen on the kinematic MRI examination of the shoulder. Axial plane MR images were acquired through the mid-glenohumeral joint in the patient after intra-articular injection of dilute gadolinium solution. In (A), the posterior labrum is an unremarkable-appearing black triangle (arrow). When placed in external rotation (B), the posterior labrum shifts posterio-medially and demonstrates a high signal at its base, consistent with a labral tear/detachment. Note the delineation of the posterior capsule along the glenoid neck in (B).

B. MECHANICAL IMPINGEMENT

Despite its common clinical occurrence, the etiologic factors responsible for the clinical syndrome of mechanical impingement are not well understood.[43-46] Kinematic MRI of the shoulder with the joint positioned in abduction has the potential to shed light on this subject, as direct evaluation of the subacromial space, the rotator cuff, and the bony structures is available (Figures 11.5, 11.13, and 11.14).

Using conventional static-view MR imaging, only indirect signs of impingement are seen as the arm is adducted and the muscles are in a state of relaxation.[42,43] Conversely, with abduction, the greater tuberosity of the humerus approaches the acromion, reducing the width of the subacromial space and potentially creating direct impingement on the supraspinatus.

While it may seem that a kinematic MRI examination would easily depict the direct causes of impingement, it has proven difficult to systematically characterize the subacromial distance during abduction. This is because the greater tuberosity rotates under the acromion during abduction. Furthermore, the degree of internal/external rotation and arm flexion also influences the acromiohumeral distance.

In an initial study using kinematic MRI of the shoulder in the oblique coronal plane, we found that the acromiohumeral distance tended to decrease with abduction, but that intersubject variability was great.[46] Using a similar system, Dufour et al.[47] have also begun to systematically characterize motion patterns in mechanical impingement (also see Chapter 12). More elaborate analyses, such as the three-dimensional modeling approaches, are likely to be useful in arriving at a more comprehensive understanding of mechanical impingement.[44,45]

V. SUMMARY, CONCLUSIONS, AND FUTURE DIRECTIONS

Performance of kinematic MRI of the shoulder using a vertically opened MR system is a highly promising technique that is presently in its early stages of development. Technical parameters continue to be optimized in terms of temporal, spatial, or contrast resolution. Nevertheless, the use of the vertically opened MR system has the advantage of being able to place the patient's arm into almost any position for the kinematic MRI procedure, allowing an examiner to approach and actually perform an MR-guided physical examination of the joint. In this paradigm, MR becomes more of an interactive examination, similar to diagnostic ultrasound. At the same time, the kinematic MRI studies often require considerable time and expertise to perform, so that cost- and time-efficiency are important considerations.

To optimize MR-guided physical examination of glenohumeral instability, the following issues must be addressed: (1) temporal resolution needs to be maximized to capture the joint during true dynamic function (i.e., at the rate of several images per second); (2) spatial resolution must be improved to provide similar detail as that available using high-field, static-view MR imaging; (3) image contrast resolution in the fast imaging regime needs to be improved, so that intra-articular contrast injection will not necessarily be required; and (4) standard approaches to MR-guided interactions between an examining physician and the patient need to be developed so that the methods can be broadly validated and used routinely in the clinical setting.

While these are challenging tasks, we are confident that with further development and experience, kinematic MRI of the shoulder will become a very useful tool in the comprehensive evaluation of patients with shoulder pain or dysfunction due to glenohumeral instability or mechanical impingement.

ACKNOWLEDGMENTS

We are grateful for the helpful contributions from the following individuals: A. G. Bergman, M.D.; K. Butts, Ph.D.; C. Cooper, R. T. (MR); B. L. Daniel, M.D.; M. F. Dillingham, M.D.; R. J. Herfkens, M.D.; D. K. Hodge, M.D.; P. K. Lang, M.D.; A. Pearle, M.D.; G. Thabit III, M.D.; and J. Vandevenne, M.D.

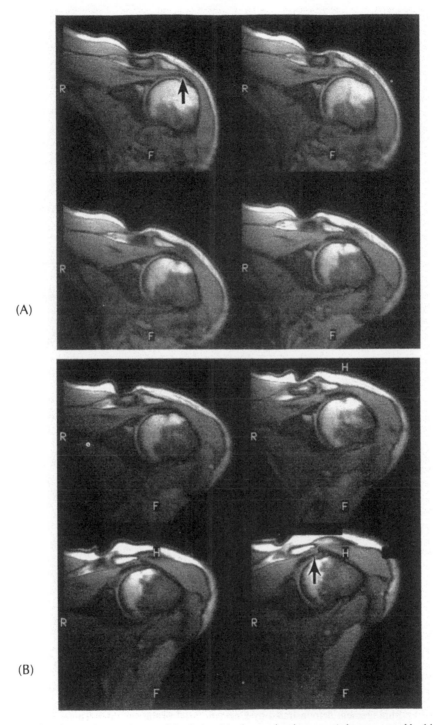

(A)

(B)

FIGURE 11.13   Normal humeral-acromial relationship (i.e., no impingement) demonstrated by kinematic MRI of the shoulder. This study was performed using a conventional open MR system. The kinematic MRI examination was conducted obtaining oblique coronal plane images, acquired at various incremental positions from adduction (A) to abduction (B). This study revealed a normal humeral-acromial relationship. Preservation of the height of the subacromial space (arrow) is observed throughout the range of motion. (Figure provided courtesy of John D. Reeder, M.D., Chief, Musculoskeletal Imaging Division, ProScan International, Cincinnati, OH.)

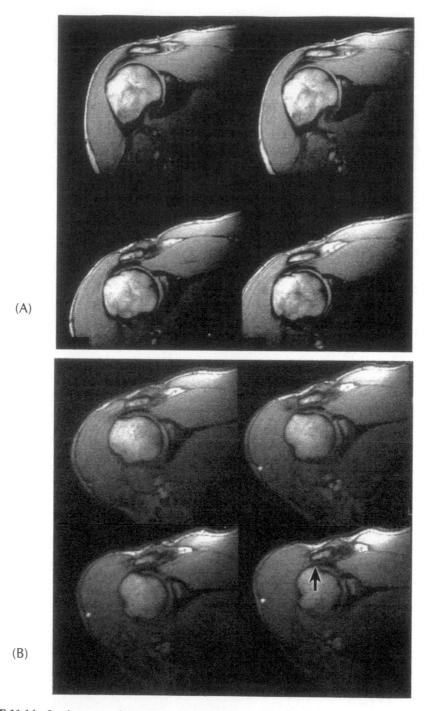

(A)

(B)

FIGURE 11.14   Impingement demonstrated by kinematic MRI of the shoulder. This study was performed using a conventional open MR system. The kinematic MRI examination was conducted obtaining oblique coronal plane images, acquired from adduction (A) to abduction (B). This study revealed marked narrowing of the subacromial space (arrow) and juxtaposition of the acromion and the greater tuberosity adjacent to the insertion of the supraspinatus tendon. Notably, the patient exhibited signs and symptoms of impingement on physical examination. (Figure provided courtesy of John D. Reeder, M.D., Chief, Musculoskeletal Imaging Division, ProScan International, Cincinnati, OH.)

REFERENCES

1. Tsai, L., Wredmark, T., Johansson, C., Gibo, K., Engström, B., and Törnqvist, H., Shoulder function in patients with unoperated anterior shoulder instability, *Am. J. Sports Med.*, 19, 469–473, 1991.
2. Matsen, F. A., Harryman, D. T., and Sidles, J. A., Mechanics of glenohumeral instability, *Clin. Sports Med.*, 10, 783–788, 1991.
3. Bankart, A., The pathology and treatment of recurrent dislocation of the shoulder-joint, *Br. J. Surg.*, 26, 23–29, 1938.
4. Perthes, G., Uber operation bei habitueller schulterluxation, *Dtsch. Z. Chir.*, 85, 199–227, 1906.
5. Bigliani, L. U., Kelkar, R., Flatow, E. L., Pollock, R. G., and Mow, V. C., Glenohumeral stability. Biomechanical properties of passive and active stabilizers, *Clin. Orthop.*, 330, 13–30, 1996.
6. Cole, B. J. and Warner, J. J. P., Anatomy, biomechanics, and pathophysiology of glenohumeral instability, in *Disorders of the Shoulder: Diagnosis and Management,* Iannotti, J. P. and Williams, G. R., Eds., Lippincott Williams & Wilkins, Philadelphia, 1999, pp. 207–232.
7. Harryman, D. T., Sidles, J. A., Clark, J. M., McQuade, K. J., Gibb, T. D., and Matsen, F. A., Translation of the humeral head on the glenoid with passive glenohumeral motion, *J. Bone Joint Surg.*, 72, 1334–1443, 1990.
8. Speer, K. P., Deng, X., Borrero, S., Torzilli, P. A., Altchek, D. A., and Warren, R. F., Biomechanical evaluation of a simulated Bankart lesion, *J. Bone Joint Surg. [Am.],* 76, 1819–1826, 1994.
9. Shaffer, B. S. and Tibone, J. E., Arthroscopic shoulder instability surgery. Complications, *Clin. Sports Med.*, 18, 737–767, 1999.
10. Bigliani, L. U., Pollock, R. G., Soslowsky, L. J., Flatow, E. L., Pawluk, R. J., and Mow, V. C., Tensile properties of the inferior glenohumeral ligament, *J. Orthop. Res.*, 10, 187–197, 1992.
11. Seeger, L. L., Yao, L., and Gold, R. H., Diagnosis of glenoid labral tears: a comparison between magnetic resonance imaging and clinical examinations [letter; comment], *Am. J. Sports Med.*, 25, 141–144, 1997.
12. Tirman, P. F., Palmer, W. E., and Feller, J. F., MR arthrography of the shoulder, *Magn. Reson. Imag. Clin. North Am.*, 5, 811–839, 1997.
13. Minkoff, J., Stecker, S., and Cavaliere, G., Glenohumeral instabilities and the role of MR imaging techniques. The orthopedic surgeon's perspective, *Magn. Reson. Imag. Clin. North Am.*, 5, 767–785, 1997.
14. Palmer, W. E. and Caslowitz, P. L., Anterior shoulder instability: diagnostic criteria determined from prospective analysis of 121 MR arthrograms, *Radiology,* 197, 819–825, 1995.
15. Palmer, W. E., Caslowitz, P. L., and Chew, F. S., MR arthrography of the shoulder: normal intraarticular structures and common abnormalities, *Am. J. Roentgenol.*, 164, 141–6, 1995.
16. Tirman, P. F., Stauffer, A. E., Crues, J. V. et al., Saline magnetic resonance arthrography in the evaluation of glenohumeral instability, *Arthroscopy*, 9, 550–559, 1993.
17. Wall, M. S. and O'Brien, S. J., Arthroscopic evaluation of the unstable shoulder, *Clin. Sports Med.*, 14, 817–839, 1995.
18. Beaulieu, C. F., Bergman, A. G., Butts, K. et al., Dynamic MR imaging of glenohumeral stability in normal volunteers, *Fifth Annual Meeting, International Society of Magnetic Resonance in Medicine,* Vol. 1, International Society of Magnetic Resonance in Medicine, Berkeley, CA, 1997.
19. Beaulieu, C. F., Hodge, D. K., Bergman, A. G. et al., Glenohumeral relationships during physiologic shoulder motion and stress testing: initial experience with open MR imaging and active imaging-plane registration, *Radiology,* 212, 699–705, 1999.
20. Tirman, P. F., Steinbach, L. S., Belzer, J. P., and Bost, F. W., A practical approach to imaging of the shoulder with emphasis on MR imaging, *Orthop. Clin. North Am.*, 28, 483–515, 1997.
21. Wintzell, G., Larsson, H., and Larsson, S., Indirect MR arthrography of anterior shoulder instability in the ABER and the apprehension test positions: a prospective comparative study of two different shoulder positions during MRI using intravenous gadodiamide contrast for enhancement of the joint fluid, *Skeletal Radiol.*, 27, 488–94, 1998.
22. Shellock, F. G., Kinematic MRI of the joints, *Semin. Musculoskeletal Radiol.*, 1, 143, 1997.
23. Shellock, F. G., Mink, J. H., Deutsch, A., and Pressman, B. D., Kinematic magnetic resonance imaging of the joints: techniques and clinical applications, *Magn. Reson. Q.*, 7, 104–135, 1991.

24. Shellock, F. G., Mink, J. H., Deutsch, A. L., and Foo, T. K., Kinematic MR imaging of the patellofemoral joint: comparison of passive positioning and active movement techniques, *Radiology*, 184, 574–577, 1992.

25. Graichen, H., Stammberger, T., Bonel, H., Karl-Hans, E., Reiser, M., and Eckstein, F., Glenohumeral translation during active and passive elevation of the shoulder — a 3D open-MRI study, *J. Biomech.*, 33, 609–613, 2000.

26. Dumoulin, C. L., Souza, S. P., and Darrow, R. D., Real time position monitoring of invasive devices using magnetic resonance, *Magn. Reson. Med.*, 29, 411–415, 1993.

27. Daniel, B. L., Norbash, A. M., Butts, K. et al., Active scan plane registration during dynamic musculoskeletal MR-imaging using an external MR-tracking coil, *Proceedings of the International Society of Magnetic Resonance in Medicine, 5th Scientific Meeting*, International Society of Magnetic Resonance in Medicine, Berkeley, CA, 1997.

28. Pearle, A. D., Daniel, B. L., Bergman, A. G. et al., Joint motion in an open MR unit using MR tracking, *J. Magn. Reson. Imag.*, 10, 8–14, 1999.

29. Poppen, N. K. and Walker, P. S., Normal and abnormal motion of the shoulder, *J. Bone Joint Surg.*, 58(A), 195–201, 1976.

30. Graichen, H., Bonel, H., Stammberger, T., Englmeier, K. H., Reiser, M., and Eckstein, F., Subacromial space width changes during abduction and rotation — a 3-D MR imaging study, *Surg. Radiol. Anat.*, 21, 59–64, 1999.

31. Howell, S. M., Galinat, B. J., Renzi, A. J., and Marone, P. J., Normal and abnormal mechanics of the glenohumeral joint in the horizontal plane, *J. Bone Joint Surg.*, 70(A), 227–232, 1988.

32. Sans, N., Richardi, G., Railhac, J.-J. et al., Kinematic MR imaging of the shoulder: normal patterns, *Am. J. Roentgenol.*, 167, 1517–1522, 1996.

33. Cardinal, E., Buckwalter, K. A., and Braunstein, E. M., Kinematic magnetic resonance imaging of the normal shoulder: assessment of the labrum and capsule, *Can. Assoc. Radiol. J.*, 47, 44–50, 1996.

34. Bonutti, P. M., Norfray, J. F., Friedman, R. J., and Genez, B. M., Kinematic MRI of the shoulder, *J. Comput. Assist. Tomogr.*, 17, 666–669, 1993.

35. Palmer, W. E., Brown, J. H., and Rosenthal, D. I., Labral-ligamentous complex of the shoulder: evaluation with MR arthrography [see comments], *Radiology*, 190, 645–651, 1994.

36. Palmer, W. E., MR arthrography of the rotator cuff and labral-ligamentous complex, *Semin. Ultrasound CT MR*, 18, 278–290, 1997.

37. Beaulieu, C. F., Dillingham, M. F., Hodge, D. K. et al., Physical examination of shoulder instability combined with MRI: initial experience in 43 patients, *Proceedings of the International Society of Magnetic Resonance in Medicine*, International Society of Magnetic Resonance in Medicine, Berkeley, CA, 2000.

38. Hodge, D. K., Beaulieu, C. F., Thabit, G. H. et al., Dynamic MR imaging and stress testing in glenohumeral instability: comparison with normal shoulders and clinical/surgical findings, *Am. J. Roentgenol.*, in press.

39. Vandevenne, J. E., Bergman, G., Beaulieu, C., Cooper, C., Butts, K., and Lang, P., MR arthrography of the shoulder: MR guided intraarticular injection followed by stress testing, *Annual Meeting of European Society of Musculoskeletal Radiology*, Bled, Slovenia, October, 1998.

40. Petersilge, C. A., Lewin, J. S., Duerk, J. L., and Hatem, S. F., MR arthrography of the shoulder: rethinking traditional imaging procedures to meet the technical requirements of MR imaging guidance, *Am. J. Roentgenol.*, 169, 1453–1457, 1997.

41. Hilfiker, P. R., Weishaupt, D., Schmid, M., Dubno, B., Hodler, J., and Debatin, J. F., Real-time MR-guided joint puncture and arthrography: preliminary results, *Eur. Radiol.*, 9, 201–204, 1999.

42. Allmann, K. H., Uhl, M., Gufler, H. et al., Cine-MR imaging of the shoulder, *Acta Radiol.*, 38, 1043–1046, 1997.

43. Neer, C. S., Impingement lesions, *Clin. Orthop.*, 173, 70–77, 1983.

44. Bigliani, L. U., Ticker, J. B., Flatow, E. L., Soslowsky, L. J., and Mow, V. C., The relationship of acromial architecture to rotator cuff disease, *Clin. Sports Med.*, 10, 823–838, 1991.

45. Brossmann, J., Preidler, K. W., Pedowitz, R. A., White, L. M., Trudell, D., and Resnick, D., Shoulder impingement syndrome: influence of shoulder position on rotator cuff impingement — an anatomic study, *Am. J. Roentgenol.*, 167, 1511–5, 1996.

46. Bergman, A. G., Rotator cuff impingement. Pathogenesis, MR imaging characteristics, and early dynamic MR results, *Magn. Reson. Imag. Clin. North Am.,* 5, 705–719, 1997.

47. Dufour, M., Lapierre, C., Moffet, H. et al., A technique for dynamic evaluation of the acromiohumeral distance of the shoulder in the seated position under open-field MRI, *Seventh Scientific Meeting, International Society Magnetic Resonance in Medicine,* International Society of Magnetic Resonance in Medicine, Berkeley, CA, 1999.

12 Kinematic MRI of the Shoulder: Assessment in the Seated Position

Marie Dufour, Hélène Moffet, Luc J. Hébert, and Christian Moisan

CONTENTS

I. INTRODUCTION

Among acute musculoskeletal disorders, shoulder pain is the second most common cause of consultation.[1-5] The use of magnetic resonance imaging (MRI) in supporting a clinical diagnosis for the shoulder joint is well established. Using the normal "tunnel-shaped" configured MR system, indirect signs of certain pathological conditions of the shoulder can be described.[2,6-9] However, early signs of subacromial lesions induced by mechanical impingement[10] cannot be easily identified.

Few investigations have addressed the kinematic behavior of the shoulder using MRI.[11-19] However, in these studies, the genuine biomechanics of the shoulder may have been hindered because the subjects did not move their arms against an external gravitational load, as is the case in activities of daily living.

For instance, a study conducted by Brossmann et al.[11] relied on a cadaveric model. The authors found impingement of the distal supraspinatus tendon between the acromion and the greater tuberosity of the humerus. Since the positioning of the shoulder was only passive, the results of the study may have been partly biased as the humerus may have behaved somewhat differently during dynamic motion. Notably, the type of specialized MRI examination that was performed was only possible on amputated cadavers, hence, reducing the clinical impact of the study.[11]

Only a few MRI studies have been performed using quantitative *in vivo* data during "free" movements of the shoulder.[15-17] Bergman et al.[15] showed that the distance between the acromion and the humeral head at the narrowest location was decreased, when considering different degrees

0-8493-0807-0/01/$0.00+$.50
© 2001 by Frank G. Shellock

of continuous nonrestrained shoulder abduction with patients in the lateral decubitus position. Allmann et al.[16] reported a smaller subacromial distance in abduction in patients with impingement compared to healthy volunteers. These subjects were studied in a supine position with the shoulders moving during active abduction.

Graichen et al.[17] demonstrated that during isometric abduction, patients with shoulder impingement syndrome showed an acromiohumeral distance significantly smaller than those obtained with healthy volunteers or with the same shoulder during relaxation. This study also was performed in patients in a supine position using a novel MRI-based technique and three-dimensional image processing.

The open-configured MR systems are ideal imaging platforms for conducting kinematic MRI procedures. The relative openness of these devices enables certain types of kinematic MRI applications that would simply not be possible within the constraints of a standard "tunnel-shaped" MR system.

Among state-of-the-art open-configuration systems,[20] the SIGNA SP/I™ (General Electric Medical Systems, Milwaukee, WI) is unique because of its vertical access opening.[21] This system offers an opportunity to investigate the behavior of the shoulder during active motions of controlled and large amplitude with the subject in an upright, seated position (see also Chapter 11).[18]

In a kinematic MRI study of shoulder impingement using the vertically opened MR system, Bergman et al.[15] reported preliminary findings obtained in 10 normal volunteer subjects. However, the study only considered subjects in the side-lying position, which may fail to reproduce the conditions in which symptoms of shoulder disorders are frequently reproduced. Later, Beaulieu et al.[18] recognized the importance of conducting kinematic MRI of the shoulder examinations in volunteer subjects and patients in an upright, seated position. The experience of this group is presented in Chapter 11 of this textbook.

Similarly, our group has addressed the limitation of examining patients in a lying position and, therefore, developed a technique for kinematic MRI of the shoulder that is performed with the patient in an upright, seated position. This chapter provides a comprehensive account of the kinematic MRI protocol that we use and describes our experience with the use of this unique diagnostic imaging technique.

II. TECHNICAL ASPECTS

A. THE MAGNETIC RESONANCE SYSTEM AND PATIENT POSITIONING

The kinematic MRI protocol was designed to assess the subject in an upright, seated position while the subject moved the shoulder joint in a controlled manner in all ranges of motion. The technique also was conceived to allow for a standardized kinematic MRI assessment of the shoulder using the *active movement technique*, permitting free shoulder girdle movements.

The basic protocol exploits the features of the vertically opened MR system (0.5 T SIGNA-SP/I) shown in Figure 12.1. The so-called "double donut" configuration and near-real-time imaging capacity of this MR system, designed primarily for interventional MR applications, is well suited for kinematic MRI studies of the musculoskeletal system. This MR system has a 56 cm vertical access gap. Within this gap, a dedicated adjustable seat may be positioned that allows the subject to sit comfortably, with the shoulder located within the 30 cm diameter imaging volume at the center of the magnet opening.

To allow for the standardization of the seated position from one case to another, a dedicated seating bench was built to fit in the central opening of the vertically opened MR system (Figure 12.1). This simple wooden bench can be adjusted to accommodate the size of each subject. In particular, it may be readily adjusted to allow for free movements of the scapula and to bring the shoulder to the nominal center of the MR magnet, as well as to place the cervical and thoracoscapular regions in a standardized position. With the subject seated in this

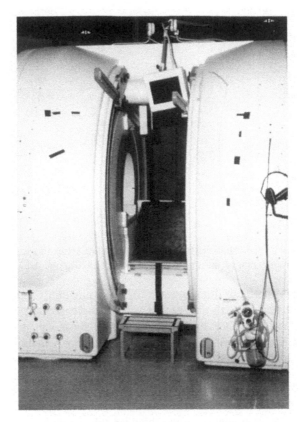

FIGURE 12.1   The vertically opened MR system (Signa SP/I, General Electric Medical Systems, WI). Note the seat in the center of the "double donut" configured magnet that permits the subject to be examined in an upright, seated position.

manner, the hip and knee joints are flexed at 100° and 90° of flexion, respectively, and the feet are supported.

B. IMAGING PARAMETERS AND PROTOCOL

The hardware components necessary to perform the kinematic MRI examination of the shoulder are shown in Figure 12.2. Figure 12.3 illustrates the setup of these components on the subject's shoulder and arm while seated in an upright position within the vertically opened MR system.

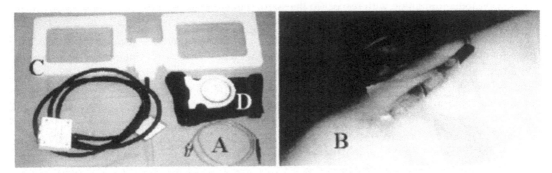

FIGURE 12.2   (Left) Hardware components used for the kinematic MRI examination of the shoulder: tip tracking coil (A), a flexible surface coil (C), and an hydrogoniometer (D). (Right) Installation of the active tip tracking coil (B) onto the subject's acromioclavicular joint line.

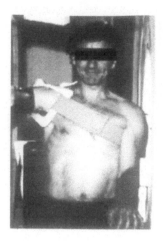 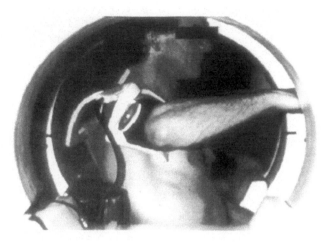

FIGURE 12.3   Frontal (left) and lateral (right) views of the subject setup and positioning at 90° of abduction for the kinematic MRI examination of the shoulder using the vertically opened MR system.

Our technique for performing the kinematic MRI examination of the shoulder uses the MR Tracking system to actively localize the acromium. The implementation and performance of the MR Tracking system are described by Dumoulin et al.[22] Basically, this device performs as a miniature untuned radiofrequency (RF)-receiving coil sensitive only to those hydrogen spins immediately surrounding it. The spatially limited sensitivity of the miniature coil leads to a direct relationship between its position within a magnetic field gradient and the frequency spectrum of its received MR signal. Fast localization in a three-dimensional space is achieved using a dedicated Hadamard multiplexed pulse sequence.

For the kinematic MRI examination of the shoulder, this active localizer coil is positioned and taped to the subject's skin over the acromioclavicular joint line (Figure 12.2). This location permits acquisition of "near-real-time" imaging of the acromion and the humeral head, simultaneously. Notably, a transmit/receive flexible RF surface coil is used to facilitate the kinematic MRI procedure (Figure 12.2).

MR imaging is performed in near-real-time mode using a fast gradient echo pulse sequence (repetition time, TR, 19.0 msec; echo time, TE, 7.2 msec; flip angle, 70°) while actively registering the tip tracking coil. A single 7 mm thick section location is acquired in an oblique coronal plane oriented parallel to the supraspinatus tendon. The resulting image acquisition rate is 2.5 sec/image, including active slice localization by the MR Tracker.

Finally, a fluid goniometer (MIE, Medical Research Ltd.) is strapped to the subject's upper arm (Figures 12.2 and 12.3). This device allows for a direct measurement of the subject's arm flexion or abduction angle with respect to the starting position (0° of flexion). The accuracy of the goniometer is 0.96 degrees.[23]

Figure 12.4 shows a typical MR image acquired in a subject at 0° of arm elevation using the aforementioned sequence. Figure 12.5 shows a kinematic MRI examination of the shoulder obtained with a healthy subject executing a movement of forward flexion from 15° to 130°. Starting from the resting position, the subject was instructed to perform two consecutive trials of anterior flexion and to maintain successive angles of 15°, 50°, 70°, 90°, 110°, and 130°. All movements were performed in neutral humerus rotation with the forearm in mid-pronation and the thumb oriented upward.

Figure 12.6 shows a typical dynamic series of images of the shoulder joint of the same healthy subject now performing an abduction movement. Here again, starting from the resting position, the subject executed two consecutive trials of abduction, maintaining arm positions of 50°, 70°, 80°, 90°, and 110°. These examples illustrate the kinematic MRI procedure performed using the *active movement technique*.

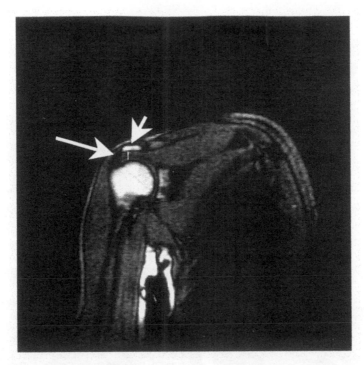

FIGURE 12.4 Typical MR image of a normal shoulder joint obtained using a "near-real-time" pulse sequence that facilitates the kinematic MRI examination of the shoulder using the *active movement technique.* The long arrow points to the subacromial space delimited above by the acromion (short arrow) and below by the humeral head. The white line defines the acromiohumeral distance.

III. KINEMATIC MRI OF THE SHOULDER: ASSESSMENT OF CHANGES IN THE ACROMIOHUMERAL DISTANCE

The kinematic MRI technique introduced here was developed to enable measurements of the acromiohumeral distance (AHD) at controlled angles of flexion and abduction. The intra- and interobserver reliability, as well as the accuracy of measurements of the AHD obtained with this new technique, have been determined in a group of healthy volunteer subjects.

First, asymptomatic candidates considered as "control subjects" underwent a standardized clinical evaluation to ensure the integrity of the upper quadrant, especially that of the shoulder girdle complex. Candidates demonstrating normal results on the physical and clinical tests were then evaluated using plain film radiography. Subsequently, only those subjects whose glenohumeral joint was diagnosed as unimpaired were included in the normal subject group (13 individuals; 7 men, 6 women).

These normal volunteer subjects underwent kinematic MRI of the shoulder using the active movement technique. To quantify the acromiohumeral distance from MR images acquired with our protocol, the AHD was defined as the smallest vertical distance measured between the external cortical lines of the acromion and the humeral head. A typical measurement of the AHD is shown in Figure 12.4.

Four measurements of the AHD were drawn at each angular position from any selected image. Measurements were carried out by two independent radiologists, each reading the images at two different times. As a result, eight measurements (two trials × two readers × two readings) of the AHD were collected for each flexion or abduction position. Thus, a mean value for the AHD of the shoulder under study at each position of flexion and abduction was calculated. Combining the measurements obtained from both readers and trials also allowed us to compute the intraclass correlation coefficients (ICC) as well as the inter-reader and intertrial measurement error.

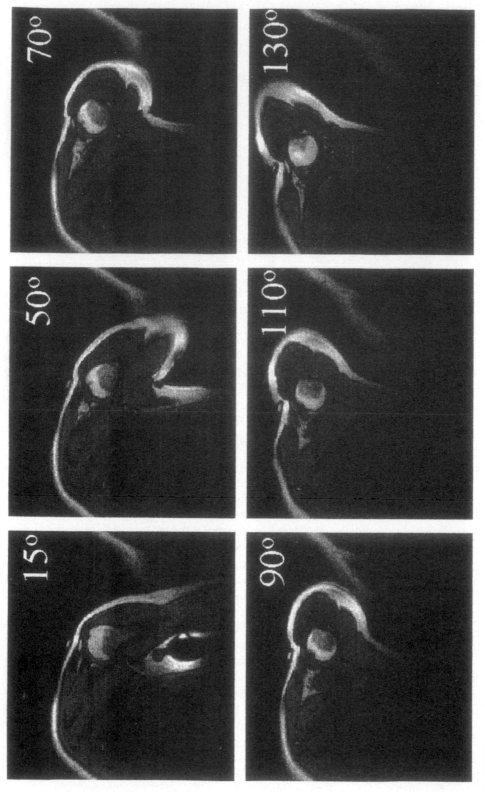

FIGURE 12.5   Series of oblique coronal plane kinematic MR images of the shoulder joint obtained between 15° and 130° of forward flexion.

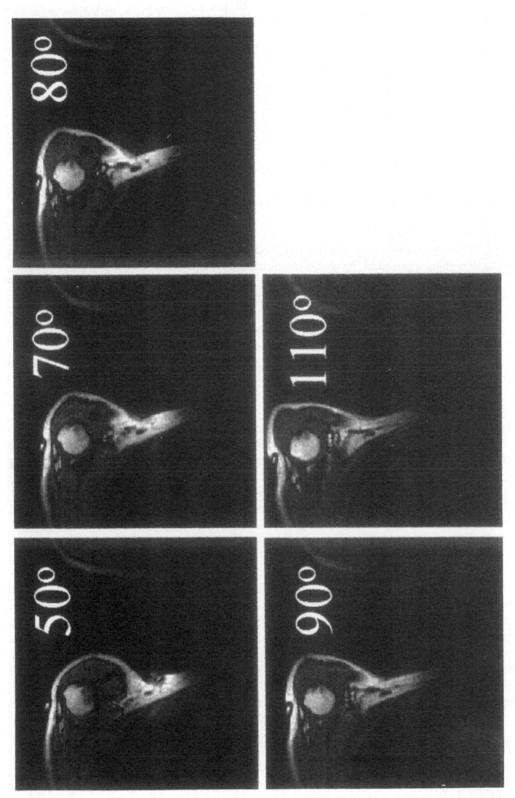

FIGURE 12.6 Series of oblique coronal plane kinematic MR images of the shoulder joint obtained between 50° and 110° of shoulder abduction.

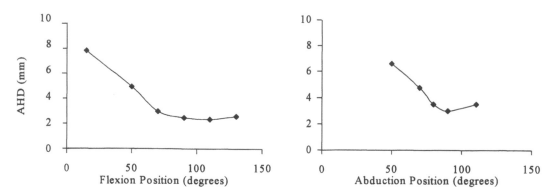

FIGURE 12.7   Average acromiohumeral distance (AHD) as a function of forward flexion angle (right) and abduction angle (left) observed for a normal subject.

Figure 12.7 illustrates typical changes in the AHD in one subject as a function of the flexion and abduction angular positions. As shown in this case, there is a decrease of the AHD as elevation of the arm increases. For this subject, the trend as well as the change in AHD are quite comparable between flexion and abduction.

Notably, the intra- and interobserver reliability of the technique were found to be very good.[24] The results also indicated minimal inter-reader error. The largest absolute difference in the evaluation of the AHD by the two radiologists was 1 mm. In abduction, independent readings of the AHD by two radiologists also were found to yield AHD measurements which agreed to within ±0.5 mm for a confidence level of 91%.

However, we observed significant variations of AHD values measured between two independent trials of movements. Indeed, independent trials were found to yield AHD measurements agreeing to ±1.5 mm for a confidence level of 92% in both flexion and abduction. A number of good reasons may be put forward to explain the intertrial variation obtained in this study. The most obvious source of variation across trials could result from the difficulty in ensuring the exact positioning of the subjects and especially in controlling for head positioning and trunk posture without hindering the natural dynamic motion of the shoulder. In addition, small protraction and retraction movements may have occurred. These motions would be expected to contribute to measurable variations of the AHD between trials.[25]

Another factor contributing to the intertrial error could be associated with the use of the tip tracking coil in locating the acromion and imaging through the acromioclavicular joint line. This component of the protocol is indeed sensitive to several factors that were not controlled during the course of our study. For instance, the accuracy with which the device can be positioned over the same location on the subject's shoulder from one trial to another is a potentially significant source of variability. In addition, although the tip tracking device is taped to the skin, small changes in its position may occur as the subject executes a flexion or abduction movement of large amplitude. Given that the miniature receiving RF-coil of the tip tracker is encapsulated in a plastic cap of 5 mm diameter, control of its location between trials within its millimeter precision could indeed be an issue. Subsequently, the determination of the appropriate oblique-coronal slice through the tip tracker location and the supraspinatus muscle is dependent on the direct appreciation of the clinician supervising the case and could easily be subject to error from one trial to the other. To understand the contributions to the observed intertrial error of the technique, a systematic study was carried out using an anthropomorphic phantom. Results of this study indicated that contributions to the intertrial uncertainty inherent to the imaging hardware and sequence are altogether smaller than 1 mm and, thus, do not dominate the intertrial error.

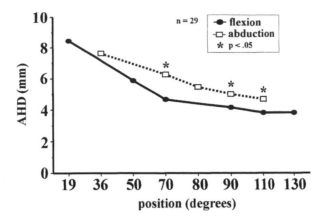

FIGURE 12.8 Mean values of the acromiohumeral distance (AHD) during forward flexion and abduction as a function of arm position. Results are from a group of 29 healthy asymptomatic shoulders. Asterisks indicate a significant difference between AHD values in flexion and abduction.

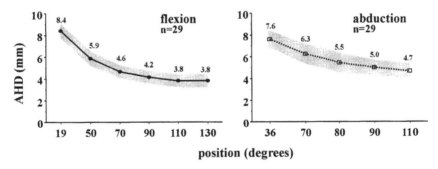

FIGURE 12.9 Mean acromiohumeral distance (AHD) as a function of forward flexion angle (left) and abduction (right). Mean values and 95% confidence intervals (gray band) were obtained from a group of 29 healthy asymptomatic shoulders.

A. REFERENCE AHD VALUES IN HEALTHY SUBJECTS

Figures 12.8 and 12.9 summarize the AHD changes associated with different shoulder movements in healthy subjects and compare the mean AHD values during forward flexion and abduction as a function of arm positions for the entire group. Figure 12.9 presents the mean AHD values against their 95% confidence intervals. As illustrated by the figures, there is a significant decrease of the mean AHD as elevation of the arm increases from rest to the maximum elevation. Although the trend is similar, the magnitude in the reduction of the AHD is greater in flexion than in abduction (from 70° to 100° of elevation). Statistical analysis of these data revealed a smaller AHD value ($p < 0.01$) at 110° of flexion (4.1 mm) and abduction (4.6 mm) compared to the other positions, with the exception of 130° of flexion and 90° of abduction positions. These latter positions were found not to differ from the AHD at 110° in their corresponding plane of movement.

IV. CLINICAL APPLICATION: SHOULDER IMPINGEMENT SYNDROME

Many etiologies are involved in the pathogenesis of shoulder pain. However, a high proportion is secondary to the so-called "shoulder impingement syndrome" or SIS.[26] Although SIS has been closely associated with lesions of the rotator cuff,[27-30] it is now recognized as a clinical entity to which one attributes pain and dysfunction resulting from irritation of the structures contained within the subacromial space. In fact, one of the factors put forward in explaining the etiology of SIS is narrowing of the subacromial space during elevation of the arm against gravity.[12,18,31]

SIS is thought to reflect the painful compression of the supraspinatus tendon, the subacromial-subdeltoid bursa and the long head of the biceps tendon between the humeral head and the acromion.[26,27] In a clinical context, signs and symptoms of SIS, such as a painful arc or impingement signs, can only be observed during free motions or at arm angles around 90° of elevation.

SIS is a clinical diagnosis that is supported with information obtained from conventional static-view MRI. However, most MRI findings appear rather nonspecific because the imaging protocol is not performed in the position and conditions in which SIS actually occurs. Thus, SIS may best be evaluated using kinematic MRI to examine the shoulder during active, unrestricted motions. Accordingly, one of our prime objectives was to develop a kinematic MRI protocol that reproduced the clinical examination routinely performed to diagnose SIS. Thus, the diagnostic imaging procedure should adequately reproduce the conditions in which the impingement is more likely to happen, thereby complementing clinical findings with objective kinematic MRI data.

Patients with a diagnosis of SIS were evaluated to investigate the use of kinematic MRI of the shoulder to assess patients with this condition. Subjects with a unilateral SIS diagnosis were assessed by the same physical therapist and considered eligible if the affected shoulder presented a positive finding in each of the three following categories: (a) painful arc during active shoulder flexion or abduction;[32] (b) positive Neer[10] or Kennedy-Hawkins[33] impingement signs; and (c) pain on resisted isometric lateral rotation, abduction, or the Jobe test.[34] According to these criteria, SIS subjects were diagnosed as having had stage I or II impingement.[10] Subjects with one of the following criteria were excluded: (a) rheumatoid, inflammatory, degenerative, and neurological diseases; (b) stroke; (c) previous surgery involving the neck and the shoulder; (d) neck pain or restricted neck motion, cervico-brachialgia or shoulder pain reproduced during active neck movements; (e) trapezius myalgia syndrome; (f) shoulder capsulitis defined as a restriction of active and passive glenohumeral movements of at least 30% of amplitude for two or more directions of shoulder movements; and (g) collaborative problems interfering with tests. The subjects also were screened by an experienced shoulder orthopedic surgeon to rule out fractures, bone abnormalities, calcification, and shoulder instability. Healthy volunteer subjects also underwent the same procedures.

Figure 12.10 shows the changes in the AHD as a function of arm position during forward flexion and abduction for six subjects with a unilateral SIS imaged using the active movement kinematic MRI examination with the patient in an upright, seated position. The data displayed in this figure allow a comparison of the changes in the AHD for SIS subjects at successive positions of abduction and flexion compared to a group of 29 control subject shoulders. Notably, from 90° of flexion and abduction, the AHD values in all six SIS subjects are located outside the 95% confidence interval band of the data obtained in the healthy shoulders.

With patients in a supine position and under static conditions, the minimal thickness of normal supraspinatus tendon has been reported to be 3 mm, as shown on MR images using a T1-weighted pulse sequence.[35] Therefore, the minimal AHD value at 90° of arm elevation in a supine, as well as in an upright, position must be greater than 3 mm to prevent compression of the supraspinatus tendon. This distance should be even more when considering the additional space required for other subacromial structures. However, such is not the case for some of our SIS subjects who presented AHD values as low as 2 mm. Similar results were reported by others[16,17] for SIS subjects who did not present a full-thickness tear of the rotator cuff.

Errors associated with determining ADH values may be related to the difficulty of MR imaging to differentiate the articular cartilage of the humeral head from surrounding structures. Since cortical bone does not contain protons, this part of the bone does not yield a significant MR signal. A widening of the hypointense signal associated with cortical bone on the MR image contributes to an artificial decrease of the space between the acromion and the humeral head. Thus, this leads to an underestimation of the AHD.

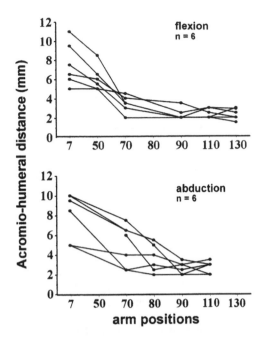

FIGURE 12.10 Changes in the acromiohumeral distance (AHD) as a function of forward flexion (top) and abduction (bottom) for six patients with a unilateral SIS diagnosis.

In a study performed with cadavers, Hodler et al.[36] reported that several of the routinely used MR sequences tend to overestimate thin cartilage and underestimate thick cartilage. MR images obtained without intra-articular contrast material are more prone to this artifact than are MR arthrographic images. However, the underlying underestimation of AHD values, or overestimation of the mechanical impingement, will apply to both normal and symptomatic shoulder groups. As a result it will not affect a comparison between controls and SIS subjects.

A second possible source of error in measuring the AHD relates to partial volume effects from cartilage as a function of orientation in the imaging plane. The use of three-dimensional image processing with MRI and computed tomography (CT) has been proposed[37] to overcome geometric distortions[38] and truncation artifacts[39] inherent to two-dimensional imaging.

Despite the potential for overestimation of the mechanical impingement when using two-dimensional MR imaging, results available in the literature support the use of this imaging technique to characterize movement-related changes of the AHD. Indeed, a close comparison of the results obtained with our protocol to those obtained on three-dimensional MR images[17,37] indicates that the mean changes observed in the AHD and their variability are quite similar for both two- and three-dimensional MR images. For example, the mean AHD reported by Graichen et al.[37] decreased from 7.9 to 5.9 mm between 30° and 150° of abduction. This is in agreement with change from 7.6 to 4.7 mm between 35° and 110° of abduction, which we observed for our group of 29 healthy shoulders.

Figure 12.11 presents data that show large intersubject differences observed in the AHD values from the SIS subjects at rest are lost in elevation positions. The AHD in SIS subjects at rest is highly and positively correlated with the magnitude of its reduction. One can easily observe that the greater the AHD value is at rest the greater its reduction with arm elevation.

Our findings show that SIS subjects with greater AHD at rest are not keeping greater AHD during arm elevation. This may be attributed to the muscles required to stabilize and move the arm. Normally, these muscles associated with the glenohumeral joint generate compressive forces that are maximal between 60° and 140° of arm elevation.[40] The muscles also ensure maximal rotation of the scapula to optimize the position of the glenoid fossa with respect to the humeral head.[41]

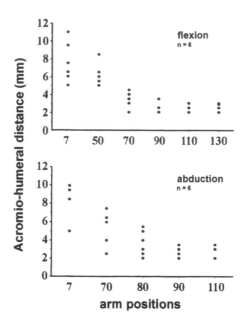

FIGURE 12.11   Changes in the acromiohumeral distance (AHD) as a function of forward flexion positions (top) and abduction positions (bottom) for six patients with a unilateral SIS diagnosis.

Therefore, muscles act to maintain a close proximity between the humeral head and the scapula leaving a very small range for AHD variations around 90° of arm elevation.

Furthermore, as shear forces are also maximal in this range,[40] there must be a balance between shear and compressive forces to avoid humeral head instability which leads to a fine tuning of AHD during arm elevation. For patients with SIS, passive anatomical factors,[10,25,42-45] such as the type of acromion or posterior capsule tightness, can further influence the relationship between the humeral head and the acromion during active shoulder motion. An early recruitment of the supraspinatus and deltoid muscles,[40] as well as the inability of the subscapularis, infraspinatus, and teres minor muscles to depress the humeral head,[30,46-47] can drive the humeral head in a superior direction, contributing to a greater reduction of the AHD during arm elevation.

V. SUMMARY AND CONCLUSIONS

In this chapter, we described a protocol for the kinematic MRI evaluation of the shoulder performed with the patient in an upright, seated position. This new approach specifically exploits the space afforded by the vertically opened MR system that is particularly well suited to accommodating the natural motion of the shoulder joint. The shoulder movements for this kinematic MRI examination are standardized in terms of positions and the plane of motion. Near-real-time MR images are acquired using the acromioclavicular joint line as an anatomic landmark for the origin of the imaging plane and the direction of the supraspinatus muscle to fix its orientation.

To date, our experience presented herein has demonstrated the feasibility and capacity of this kinematic MRI technique to monitor active movement-related changes of the AHD in healthy subjects as well as in patients diagnosed with impingement syndrome. Our results have confirmed that AHD values obtained with this protocol are reliable.

The kinematic MRI examination of the shoulder with the patient in an upright, seated position leads to a better understanding of the biomechanics of the shoulder. We have shown a clear application of the technique in SIS subjects where the AHD observed at the critical positions for shoulder impingement provides an outcome measure to discriminate between shoulders with and without impingement.

Further use of this technique should add to known radiological-clinical correlation and lead to a better understanding of the pathogenesis of the SIS and other shoulder disorders, such as shoulder instability. Kinematic MRI of the shoulder also provides an instrument of choice for a large array of research interests aimed at better understanding the normal and pathological biomechanics of the shoulder joint. In conjunction with other outcome measures such as muscle strength, three-dimensional movements of the scapula, and glenohumeral range of motion, kinematic MRI of the shoulder should find further clinical applications, especially in validating the response to rehabilitation or medical interventions.

REFERENCES

1. Anderson, J. A. D., Shoulder pain and tension neck and relation to work, *Scand. J. Work Environ. Health*, 10, 435, 1984.
2. Cole, D. C. and Hudak, P., Prognostic of non-specific work-related musculoskeletal disorders of the neck and upper extremity, *Am. J. Ind. Med.*, 29, 657, 1996.
3. Ekberg, K. et al., Case-control study of risk factors for disease in the neck and shoulder occupational area, *Occup. Environ. Med.*, 51, 262, 1994.
4. Sommerich, C. M., McGlothlin, J. D., and Marras, W. S., Occupational risk factors associated with tissue disorders of the shoulder: a review of recent investigations in the literature, *Ergonomics*, 36, 697, 1993.
5. Royal College of General Practitioners Surveys, Morbidity statistics from general practice, O.o.P.C.a., London, 1986.
6. Kieft, G., Bloem, J., Rozing, P., and Oberman, W., Rotator cuff impingement syndrome: MR imaging, *Radiology*, 166, 211, 1988.
7. Miniaci, A. and Salonen, D., Rotator cuff evaluation: imaging and diagnosis, *Orthop. Clin. North Am.*, 28, 43, 1997.
8. Seeger, L., Gold, R., Bassett, L., and Ellman, H., Shoulder impingement syndrome: MR findings in 53 shoulders, *Am. J. Roentgenol.*, 150, 343, 1988.
9. Zlatkin, M., Dalinka, M., and Kressel, H., *Magn. Reson. Quarterly*, 5, 3, 1989.
10. Neer, C. S., Impingement lesions, *Clin. Orthop.*, 173, 70, 1983.
11. Brossmann, J., Preidler, K., Pedowitz, R., White, L., Trudell, D., and Resnick, D., Shoulder impingement syndrome: influence of shoulder position on rotator cuff impingement — an anatomic study, *Am. J. Roentgenol.*, 167, 1511, 1996.
12. San, N., Richardi, G., Raillac, J., and Assoun, J., Kinematic MR imaging of the shoulder: normal patterns, *Am. J. Roentgenol.*, 167, 1517, 1996.
13. Cardinal, E., Buckwalter, K. A., and Braunstein, E. M., Kinematic magnetic resonance of the normal shoulder: assessment of the labrum and capsule, *Can. Assoc. Radiol. J.*, 47, 44, 1996.
14. Bonnutti, P. M., Norfray, J. F., Friedman, R. J., and Genez, B. M., Kinematic MRI of the shoulder, *J. Comput. Assist. Tomogr.*, 17, 666, 1993.
15. Bergman, A. G. et al., Shoulder impingement: motion evaluation of abduction in 10 normal volunteers using a 0.5 T MRT system, in *Proceedings of the International Society for Magnetic Resonance in Medicine, Book of Abstracts*, Vol. 3, Berkeley, 1997, p. 1006.
16. Allmann, K.-H. et al., Cine-MR imaging of the shoulder, *Acta Radiol.*, 38, 1043, 1997.
17. Graichen, H. et al., Three-dimensional analysis of the width of the subacromial space in healthy subjects and patients with impingement syndrome, *Am. J. Roentgenol.*, 172, 1081, 1999.
18. Beaulieu, C. F., Hodge, D. K., Bergman, A. G. et al., Glenohumeral relationships during physiologic shoulder motion and stress testing: initial experience with open MR imaging and active imaging-plane registration, *Radiology*, 212, 699–705, 1999.
19. Graichen, H., Stammberger, T., Bonel, H., Hauber, M., Englmeier, K.-H., Reiser, M., and Eckstein, F., Magnetic resonance based motion analysis of the shoulder during elevation, *Clin. Orthop. Relat. Res.*, 370, 154, 2000.

20. Zhao, Z. P., Overview of interventional MRI magnets, in *Interventional MRI*, Lufkin, R. B., Ed., Mosby, New York, 1999, p. 3.

21. Schenck, J. et al., Superconducting open-configuration MR imaging system for image-guided therapy, *Radiology*, 195, 805, 1995.

22. Dumoulin, C. L., Souza, S. P., and Darrow, R. D., Real-time position monitoring of invasive devices using magnetic resonance, *Magn. Reson. Med.*, 29, 411, 1993.

23. Hébert, L. J., Moffet, H., McFadyen, B. J., and St.-Vincent, G., A method of measuring three-dimensional scapular attitudes using the optotrak probing system, *Clin. Biomech.*, 15, 1, 2000.

24. Moffet, H. et al., Variation in sub-acromial distance measured by magnetic resonance imaging during shoulder flexion and abduction movements, *Can. J. Rehabil.*, 11, 265, 1998.

25. Solem-Bertoft, E., Thomas, K. A., and Westerberg, G. E., The influence of scapular retraction and protraction on the width of the subacromial space — an MRI study, *Clin. Orthop.*, 296, 99, 1993.

26. Fu, F. H., Harner, C. D., and Klein, A. H., Shoulder impingement syndrome: a critical review, *Clin. Orthop. Relat. Res.*, 269, 162, 1991.

27. Boublik, M. and Hawkins, R. J., Clinical examination of the shoulder complex, *J. Orthop. Sports Phys. Ther.*, 18, 379, 1993.

28. Jobe, F. W. and Pink, M., Classification and treatment of shoulder dysfunction in the overhead athlete, *J. Orthop. Sports Phys. Ther.*, 18, 427, 1993.

29. Jobe, F. W. and Bradley, J. P., The diagnosis and non-operative treatment of shoulder injuries in athletes, *Clin. Sports Med.*, 8, 419, 1989.

30. Neer, C. S. and Welsh, R. P., The shoulder in sport, *Orthop. Clin. North Am.*, 8, 379, 1977.

31. Zucherman, J. D., Kummer, F. J., Cuomo, F., Simon, J., Fosenblur, S., and Katz, N., The influence of coracoacromial arch anatomy on rotator cuff tears, *J. Shoulder Elbow Surg.*, 1, 4, 1992.

32. Hawkins, R. J. and Abrahams, J. S., Impingement syndrome in the absence of rotator cuff tear (stage 1 and 2), *Orthop. Clin. North Am.*, 18, 373, 1987.

33. Hawkins, R. J. and Kennedy, J. C., Impingement syndrome in athletes, *Am. J. Sports Med.*, 8, 151, 1980.

34. Magee, D., The shoulder, in *Orthopaedic Physical Assessment*, W.B. Saunders, Philadelphia, 1992, p. 175.

35. Bergman, A. G., Rotator cuff impingement: pathogenesis, MR imaging characteristics, and early dynamic MR results, *Magn. Reson. Imag. Clin. North Am.*, 5, 705, 1997.

36. Hodler, J., Loredo, R. A., Longo, C., Trudell, D., Yu, J. S., and Resnick, D., Assessment of articular cartilage thickness of the humeral head: MR-anatomic correlation in cadavers, *Am. J. Roentgenol.*, 165, 615, 1995.

37. Graichen, H. et al., A technique for determining the spatial relationship between the rotator cuff and the subacromial space in arm abduction using MRI and 3D image processing, *Magn. Reson. Med.*, 40, 640, 1998.

38. Lochmuller, E. M., Maier, U., Anetzberger, H., Habermeyer, P., and Muller-Gerbl, M., Determination of subacromial space width and inferior acromial mineralization by 3D CT. Preliminary data from patients with unilateral supraspinatus outlet syndrome, *Surg. Radiol. Anat.*, 19, 329, 1997.

39. Frank, L. R., Brossmann, J., Buxton, R. D., and Resnick, D., MR imaging truncation artifacts can create a false laminar appearance in cartilage, *Am. J. Roentgenol.*, 168, 547, 1996.

40. Sarrafian, S. K., Gross and functional anatomy of the shoulder, *Clin. Orthop. Relat. Res.*, 173, 9, 1983.

41. Bagg, D. S., and Forest, W. J., A biomechanical analysis of scapular rotation during arm abduction in the scapular plane, *Am. J. Phys. Med. Rehabil.*, 67, 238, 1988.

42. Rathburn, J. B. and MacNab, I., The microvascular pattern of the rotator cuff, *J. Bone Joint Surg. [Br.]*, 52B, 540, 1970.

43. Schneeberger, A., Nyffeler, R., and Gerber, C., Structural changes of the rotator cuff caused by experimental subacromial impingement in the rat, *J. Shoulder Elbow Surg.*, 7, 375, 1999.

44. Norwood, L. A., Barrack, R., and Jacobson, K. E., Clinical presentation of complete tears of the rotator cuff, *J. Bone Joint Surg. [Am.]*, 71, 499, 1989.

45. Tyler, T. F., Roy, T., Nicholas, S. J., McHugh, M. P., and Glein, G. W., Posterior capsule tightness and motion loss in patients diagnosed with shoulder impingement syndrome, *J. Orthop. Sports Phys. Ther.*, 30, 1, 2000.

46. Sharkey, N. A. and Marder, R. A., The rotator cuff opposes superior translation of the humeral head, *Am. J. Sports Med.,* 23, 270, 1995.

47. Payne, L. Z., Deng, X.-H., Craig, E. V., Torzilli, P. A., and Warren, R. F., The combined dynamic and static contributions to subacromial impingement, *Am. J. Sports Med.*, 25, 801, 1997.

Part VI

Temporomandibular Joint

13 The Temporomandibular Joint: Functional Anatomy and Kinesiology

Sally Ho

CONTENTS

I. INTRODUCTION

Functioning as a paired structure, the human temporomandibular joint (TMJ) serves to connect the mandible with the rest of the skeletal system. The TMJ is capable of performing various movements, including opening, closing, protrusion, retrusion, and medial and lateral deviation. However, opening and closing movements of the jaw are the most fundamental tasks, with this motion occurring approximately 1500 to 2000 times during a person's daily oral function.

As a result of its close proximity to the cranial nerves, facial structures, and the cervical spine, TMJ dysfunction can manifest as numerous symptoms, including headaches, dizziness, vertigo,

0-8493-0807-0/01/$0.00+$.50
© 2001 by Frank G. Shellock

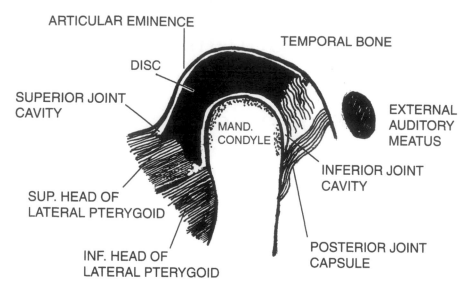

ARTICULAR EMINENCE

TEMPORAL BONE

DISC

SUPERIOR JOINT
CAVITY

MAND.
CONDYLE

EXTERNAL
AUDITORY
MEATUS

INFERIOR JOINT
CAVITY

SUP. HEAD OF
LATERAL PTERYGOID

INF. HEAD OF
LATERAL PTERYGOID

POSTERIOR JOINT
CAPSULE

FIGURE 13.1   Anatomy of the temporomandibular joint (TMJ). The TMJ is located anterior to the external ear and is classified as a diarthrodial synovial joint. It consists of the articulation between the mandibular condylar process and articular eminence of the cranium.

earache/fullness, tinnitus, joint noises and pain, malocclusions, toothaches, speech disturbances, and swallowing difficulty. Epidemiological studies have indicated that approximately 50% of the adult population will suffer at least one sign of TMJ dysfunction.[1-3] Additionally, population-based studies have reported 1% to 22% of the general population suffer severe TMJ dysfunction depending on the criteria used.[4]

A basic understanding of the normal structure and function of this complex joint is necessary for assessing the underlying process of pain and dysfunction. Thus, this chapter describes the normal functional anatomy, normal kinesiology, and pathokinesiology of the TMJ.

II. FUNCTIONAL ANATOMY

The TMJ is located anterior to the external ear and is classified as a diarthrodial synovial joint. It consists of the articulation between the mandibular condylar process and the articular eminence of the cranium (Figure 13.1). The articulating surfaces are covered by fibrocartilage, which has the ability to undergo a great deal of remodeling. A fibrocartilage disc covers the mandibular condyle, dividing the joint into superior and inferior joint cavities. These two joint cavities are both lined with synovial tissue.

A. OSSEOUS STRUCTURES: THE TEMPORAL BONE AND MANDIBULAR CONDYLE

The squamous part of the temporal bone, which forms the roof of the TMJ, consists of four parts. From posterior to anterior, there is the post-glenoid spine, the mandibular fossa, the articular eminence, and the articular tubercle (Figure 13.2). These structures are situated immediately anterior to the external auditory meatus. The mandibular fossa consists of thin, translucent bone; therefore, it is not appropriate for articular function.

By comparison, the articular eminence consists of trabecular bone and therefore provides the primary articular surface for the TMJ. The slope of the articular eminence usually ranges between 30 and 60 degrees. Slopes of less than 30 degrees are considered flat, and slopes greater than 60 degrees are considered steep. A flat slope predisposes the mandibular condyle to excessive anterior translation, resulting in anterior displacement of the articular disc.

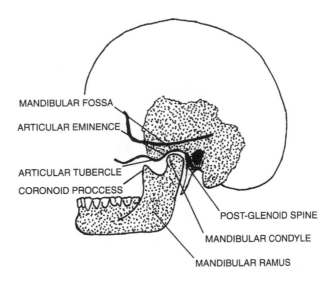

FIGURE 13.2   Osseous structures of the temporomandibular joint, from posterior to anterior, there is the post-glenoid spine, the mandibular fossa, the articular eminence, and the articular tubercle.

The floor of the TMJ is formed by the mandibular condyle. The adult condylar head is usually elliptical in shape, but may vary from convex to concave.[5] The medial and lateral poles of the condyle provide the location for the attachment of the medial and lateral collateral ligaments. Inferior to the condylar head is the condylar neck where the inferior fibers of the lateral pterygoid insert. The ramus of the mandible projects superiorly from the condylar neck and becomes the coronoid process, attachment site of the temporalis muscle. Inferiorly, the ramus becomes the body of the mandible which houses the mandibular teeth (Figure 13.2).

B. INTRACAPSULAR STRUCTURES: ARTICULAR DISC AND RETRODISCAL PAD

The articular disc consists of fibrocartilagenous tissue which has a higher proportion of dense collagen fibers than hyaline fibers. As a result, this structure is able to withstand high-level stress and undergo remodeling.[6,7] The articular disc is biconcave in shape and separates the joint space into superior and inferior compartments. The three major portions of the disc are the pes meniscus (anterior zone), pars gracilis (intermediate zone), and pars posterior (posterior zone) (Figure 13.3).

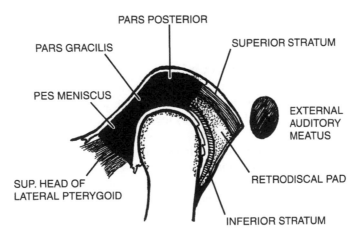

FIGURE 13.3   Sagittal view of the temporomandibular joint. Note the three major portions of the disc: the pes meniscus (anterior zone), pars gracilis (intermediate zone), and pars posterior (posterior zone).

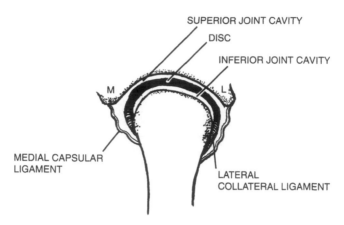

FIGURE 13.4 Frontal (coronal) view of the left temporomandibular joint.

Both the pes meniscus and pars posterior have a vascular supply and neural innervation. The intermediate pars gracilis is avascular and aneural, yet possesses the most dense fibrous tissue. It is ideally positioned for its role as a pressure-bearing surface. The pars gracilis receives its nutrition from synovial fluid.[6]

Functionally, the disc lies between the convex surface of the mandibular condyle and the convex surface of the articular eminence. This structure provides joint congruency throughout the range of motion, transmits force, and protects and lubricates the articulating surfaces. The anterior portion of the disc is attached to the superior fibers of the lateral pterygoid muscle. The posterior-superior portion of the disc is attached to the posterior stratum and the posterior-inferior portion of the disc is attached to the inferior stratum. The stratum is connective tissue which forms the bilamina area. Medially and laterally, the disc attaches to the medial/lateral poles of the condylar head through the medial and lateral collateral ligaments[5] (Figures 13.3 and 13.4). The disc also attaches to the posterior capsule. Since the disc does not attach to the capsule medially or laterally, translation between the disc and the condyle in the medial and lateral direction may occur.[6]

The retrodiscal pad is composed of connective tissue that lies between the superior and inferior stratum. This structure has its own blood supply and innervation and, therefore, is often a source of pain and inflammation. Using kinematic MRI, synovial fluid may be seen being pumped in and out of the retrodiscal tissue with opening and closing of the mouth. Such fluid dynamics provide lubrication and nutrition of the articular surfaces.[8]

C. Capsular and Extracapsular Structures: The Joint Capsule and Ligaments

Capsular tissue covers the TMJ superiorly, inferiorly, anteriorly, and posteriorly. Superiorly, the capsule attaches to the borders of the mandibular fossa and the articular eminence. Inferiorly, it attaches to the neck of the condyle and posteriorly, to the disc.[9] The capsule encompasses the joint space and retains synovial fluid produced by the synovium. The capsule is highly vascularized and innervated.

The synovium lines the superior and the inferior joint cavity and produces lubrication during joint function. When the synovial membrane is disturbed, such as in the condition of articular disc displacement, the impairment of the synovial function may lead to degenerative joint changes.[8]

The ligaments of the TMJ are extremely strong. Their primary functions are to check the different oral movements and restrict movement generated by muscle or external force, especially the translation of the mandible.[10] The temporomandibular ligament supports the lateral wall of the capsule. The oblique portion of the temporomandibular ligament arises from the lateral surface of

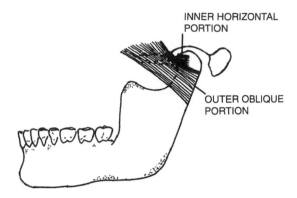

FIGURE 13.5 Lateral view of the left temporomandibular ligament.

the articular tubercle and the zygomatic process and inserts on the posterolateral surface of the condylar neck (Figure 13.5). Its function is to limit rotation of the condyle during jaw opening. The horizontal portion of the temporomandibular ligament arises from the lateral surface of the articular tubercle and the zygomatic process and inserts on the lateral pole of the condyle and the posterior part of the disc (Figure 13.5). This structure limits posterior displacement of the condyle, thereby protecting the retrodiscal pad. The temporomandibular ligament also prevents the lateral pterygoid muscle from excessive lengthening through its attachment to the disc.[6]

The collateral ligaments attach the medial and lateral borders of the articular disc to the medial and the lateral poles of the condyle, respectively (Figure 13.4). Their function is to restrict excessive medial-lateral motion of the disc, so the disc can move with the condyle as the condyle translates anteriorly and posteriorly.

The stylomandibular ligament arises from the styloid process and inserts into the posterior border and the angle of the mandibular ramus (Figure 13.6). Its function is to limit excessive protrusion of the mandible. The sphenomandibular ligament arises from the spine of the sphenoid bone and inserts into the middle surface of the inferior ramus (Figure 13.6). This ligament prevents joint separation and excessive forward translation of the mandible.[7]

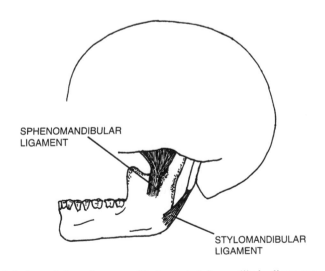

FIGURE 13.6 Medial view of the sphenomandibular and stylomandibular ligaments.

D. INNERVATION

The TMJ is innervated by the three branches of the mandibular division of the fifth cranial nerve. The posterior deep temporal and masseteric nerves supply the anterior and medial regions of the joint, whereas the auriculotemporal nerve supplies the posterior and lateral regions of the joint. The auriculotemporal nerve is the major nerve innervating the posterolateral capsule, the retrodiscal pad, the capsular blood vessels, and the temporomandibular ligament. This nerve also sends a few branches to innervate the tympani membrane, the external auditory meatus, the lateral surface of the superior half of the auricle, and the skin of the temple and scalp.[11-13]

The trigeminal nerve innervates the masicatory musculature and provides the sensory innervation of the oral and facial structures. Neurons from the trigeminal nerve share the same neuron pool as cranial nerves VII, IX, X, XI and the upper cervical neurons (cervical nerves I, II, and III).[14] This helps explain how pain from the cervical region can be referred to the trigeminal region.[15]

III. NORMAL KINESIOLOGY

The resting position of the mandible is defined as the position where all movements begin and end and all associated muscles experience minimum tension.[16,17] When the mandible is at its resting position, a small space exists between the upper and lower arch of the teeth. This is defined as the "freeway space." The average freeway space is approximately 3 mm between the upper and lower central incisors. To maintain the upright postural position of the mandible there is tonic contraction of the masticatory muscles. This contraction places the condylar head at the posterior-superior slope of the articular eminence.

There are two major arthrokinematic movements within the TMJ, rotation and translation. Rotation occurs within the inferior joint space, while translation occurs within the superior space.[9,18] These component arthrokinematic motions are essential for the osteokinematic movements of the mandible. The osteokinematic movements of the TMJ include depression, elevation, protrusion, retrusion, and lateral deviation. These movements are essential for the functional tasks of chewing, swallowing, and speech.

A. MANDIBULAR DEPRESSION AND ELEVATION (JAW OPENING/CLOSING)

The normal opening distance as measured from the upper central incisor to the lower central incisor is from 40 to 45 mm for men, and 45 to 50 mm for women.[16,19] During the initial phase of jaw opening (i.e., the first 25 mm), the mandibular condyle rotates anteriorly and the disc remains stationary.[20] This puts the disc in a relatively posterior position with respect to the condyle.

After 25 mm of opening, anterior translation of the condylar head occurs in the upper joint compartment.[5,21] As a result of the firm attachment of the disc to the mandibular condyle, the condyle and the disc translate anteriorly as a unit. During this phase of motion, the disc also rotates posteriorly relative to the mandibular condyle owing to the pull of the posterior stratum. This rotation keeps the non-innervated middle portion of the disc between the articular surfaces.

During jaw closing, the disc and the mandibular condyle translate posteriorly while the disc rotates anteriorly. Anterior rotation of the disc occurs as a result of contraction of the superior head of the lateral pterygoid muscle and progressive relaxation of the superior stratum. As with jaw opening, the non-innervated part of the disc is maintained between the articular surfaces during closing.

B. MANDIBULAR PROTRUSION AND RETRUSION

Protrusion occurs when the lower teeth move forward beyond the upper teeth. During protrusion, the mandibular condyle and the articular disc move downward and forward. This motion occurs along the articular eminence about a transverse axis.[16] To balance the movement and prevent the mandible from dropping, the muscles of elevation and the depressor-retrusors have to contract synchronically. The normal range of jaw protrusion from the neutral position is approximately 6 to 9 mm.[6]

During jaw retrusion, the mandibular condyle and the articular disc translate posteriorly and the mandible is maintained in the horizontal position by the synergistic action of the elevators and the depressors. The normal range of jaw retrusion from the neutral position is approximately 3 mm.[6]

C. Mandibular Lateral Deviation

During lateral movement of the mandible, the ipsilateral condyle (working condyle) rotates and spins forward, downward, and medially, while the contralateral condyle (balancing condyle) translates horizontally towards the working condyle. The normal range of lateral deviation is usually one fourth of the opening range or one full width of one upper central incisor.[19,22]

D. Muscular Action

The temporalis muscle is a large fan-shaped muscle that originates from the entire temporal fossa and inserts onto the coronoid process and the anterior border of the mandibular ramus (Figure 13.7). The major function of the temporalis muscle is elevation and ipsilateral deviation of the mandible.[16,23,24] The posterior fibers of the temporalis retract the mandible from the resting position, whereas all fibers retract the mandible from a protruded position.

The masseter muscle is the most powerful muscle of the body. Its superficial portion originates from the zygomatic arch and inserts on the outer surface of the inferior mandibular ramus (Figure 13.8). Its smaller, deeper portion originates from the entire length of the zygomatic arch and inserts in the lateral surface of the coronoid process and the superior half of the ramus. The major function of the masseter is to initiate elevation of the mandible and to add force during the chewing of hard food, clenching, and bruxing. The superficial portion contributes to protrusion of the mandible, while the deeper portion retracts the mandible.

The superior head of the lateral pterygoid muscle originates from the greater wing of the sphenoid bone and inserts on the articular disc (Figure 13.9). This muscle is responsible for the elevation of the mandible and pulling the disc forward during closing of the mouth. However, Eggleton and Langton[8] reported that the superior fibers of the lateral pterygoid function to decelerate and prevent invagination of the joint capsule during mandibular elevation. Thus, the superior fibers of the lateral pterygoid muscle may not have an active role in anterior disc displacement.[8,25]

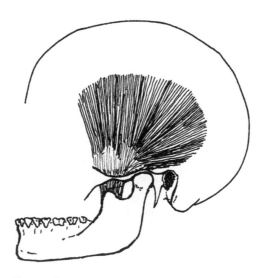

FIGURE 13.7   The temporalis muscle.

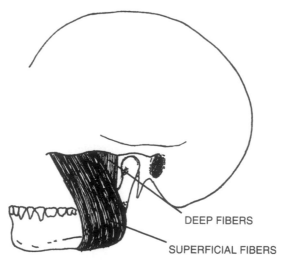

FIGURE 13.8   The masseter muscle.

The inferior head of the lateral pterygoid muscle originates from the lateral surface of the lateral pterygoid plate and inserts on the anterior surface of the condylar neck (Figure 13.9). This portion of the muscle is responsible for mandibular depression, protrusion, and lateral deviation.

The medial pterygoid muscle originates from the medial surface of the lateral pterygoid plate of the palatine bone and inserts onto the inner mandibular surface (Figure 13.9). It elevates, protrudes, and contralaterally deviates the mandible.

The suprahyoid muscles connect the mandible with the hyoid bone. This muscle group includes the paired digastrics, mylohyoids, geniohyoids, and the stylohyoids. The posterior portion of the digastrics originates from the styloid notch (just medial to the mastoid process) and inserts onto the intermediate tendinous attachment to the hyoid bone (Figure 13.10). Bilateral contraction of the posterior portion will depress the mandible during opening when the hyoid bone is fixed, and assist in the stabilization of the mandible during swallowing. The posterior digastrics also retract the mandible.

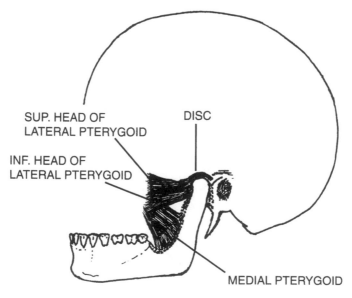

FIGURE 13.9   The medial and lateral pterygoid muscles.

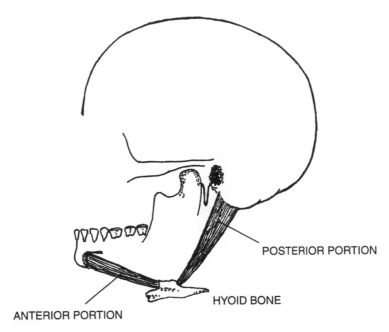

FIGURE 13.10   The digastric muscles.

The anterior portion of the digastrics originates from the lingular fossa adjacent to the midline of the mandible and inserts onto the intermediate tendinous attachment to the hyoid bone (Figure 13.10). Bilateral contraction of the anterior digastrics will elevate the hyoid bone.

The mylohyoid originates from the entire length of the mandible and inserts on the hyoid bone to form the floor of the mouth (Figure 13.11). The mylohyoid elevates the floor of the mouth, depresses the mandible when the hyoid is fixed, and elevates the hyoid when the mandible is fixed.

The geniohyoid lies above the mylohyoid, arises from the inner border of the mandible, and inserts on the hyoid bone (Figure 13.11). The function of the geniohyoid, like the digastric, is to pull the mandible downward and backward when the hyoid is fixed (i.e., during opening and retrussive movements). The geniohyoid also assists in elevation of the hyoid bone.

The stylohyoid arises from the styloid process and inserts on the hyoid bone. Its function is to assist in depression of the mandible during the initial phase of opening, as well as retract and elevate the hyoid bone when the mandible is fixed.

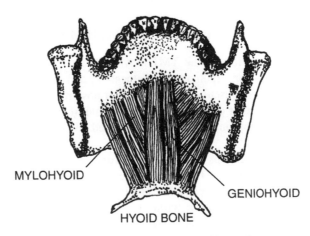

FIGURE 13.11   Superior view of the mylohyoid and geniohyoid muscles.

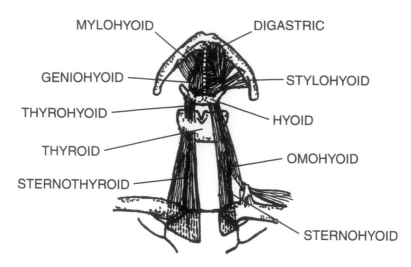

FIGURE 13.12   Infrahyoid muscles (From Iglarsh, Z. A. and Snyder-Mackler, L., The temporomandibular joint and the cervical spine, in *Clinical Orthopedic Physical Therapy*, Richardson, J. K. and Iglarsh, Z. A., Eds., W.B. Saunders, Philadelphia, 1994, chap. 1. With permission.)

The infrahyoids cover the anterior and lateral aspects of the larynx, trachea, and thyroid gland (Figure 13.12). These muscles include the sternohyoid, thyrohyoid, sternothyroid, and omohyoid. They function together to stabilize the hyoid bone and to provide a firm base for the suprahyoids to act on the mandible and the tongue.

The important aspects of muscular function of the TMJ can be summarized as follows:

1. Elevation of the mandible: masseter, temporalis, medial pterygoid, and superior head of the lateral pterygoid
2. Depression of the mandible: inferior head of the lateral pterygoid, digastric, mylohyoid, geniohyoid, and stylohyoid
3. Protrusion: masseter (superficial portion), medial pterygoid, and inferior head of the lateral pterygoid.
4. Retrusion: posterior fiber of temporalis, digastric, and suprahyoids.
5. Lateral deviation: ipsilateral termporalis, contralateral medial and lateral pterygoids.

IV. PATHOKINEMATICS AND PATHOKINESIOLOGY

Disruption of the normal function of the TMJ may be the result of mechanical causes (e.g., congenital anomaly, malocclusion, trauma, disc dislocation, and joint locking) or nonmechanical causes (e.g., myositis, synovitis, muscular imbalance, poor posture). It is widely acknowledged that the etiology of temporomandibular dysfunction (TMD) is multifactorial. TMD may manifest clinically as multiple signs and symptoms, such as pain, limited jaw opening, joint noises, headaches, neck pain, and muscle spasm.

There are two major subgroups of TMD: disorders of the TMJ and disorders of the masticatory musculature/soft tissue. Disorders of the TMJ (i.e., internal derangement) are the result of disharmony of the disc-condyle relationship. This condition is characterized by joint noise and/or limited jaw opening with or without associated pain. On the other hand, muscular/soft tissue involvement is often characterized by pain, spasm, limited opening, and altered mandibular dynamics.

A. INTERNAL DERANGEMENT (DISC DISPLACEMENT)

As mentioned previously, normal motion of the TMJ requires precise rotatory control of the disc-condyle complex. In the case of internal derangement, there is anatomical disharmony. During jaw opening and closing, the rhythmic movement of the condyle along the eminence is disturbed as a result of displacement of the disc from its normal position. In most cases, the disc is displaced anterior and medial to the mandibular condyle. In rare occasions, the disc may be displaced posteriorly.

Common reasons for disc displacement include direct blow to the jaw (trauma), whiplash injury, iatrogenic stretching during dental or surgical procedures, repetitive microtrauma from parafunctional behavior, and degenerative joint disease. Spasm of the superior lateral pterygoid may also alter timing of the disc movement and produce reciprocal obstruction during jaw closing.[26] Furthermore, loss of disc contour and elongation of the discal collateral ligaments may interfere with normal translation.

The symptoms of disc displacement typically occur as the mandibular condyle tries to translate anteriorly during opening or translate posteriorly during closing. Clinically, patients may report pain, a sticking and catching sensation, and clicking or popping. On examination, abnormal or deviation of the midline incisal path during jaw opening may be observed.

When the articular disc is displaced, locking of the TMJ often occurs. Transient locking of the TMJ may occur at any range during opening; however, midrange locking is seen in most patients.[27] Frequent intermittent locking may eventually lead to continuous locking.

Closed-lock is defined by the inability to open the mouth beyond 27 mm, as is typically associated with an anteriorly displaced disc.[28] Open-lock is defined as the inability to close the mouth from an opened position. This condition is typically caused by a posteriorly displaced disc which prevents the condyle from returning to its original position upon closure.[29]

Disc displacement and dysfunction can be organized into four categories: (1) anteriorly displaced disc with reduction, (2) anteriorly displaced disc without reduction, (3) posteriorly displaced disc, and (4) subluxation/hypermobility. Each will be discussed in detail below.

1. Anteriorly Displaced Disc with Reduction

This is the most common form of derangement and occurs when the disc is positioned anteriomedial to the mandibular condyle.[19] The anteriorly displaced disc can be the result of biomechanical abnormality (posterior bite collapse which shifts the condyle posteriorly), macrotrauma (disc displacement due to whiplash injury, sports injury, etc.), and microtrauma (bruxing, clenching, chronic gum chewing that causes masticatory muscle imbalance).[29] When the disc is displaced anteromedial to the mandibular condyle, there may be connective tissue changes, disc distortion, ligament elongation, and joint adaptation.

During mouth opening, there is interference with the smooth translation of the condylar head and one may hear a clicking noise indicating relocation of the disc with respect to the condyle. During closing, the disc displaces anteromedial to the condyle and produces the second clicking sound. This is defined as reciprocal clicking[30,31] (Figure 13.13).

The structure that is responsible for relocating the disc during opening is the posterior superior stratum. When there is still sufficient integrity of this connective tissue, it will "snap" the disk back into place as a result of tension developed during the translation phase.

Clinically, an early opening click occurs at 10 to 20 mm of opening, an intermediate click occurs at 20 to 30 mm of opening, and a late click occurs at 40 to 50 mm. The prognosis for a late click is worse than that associated with other abnormalities because of the progressive stretching of the posterior ligament.[32]

2. Anteriorly Displaced Disc without Reduction

In this condition, the disc is displaced anteriomedial to the mandibular condyle and does not reduce during jaw opening (Figure 13.14). Therefore, there is only an audible opening click as the condyle

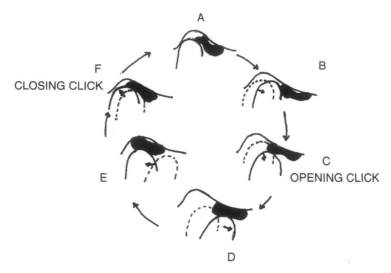

FIGURE 13.13   Schematic showing reciprocal clicking related to movements of the TMJ: (A) the disc is displaced anteriorly in the mouth-closed position; (B) the disc remains in front of the condyle as the condyle translates anteriorly during the initial phase of opening; (C) the condyle snaps underneath the disc as anterior translation continues and creates an opening click; (D) the condyle and disc continue to translate anteriorly during the opening phase; (E) the condyle and disc translate posteriorly during the closing phase; (F) at the end of closing, the disc displaces anteriorly as the condylar head translates postero-superiorly, creating a second click. (From Farra, W. B. and McCarty, W. L., *A Clinical Outline of Temporomandibular Joint Diagnosis and Treatment,* Normandie Publications, Montgomery, 1982, 54. With permission.)

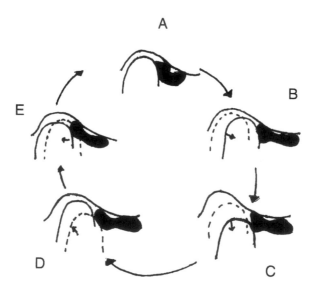

FIGURE 13.14   Schematic showing anteriorly displaced disc without reduction: (A) the disc is displaced anteriorly in the closed-mouth position; (B) as the condylar head translates anteriorly during opening, it may contact the disc and produce a clicking sound; (C) the disc becomes thickened or folded and remains in front of the condyle throughout the entire opening cycle; (D) the disc remains in front of the condyle during the closing cycle, too; (E) at the end of closing, the disc still remains in front of the condyle and does not reduce to its normal position superior to the condylar head. In this condition, reciprocal clicking does not occur. (From Farra, W. B. and McCarty, W. L., A *Clinical Outline of Temporomandibular Joint Diagnosis and Treatment,* Normandie Publications, Montgomery, 1982, 55. With permission.)

translates anteriorly and compresses the disc. Limited jaw opening and deviation toward the ipsilateral side during opening and protrusion is typically noted.[22] There is no clear explanation as to why a displaced disc is reducible or nonreducible; however, ligament integrity may play an important role.

In general, disc displacement with reduction may progress to the stage where there is no reduction. Over a period of time, chronic disc displacement is often accompanied by degeneration,[18,33,34] and occasionally disc perforation.[28,33] Perforation occurs when the disc is displaced and the posterior attachment or the disc tissue is disrupted, causing a tear or hole.[18] Mechanical wear and loss of synovial fluid are common reasons for disc perforation.[35]

3. Posteriorly Displaced Disc

Posterior displacement of the disc in relationship to the mandibular condyle can occur; however, the incidence is extremely rare.[32,36] One possible cause of a posteriorly displaced disc is laxity of the stylomandibular and/or sphenomandibular ligaments which allows excessive anterior translation of the condylar head during opening.

At the end of the opening, an audible click is produced as the condylar head passes the anterior band of the disc.[5] Upon full closure, the condylar head is prevented from returning to its original position by the posteriorly displaced disc.[29] This condition usually occurs after extreme yawning or a prolonged dental procedure.

4. Subluxation/Hypermobility

Subluxation or hypermobility occurs when there is an excessive amount of condylar translation during opening (i.e., the condyle translates beyond the articular tubercle). Clinically, excessive opening often is noted with jaw deflection to the contralateral side. Normally, there may be a single clicking noise occurring near maximum gape[37] or at the beginning of closing.[22] This is an indication that the joint is spontaneously reduced.[19] Anatomical predisposition for subluxation includes a flattened condylar head or a decrease in the slope of the articular eminence.

B. MASTICATORY MUSCLE DISORDER AND MYOFASCIAL PAIN

1. Masticatory Muscle Disorders

TMJ dysfunction can be myogenic and typically includes the masticatory musculature and other soft tissues. The masticatory muscle disorders may be caused by protective muscle splinting, muscle spasm, and muscle inflammation. Protective muscle splinting is the result of central nervous system-induced hypertonicity that occurs as a result of protection against injury or muscular fatigue. Muscle spasm may be the result of protective muscle splinting or reaction to myofascial pain syndrome. Muscle inflammation may be caused by disease process or as a result of continuous myospasm.[26] Several conditions leading to muscular disorders of the TMJ include trismus, myositis, myalgia, dyskinesia, and parafunctional habits.[27] One or more of the masticatory muscles may be involved, creating imbalanced action of the entire system. For example, if the lateral pterygoid is in spasm during jaw closing, it may affect movement of the disc and create abnormal joint dynamics.

2. Myofascial Pain Disorder Syndrome (MPDS)

MPDS is the most common cause of TMJ dysfunction and is defined by pain originating from myofascial structures. MPDS is normally characterized by trigger points which cause local tenderness and referred pain.[38,39] The clinical manifestation of MPDS includes, but is not limited to: headaches, facial pain, neck pain, tinnitus, dizziness, vertigo, joint noises, limited opening.[35] MPDS may be the cause of disc displacement, secondary to disc displacement, or non-disc related. The non-disc related causes include muscular tension, stress, and poor posture.[40]

C. THE INFLUENCE OF FORWARD HEAD POSTURE ON TMJ FUNCTION

The cervical spine and the TMJ are functionally interrelated as a result of their close proximity and musculo-ligamentous connections. Thus, the abnormal function of one system can substantially affect the function of the other.[11,41-43]

There have been numerous published studies demonstrating the influence of the cervical spine "posture" on TMJ function.[17,19,44-50] For example, Higbie et al.[51] studied the effect of posture on mandibular opening. The greatest range of motion was found in the forward head position (obviously, changes in the position of the cervical spine translate into changes in the position of the head), followed by the neutral position, with the smallest range of motion associated with the retracted head position. Therefore, Higbie et al.[51] concluded that cervical spine/head position is an important factor in determining the amount of vertical mandibular opening in healthy adults.

Braun[52] and Lee et al.[53] reported that patients with TMD demonstrated a greater forward cervical spine/head position than individuals without TMD. With a forward cervical spine/head posture, the upper cervical spine has to be held in a hyperextended position to allow for adequate visual function. To support the weight of the head in this mechanically disadvantaged position, the posterior cervical muscles have to exert more tension through excessive contraction. This continuous increase in tension of the posterior cervical muscles causes compression of the greater occipital nerve in the suboccipital region, which refers pain in the TMJ/head area. The increased tension of the posterior cervical muscles also causes the cranium to rotate posteriorly, thereby interfering with the cranium-mandibular alignment. Under these circumstances, the mandible is held either in a closed position by increased tension of the masseter/temporalis muscles, or in an opened-mouth position by the pull of gravity or the increased activity of the suprahyoid muscles. This sequence of events can set off a vicious cycle of masticatory muscle imbalance. Resulting compensatory movement may eventually affect the capsule, the disc mechanism, and the overall function of the TMJ.

V. SUMMARY AND CONCLUSIONS

The temporomandibular joint is a uniquely complex synovial joint. Anatomically, it is connected with the cervical spine/head structures and its movements are affected by the contacting tooth surfaces. Kinematically, it has six degrees of freedom which allow diverse daily oral function. Clinically, symptom manifestation is multifactorial and multifaceted. Any disruption of the normal relationship of the entire system can set off chain reactions and lead to numerous symptoms.

REFERENCES

1. Clark, G. T. and Mulligan, R., A review of the prevalence of temporomandibular dysfunction, *Gerontology*, 3, 231, 1984.
2. Clark, G. T., Diagnosis and treatment of painful temporomandibular disorders, *Dent. Clin. North Am.*, 31, 654, 1987.
3. Okeson, J. P. and Kanter, R. J., Temporomandibular disorders in the medical practice, *J. Family Practice*, No. 4, 1966.
4. Carlson, G. E. and LeReschel, L., Epidemiology of temporomandibular disorders, in *Temporomandibular Disorders and Related Pain Conditions*, Sessle, B. J., Bryant, P. S., and Dionne, R. A., Eds., Progress in Pain Research and Management, IASP Press, Seattle, 1995, p. 211.
5. Gage, J. P., Mechanisms of disc displacement in the temporomandibular joint, *Austr. Dent. J.*, 34, 427, 1989.
6. Perry, J. F., The temporomandibular joint, in *Joint Structure and Function — A Comrehensive Analysis*, Norkin, C. C. and Levangie, P. K., Eds., F.A. Davis, Philadelphia, 1992, chap. 6.
7. Hesse, J. R. and Hansson, T. L., Factors influencing joint mobility in general and in particular respect of the craniomandibular articulation: a literature review, *J. Craniomand. Disorders*, 2, 19, 1989.

8. Eggleton, T. M. and Langton, D. P., Clinical anatomy of the temporomandibular complex, in *Temporomandibular Disorders, Clinics in Physical Therapy,* Kraus, S. L., Ed., Churchill Livingstone, New York, 1994, chap. 1.

9. Bourbon, B., Craniomandibular examination and treatment, in *Saunders Manual of Physical Therapy Practice,* Meyers, R.S., Ed., W.B. Saunders, Philadelphia, 1995, chap. 28.

10. Kang, Q. S., Updike, D. P., and Salathe, E. P., Kinematic analysis of the human temporomandibular joint, *Ann. Biomech. Eng.,* 21, 699, 1993.

11. Grieve, G. P., *Common Vertebral Joint Problems,* Churchill Livingstone, New York, 1995, p. 22.

12. Davis, D., *Gray's Anatomy Descriptive and Applied,* 34th edition, Longmans Green, London, 1967.

13. Greenfield, B. and Wyke, B., Reflex innervation of the temporomandibular joint, *Nature,* 211, 940, 1966.

14. Austin, D. G., Special considerations in orofacial pain and headache, *Dent. Clin. North Am.,* 41, 325, 1997.

15. McNeill, C., *Temporomandibular Disorders — Guidelines for Classification, Assessment, and Management,* Quintessence Publishing, Carol Stream, 1993, p. 11.

16. Hertling, D., The temporomandibular joint, in *Management of Common Musculoskeletal Disorders — Physical Therapy Principles and Methods,* Hertling, D. and Kessler, R. M., Eds., J. B. Lippincott, Philadelphia, 1996, p. 444.

17. Kraus, S. L., Cervical spine influence on the management of temporomandibular disorders, in *Temporomandibular Disorders, Clinics in Physical Therapy,* Kraus, S. L., Ed., Churchill Livingstone, New York, 1994, chap. 11.

18. Dolwick, M. F., The temporomandibular joint: normal and abnormal anatomy, in *Internal Derangements of the Temporomandibular Joint,* Helms, C. A., Katzerg, R. W., and Dolwick, M. F., Eds., Radiology Research and Education Foundation, San Francisco, 1983, p. 1.

19. Rocabado, M. and Iglarsh, Z. A., *Musculoskeletal Approach to Maxillofacial Pain,* J.B. Lippincott, Philadelphia, 1991, p. 495.

20. Shellock, F. G., Mink, J. H., Deutsch, A., and Pressman, B. D., Kinematic magnetic resonance imaging of the joints: techniques and clinical applications, *Magn. Reson. Quarterly,* 7, 104, 1991.

21. Yustin, D. C., Reiger, M. R., McGuckin, R. S., and Connelly, M. E., Determination of the existence of hinge movements of the temporomandibular joint during normal opening by cine-MRI and computer digital addition, *J. Prosthodontics,* 2, 190, 1993.

22. Kraus, S. L., Temporomandibular joint, in *Evaluation, Treatment and Prevention of Musculoskeletal Disorders,* Saunders, H. D., Ed., Anderberg-Lund Printing, Minneapolis, 1986, chap. 7.

23. Peters, R. A. and Gross, S. G., Functional anatomy and biomechanics of the temporomandibular joint, in *Clinical Management of Temporomandibular Disorders and Orofacial Pain,* Peters, R. A. and Gross, S. G., Eds., Quintessence Publishing, Carol Stream, 1995, chap. 1.

24. Iglarsh, Z. A. and Snyder-Mackler, L., Temporomandibular joint and the cervical spine, in *Clincal Orthopedic Physical Therapy,* Richardson, J. K. and Iglarsh, Z. A., Eds., W.B. Saunders, Philadelphia, 1994, chap. 1.

25. Tanaka, T. T., Advanced Dissection of Temporomandibular Joint. Instructional Video, Clinical Research Foundation, Chula Vista, CA, 1988.

26. Bell, W. B. and Domenech, M. A., *Temporomandibular Disorders: Classification, Diagnosis, Management,* Year Book Medical, Chicago, 1990, chaps. 9, 10.

27. Clark, G. T., Adachi, N. Y., and Doran M. R., Physical medicine procedures affect temporomandibular disorders: a review, *J. Am. Dent. Assoc.,* 121, 151, 1990.

28. McCarty, W. L., Internal derangement of the temporomandibular joint, in *Surgery of the Temporomandibular Joint,* Keith, D. A., Ed., Blackwell Scientific Publications, Cambridge, 1992, 180.

29. Clark, G. T., Temporomandibular Joint Disorder Classification, Thesis, Department of Biokinesiology and Physical Therapy, University of Southern California, Dec. 4, 1997.

30. Friedman, M. H. and Weisberg, J., The temporomandibular joint, in *Orthopedic and Sports Physical Therapy,* Gould, J. A. and Davies, G. J., Eds., C.V. Mosby, St. Louis, 1985, chap. 24.

31. Farra, W. B. and McCarty, W. L., *A Clinical Outline of Temporomandibular Joint Diagnosis and Treatment,* Normandie Publications, Montgomery, 1983, chap. 4.

32. McCarty, W., Diagnosis and treatment of internal derangements of the articular disc and mandibular condyle, in *Temporomandibular Problems: Biologic Diagnosis and Treatment,* Solberg, W. K. and Clark, G. T., Eds., Quintessence Publishing Company, Chicago, 1980.

33. Bays, R. A., TMD: signs and symptoms, in *Current Controversies in Temporomandibular Disorder, Proceedings of the Craniomandibular Institutes's 10th Annual Squaw Valley Winter Seminar,* McNeill, C., Ed., Quintessence Publishing Company, Carol Stream, 1992, p. 38.

34. Oberg, T., Carlsson, G. E., and Fajers, C. M., The temporomandibular joint. A morphologic study on human autopsy material, *Acta Odontol. Scand.,* 29, 349, 1971.

35. Miles, D., Disorders of the temporomandibular joint, in *Oral and Maxillofacial Radiology: Radiologic/Pathologic Correlatations,* Miles, D. A., VanDis, M. L., Kaugars, G. E., and Lovas, J. G., Eds., W.B. Saunders, Philadelphia, 1991, p. 261.

36. Behr, M., Held, P., Leibrock, A., Fellner, C., and Handel, G., Diagnostic potential of pseudo-dynamic MRI (cine-mode) for evaluation of internal derangement of the temporomandibular joint, *Eur. J. Radiol.,* 23, 212, 1996.

37. Prinz, J. F., Physical mechanisms involved in the genesis of TMJ sounds, *J. Oral Rehabil.,* 25, 706, 1998.

38. International Association for the Study of Pain Subcommittee on Taxonomy, Classification of chronic pain, descriptions of chronic pain syndromes and definition of pain terms, *Pain (Suppl.),* 3, S1, 1986.

39. Travell, J. G. and Simons, D. G., *Myofascial Pain and Dysfunction — The Trigger Point Manual,* Williams & Wilkins, Baltimore, 1983.

40. Haddox, J. D., Psychological and medical management of myofascial pain, in *Temporomandibular Disorders, Clinics in Physical Therapy,* Kraus, S. L., Ed., Churchill Livingstone, New York, 1994, chap. 13.

41. Friedman, M. H. and Weisberg, J., Description and etiology of temporomandibular joint dysfunction, in *Temporomandibular Disorders: Diagnosis and Treatment,* Friedman, M. H. and Weisberg, J., Eds., Quintessence Publishing, Chicago, 1985, chap. 3.

42. Kraus, S. L., Physical therapy management of temporomandibular disorder, in *Temporomandibular Disorders, Clinics in Physical Therapy,* Kraus, S. L., Ed., Churchill Livingstone, New York, 1994, chap. 7.

43. Schneider, K., Zernicke, R. F., and Clark, G. T., Modeling of jaw-head-neck dynamics during whiplash, *J. Dent. Res.,* 68, 1360, 1989.

44. Clark, G. T., Green, E. M., Dornan, R. M., and Flack, V. F., Craniocervical dysfunction levels in a patient sample from a temporomandibular joint clinic, *J. Am. Dent. Assoc.,* 115, 251, 1987.

45. Kraus, S. L., Influences of the cervical spine on the stomatognathic system, in *Orthopedic Physical Therapy,* Donatelli, R. and Wooden, M. J., Eds., Churchill Livingstone, New York, 1989, p. 59.

46. Friedman, M. H. and Weisberg, J., Application of orthopedic principles in evaluation of the temporomandibular joint, *Phys. Ther.,* 62, 597, 1982.

47. Browne, P. A., Clark, G. T., Kuboki, T., and Adachi, N. Y., Concurrent cervical and craniofacial pain: a review of empiric and basic science evidence, *Oral Surg. Oral Med. Oral Pathol. Oral Radiol. Endodontics,* 86, 633, 1998.

48. Rocabado, M., Johnston, B. E., Jr., and Blaken, M. G., Physical therapy and dentistry: an overview, *J. Craniomand. Pract.,* 1, 47, 1982.

49. Mohl, N. D., The role of head posture in mandibular function, in *Abnormal Jaw Mechanics,* Solberg, W. K. and Clark, G. T., Eds., Quintessence Publishing, Chicago, 1984, p. 97.

50. Wright, F. B., Domench, M. A., and Fischer, J. R., Jr., Usefulness of posture training for patients with temporomandibular disorders, *J. Am. Dent. Assoc.,* 131, 202, 2000.

51. Higbie, E. J., Seidel-Cobb, D., Taylor, L. F., and Cummings, G. S., Effect of head position on vertical mandibular opening, *J. Orthop. Sports Phys. Ther.,* 29, 127, 1999.

52. Braun, B. L., Postural difference between asymptomatic men and women and craniofacial pain patients, *Arch. Phys. Med. Rehabil.,* 72, 653, 1991.

53. Lee, W. Y., Okeson, J. P., and Lindroth, J., The relationship between forward head posture and temporomandibular disorders, *J. Orofacial Pain,* 9, 161, 1995.

14 Kinematic MRI of the Temporomandibular Joint

Frank G. Shellock

CONTENTS

I. INTRODUCTION

Internal derangement of the temporomandibular joint (TMJ) occurs in a high percentage of the adult population and is associated with marked pain and functional abnormalities.[1-26] Thus, identification and characterization of TMJ disorders is of great interest, particularly since objective documentation of internal derangement is often required by third-party payors before long-term therapy or surgical intervention is approved.[19]

The first magnetic resonance imaging (MRI) procedures developed to assess the TMJ were described in the mid-1980s.[1,2] This MRI application evolved rapidly to become the diagnostic imaging procedure of choice for assessment of all types of TMJ disorders.[3-44] Compared with other radiographic techniques, MRI is unsurpassed for depicting the important soft tissue and osseous components of the TMJ, including the disc, mandibular condyle, glenoid fossa, articular eminence, hyaline cartilage, marrow, and associated muscular structures.

Initially, only static views were attainable using MRI. Because the inability to obtain a functional assessment of jaw biomechanics and disc-condyle complex coordination was considered to be a limitation of MRI, Burnett et al.[27] developed a kinematic MRI technique to examine the function of the TMJ. With further refinements of kinematic MRI methodology,[11,28,31] this imaging application emerged as a routine method of determining the functional aspects of the TMJ.[11,15,18,19,28-35]

A comprehensive evaluation of the patient with TMJ dysfunction is currently accomplished using static view and kinematic MRI procedures to obtain both anatomical and functional information.

0-8493-0807-0/01/$0.00+$.50
© 2001 by Frank G. Shellock

This chapter will describe the technical aspects of kinematic MRI and the clinical applications of this technique to assess TMJ disorders.

II. TECHNIQUE

A. THE MAGNETIC RESONANCE SYSTEM

Initially, kinematic MRI for the TMJ was developed using a conventional "tunnel-shaped," high-field-strength (1.5 Tesla) MR system.[27] Considering the anatomic features of this joint and the space required for movement, wide-bore or "open" configured MR systems do not offer any advantage for the kinematic MRI examination. Notably, the comparatively higher signal-to-noise associated with the use of a high-field-strength MR system provides a technically more acceptable study because of the spatial resolution required to resolve the relatively small anatomic details of this joint. Mid- or low-field strength MR systems may be used for kinematic MRI examinations of the TMJ as long as the proper adjustments are made to the imaging protocol that are necessary to achieve high spatial resolution (e.g., increasing the number of signal averages, reducing the bandwidth).[19]

B. POSITIONING DEVICES AND RADIOFREQUENCY COILS

Most kinematic MRI studies of the TMJ have been accomplished using the incremental, passive positioning technique. Various types of positioning may be used for this kinematic MRI procedure, whereby the goal is to open the mouth in specific, predetermined increments.[11,27-30,33,34] Dental wedges, bite blocks, a patient-activated incrementing device, and a hydraulic jaw opener have all been used for this purpose.

Active movement or true "dynamic" MRI studies have been performed on the TMJ using fast gradient echo imaging techniques.[31] However, because of the inherent artifacts generally associated with the use of gradient echo pulse sequences,[1,28,29,37] the active movement technique is not commonly used for kinematic MRI in the clinical setting.

The most widely used, commercially available apparatus for kinematic MRI is the Burnett TMJ Positioning Device (Medrad, Pittsburgh, PA).[27] This plastic device has a ratchet and gearing mechanism that allows 1 mm incremental opening or closing of its "jaws" when the handle is depressed (Figure 14.1). The Burnett TMJ Positioning Device was specifically designed to be operated by the patient while inside the MR system.[27] The device has a quick release mechanism and disposable mouthpieces for patient protection and safety. Thus, the Burnett TMJ Positioning Device allows the MRI technologist to guide the patient during the incrementing procedure and subsequent acquisition of MR images required for the kinematic MRI examination.

Because the degree of mouth opening is different for each patient, the range of motion must be determined using the Burnett TMJ Positioning Device prior to the kinematic MRI examination. The fully closed device (i.e., the "start" position) is placed into the patient's mouth and then opened incrementally until the fully opened mouth position is reached. This is done without forcing the joint or causing pain. The millimeter incrementing gauge on the positioning device indicates the extent of the range of motion for the patient. Information pertaining to the patient's range of motion is used to guide the kinematic MRI examination, insofar as mouth opening positions are progressively imaged at 20% increments.

Obtaining high-resolution detail of the anatomy of the TMJ is crucial for an optimal evaluation.[1-3,5,6,11,14,18,19] Acquisition of MR images with a high signal-to-noise is accomplished using a surface or local radiofrequency (RF) coil.[18,19] Obviously, the position of the TMJ is ideally suited for surface RF coil imaging because the anatomy of interest is located close to the skin in a confined area.[6,18,19]

For static view or kinematic MRI examinations of the TMJ, a 3-inch circular or loop surface RF coil is typically used, centering the coil slightly anterior to the external auditory canal. Alternatively, because the TMJ is easily palpated, an open-configured surface coil may be centered on the anatomic region of interest, making this a technically simple procedure to perform.[18,19]

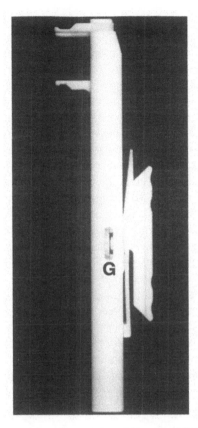

FIGURE 14.1 Nonferromagnetic device used to perform kinematic MRI examination of the TMJ using the incremental, passive positioning technique (Burnett TMJ Positioning Device, Medrad, Inc., Pittsburgh, PA). Movement of the device is controlled by the patient using the handle mechanism. A gauge (G) indicates the relative extent of mouth opening. This device has disposable mouthpieces.

Since there is bilateral articulation with the cranium, the right and left temporomandibular articulations must function together. Therefore, it is not surprising that there is a high incidence of bilateral abnormalities in patients with TMJ disorders.[1,6,11] Even though the patient may only present with unilateral symptoms, each TMJ is affected by the contralateral side. Thus, a thorough assessment of the patient for TMJ dysfunction requires MR imaging of both joints.

From an examination time consideration, it is advisable to perform MRI on both joints simultaneously.[11,18,19] Furthermore, for the kinematic MRI examination, simultaneous imaging of bilateral TMJs permits MR images to be obtained for a direct comparison between the joints at the same relative degree of mouth opening. Side-to-side differences in translation or asymmetrical motion of the TMJ may be optimally visualized utilizing this technique.[11,18,28,29]

Simultaneous, bilateral MR imaging of the TMJ can be accomplished easily using various types of coil configurations, including: (1) dual 3-inch, circular surface coils; (2) phased-array coils; or (3) a quadrature head coil.[8,11,18,19,29] Because unwanted patient motion during MRI is problematic from an image quality consideration, a variety of commercially available coil holders and patient stabilization systems have been developed and are recommended for use during static view and kinematic MRI procedures.

C. IMAGING PARAMETERS AND PROTOCOL

The TMJ consists of tissues with mostly short T2 times. Therefore, it is best to use pulse sequences with short-echo times (short TEs) when imaging the TMJ to properly visualize anatomic details.

The repetition time (TR) is not as critical insofar as MR images obtained using either T1-weighted (i.e., short TE, short TR) or proton density weighted (i.e., short TE, long TR) sequences will provide acceptable tissue contrast characteristics for proper assessment of this joint.[1,2,6,9,14,18,19]

For the kinematic MRI study, images are typically obtained using a T1-weighted, spin echo pulse sequence to best depict the disc-condyle complex through the range of motion of this joint.[11,18,28,29] Partial flip angle or gradient echo pulse sequences have also been used for kinematic MRI, but these techniques have intrinsically poor spatial resolution and are more susceptible to artifacts when metallic implants or dental appliances are present.[11,18,28,29,31] Furthermore, since the kinematic MRI examination is routinely performed using an incremental, passive positioning technique, there is no justification for using a gradient echo pulse sequence over a T1-weighted, spin echo sequence when one considers the relatively small amount of time that is saved. Finally, the T1-weighted, spin echo images acquired for the kinematic MRI study are of sufficient quality to demonstrate anatomic features of the joint as well as being useful for the assessment of TMJ function.[11,18,28,29]

The kinematic MRI procedure begins by acquiring images in the axial plane which are used to show the relative orientation of the mandibular condyles. The mandibular condyles are generally positioned at oblique angles in both the sagittal and coronal planes.[39-44] Investigations have demonstrated that the best orientation for images of the TMJ is with reference to the long axis of the condylar head,[39-44] because a significant number of both normal individuals and patients have abnormally configured condyles. Therefore, section locations used for kinematic MRI of the TMJ should be selected perpendicular (i.e., oblique sagittals) to the long axis of the condylar head, as viewed on the axial plane localizer scan (Figure 14.2). This permits imaging of the anatomic regions of interest and minimizes the overall examination time.

In consideration of the above requirements, the basic protocol for kinematic MRI of the TMJ using a high-field-strength MR system is as follows: T1-weighted, spin echo pulse sequence (i.e., TE, 20 msec/TR, 300 msec); oblique sagittal plane; section thickness, 3 mm; number of section

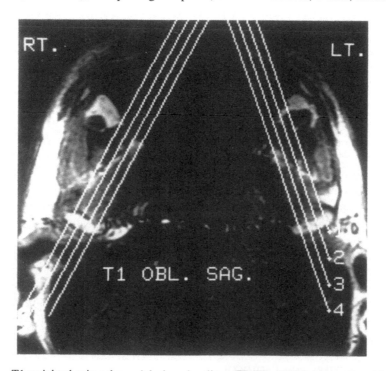

FIGURE 14.2 T1-weighted spin echo, axial plane localizer (TR/TE, 400/20 msec; slice thickness, 5 mm) used to orient section perpendicular to the condylar heads to obtain oblique sagittal plane images. Note the areas of lateral high signal intensity resulting from the dual 3 in. surface coils used for this examination.

locations imaged, 3 to 4 through each condyle (Figure 14.2); field of view, 10 to 12 cm; matrix size, 128 × 256; number of excitations, 2.

The three to four images selected through each TMJ in the oblique sagittal plane should be imaged in the following mouth positions (i.e., a total of seven series is acquired):

Series One, closed-mouth view (i.e., maximum intercuspation of the teeth)
Series Two, partially closed mouth with the positioning device in place (note that the distance
    the patient's mouth is opened at this increment is dependent on the length of the incisors)
Series Three, first 20% increment (distance based on 20% of range of motion for the patient)
Series Four, second 20% increment
Series Five, third 20% increment
Series Six, fourth 20% increment
Series Seven, fifth 20% increment

Using this kinematic MRI protocol, standardized and consistent information may be obtained in an acceptable time in the clinical setting.

MR images may be viewed individually or displayed as a "cine-loop" using standard software commonly found on most MR systems. For the cine-loop display, images obtained at the same section location and which show the anatomy of the TMJ are sequentially "paged" forward and backward. This permits rapid viewing of multiple images at different section locations and also tends to optimally show subtle abnormalities.

D. Interpretation of the Kinematic MRI Examination

Interpreting kinematic MRI examinations of the TMJ requires an understanding of normal movement and the interaction of associated osseous and soft tissue structures, as the mouth incrementally moves from a closed to a fully opened position. Functional abnormalities of the TMJ manifest as deviations from the normal movement pattern.

1. Normal Kinematic MRI of the TMJ

Visualized in the oblique sagittal plane, closed-mouth view, the disc appears as a "bow-tie" or "drumstick" shaped structure (Figure 14.3). The normal position of the disc is such that the posterior band is in a 12 o'clock position (±10%) relative to the condylar head.[3,6,18,19,26] Any deviation of the disc from this position is considered abnormal (Figures 14.4 and 14.5).

As the mouth opens, the condyle rotates and then translates anteriorly, with the apex of the condyle moving onto the intermediate zone of the disc.[6,11,18,19,28] With further mouth opening, the condyle remains positioned on the intermediate zone as the condyle continues to translate anteriorly until it reaches the base of the articular eminence or slightly anterior to this position. In the fully opened mouth position, the condyle may move onto the anterior band of the disc.

Notably, the retrodiscal laminae (i.e., the thin bands of fibroelastic tissue that attach posteriorly to the disc) should never serve as weight-bearing surfaces during normal TMJ function.[18] The normal movement pattern as shown using kinematic MRI is characterized by a combination of rotational and translational motions, with translation being the dominant movement in the superior joint space[18] (Figure 14.6).

III. CLINICAL APPLICATIONS

Kinematic MRI provides useful diagnostic information for a variety of TMJ abnormalities of varying degrees of severity, including those associated with functional derangement, reduced range of motion, malocclusion, mandibular shift, and hypermobility.[3,6,11,18,19,23,26,28,29-35]

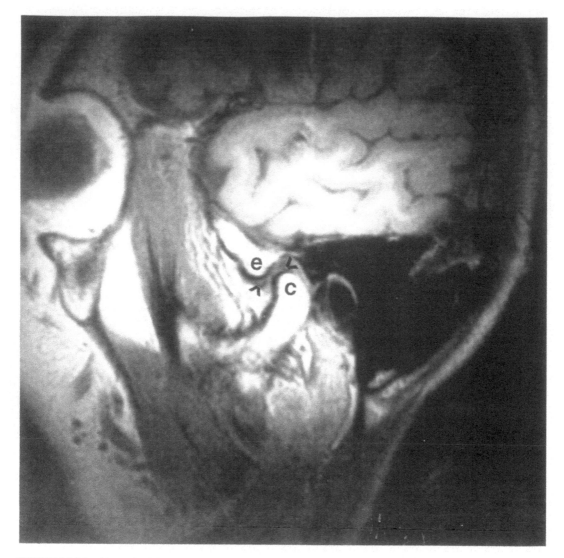

FIGURE 14.3   Normal TMJ. MR image obtained in an oblique sagittal plane using a T1-weighted, spin echo pulse sequence (closed mouth view). Note the normal position of the "bow-tie" shaped disc (arrow heads) interposed between the osseous anatomy (e, articular eminence; c, condylar head). The posterior bank of the disc is in a 12 o'clock position relative to the condylar head.

A. Anterior Displacement of the Disc with Reduction

Anterior displacement of the disc with reduction is considered to be a relatively minor form of TMJ dysfunction. This functional abnormality is present when there is 10% greater than the anterior position of the posterior band of the disc relative to the condylar apex with the mouth (Figure 14.7). As the mouth opens, the condyle translates anteriorly, beneath the disc, thereby "recapturing" the disc.[18,28,29]

Reduction of an anteriorly displaced disc may occur at any point; however, it usually occurs during the initial 30% of the range of motion for the TMJ. The anteriorly displaced disc that reduces "early" in the range of motion is considered less severe than one that reduces "late." The range of motion for the TMJ is usually with normal limits for patients with this functional disorder, and they are typically treated using conservative treatment techniques.[18]

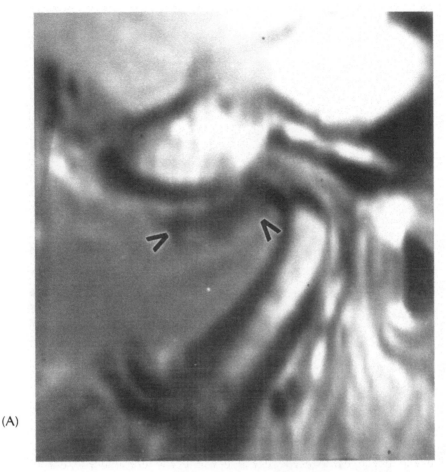

(A)

FIGURE 14.4   (A) Anterior displacement of the disc. MR image obtained in an oblique sagittal plane using a T1-weighted, spin echo pulse sequence (closed mouth view). Note the severely disrupted shape of the disc (arrow heads). (B) Perforation of the disc. MR image obtained in an oblique sagittal plane using an inversion recovery, fast spin echo pulse sequence (IR-FSE; closed mouth view). Fluid in the joint space outlines the perforated disc. Additionally, there is severe subchondral sclerosis of the condylar head.

Using kinematic MRI of the TMJ, it is possible to ascertain the relative position of the mandible when reduction of the disc occurs. This has important therapeutic implications. For example, anterior displacement of the disc is frequently treated using splint therapy.[45] The splint functions to position the mandible and condyle more anteriorly, resulting in recapture of the displaced disc and relaxation of the associated musculature, which frequently is in spasm.[19] The size of the splint must be adjusted to treat an "early" versus a "late" reduction of the disc. If splint therapy is not properly applied, internal derangement of the TMJ may progress or, at the very least, may not be corrected. Kinematic MRI of the TMJ may be performed without and with the splint in place to accurately guide the use of this conservative treatment technique.[19]

B. ANTERIOR DISPLACEMENT OF THE DISC WITHOUT REDUCTION

A more severe form of internal derangement of the TMJ is anterior displacement of the disc without reduction (Figures 14.8 to 14.10). In this form of TMJ dysfunction, the posterior band of the disc is, again, in a greater than 10% anterior position relative to the condylar apex with the mouth in a closed position. As the mouth opens, however, the condyle does not recapture the disc.[18,19,28,29]

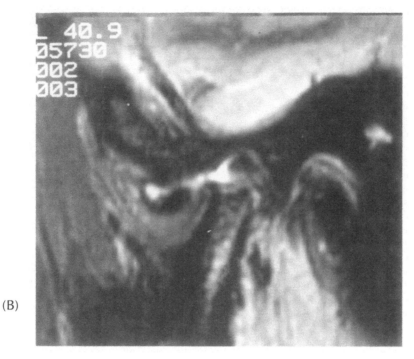

(B)

FIGURE 14.4   (continued).

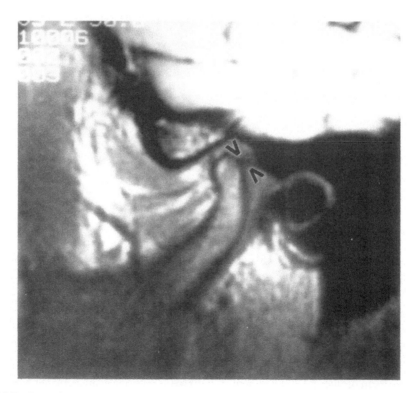

FIGURE 14.5   Posterior displacement of the disc. MR image obtained in an oblique sagittal plane using a T1-weighted, spin echo pulse sequence (closed-mouth view). The entire disc (arrow heads) is located posterior to the condylar head. This form of disc displacement is rare.

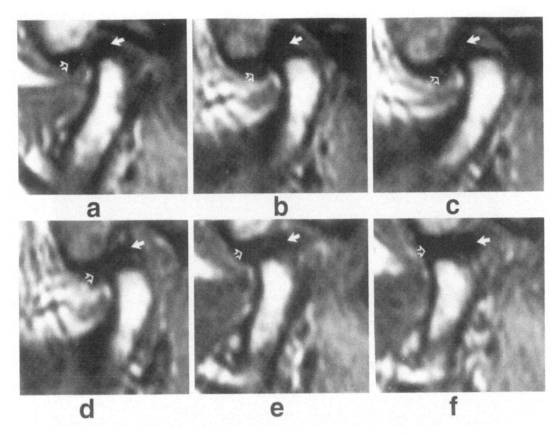

FIGURE 14.6   Normal kinematic MRI of the TMJ. MR images obtained in oblique sagittal plane using a T1-weighted, spin echo pulse sequence. Images performed with subject's mouth closed (a), with positioning device in lowest increment placed in mouth (b), and at 20% increments of the total range of motion (c, d, e, f). In the closed-mouth position (a), the posterior band of the disc is in a 12 o'clock position relative to the condylar head. As the mouth progressively opens (b to f), the condyle moves onto the intermediate zone of the disc. This relationship between the disc and condyle is maintained throughout the remaining range of motion of the joint, as the condyle translates anteriorly (bold arrow, posterior band of disc; open arrow, anterior band of disc).

The kinematic MRI examination typically demonstrates a markedly displaced disc on the closed-mouth view that has a distorted shape. As the mouth opens and the condyle translates anteriorly, the disc is pushed in front of the condylar head causing the disc to become progressively more deformed (Figures 14.8 to 14.10).

This type of TMJ dysfunction is typically associated with a limited range of motion that is caused by limited anterior translation of the abnormal disc. Severe laxity or tearing of the attachments to the posterior band of the disc is typically present.

With more advanced stages of anterior displacement of the disc without reduction, degenerative abnormalities such as osteophytes, fibrosis, and arthritis may be found[3,6,10,12,13,17-20,23,25,28,29,35] (Figure 14.10). Persistent, chronic abnormalities have been reported to be associated with facial remodeling.[13] Thus, there is a substantial reason not only to determine the presence of TMJ dysfunction, but also to characterize the relative severity of the disorder.[13,18,19]

Treatment of the patient with anterior displacement of the disc without reduction typically requires surgical intervention. Using the kinematic MRI procedure to differentiate between the disc that has a late reduction and the disc that does not recapture in a fully opened mouth position is especially useful for staging the severity of the disorder and treatment planning.

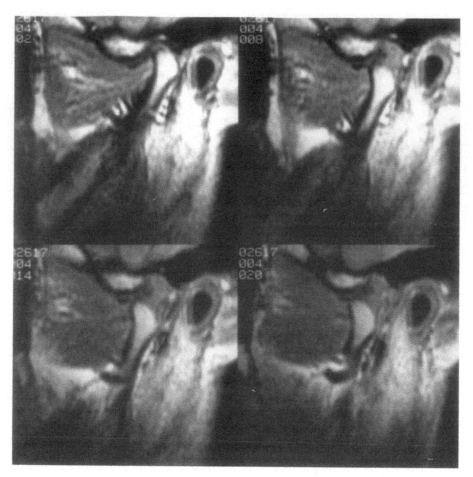

FIGURE 14.7   Anterior displacement of the disc with early reduction. MR images obtained in oblique sagittal plane using a T1-weighted, spin echo pulse sequence. This kinematic MRI examination shows the posterior band of the disc anteriorly displaced relative to the condylar head in the closed-mouth view. The anterior displacement of the disc (top left) is quickly recaptured (i.e., the condylar head moves onto the intermediate zone of the disc) as the mouth incrementally opens and the condyle translates anteriorly (top right, bottom left, bottom right).

C. HYPERMOBILITY

Excessive range of motion of the TMJ (i.e., hypermobility) may be detected using kinematic MRI (Figure 14.11). Hypermobility is present if the condylar head translates past the articular eminence with the mouth fully opened. This abnormality is a predisposition to internal derangement of the TMJ.[19] Laxity or partial tears of the anterior and/or posterior soft tissue structures may be found in joints that exhibit hypermobility.

D. ASYMMETRICAL MOTION

Because the mandible has a bilateral articulation with the cranium, both TMJs should function synchronously. As the mouth opens, both condylar heads should initially rotate then translate anteriorly. Thus, this movement pattern should occur for both TMJs, simultaneously. Any disordered, asynchronous movement comparing the right TMJ to the left TMJ is regarded as an abnormality.[11,18,19,28,29]

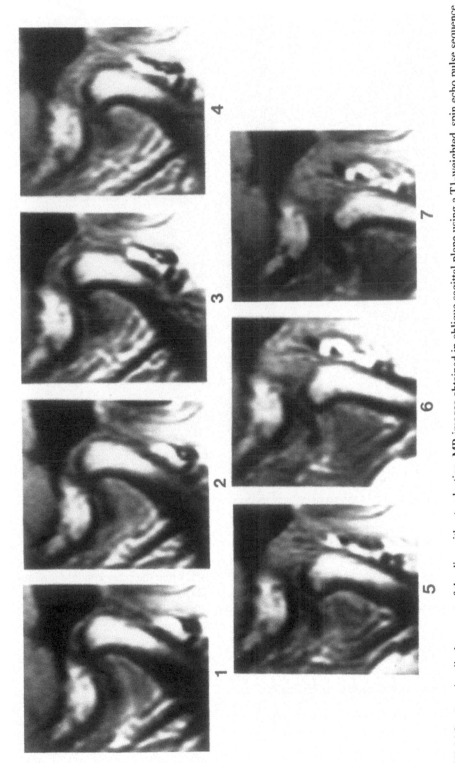

FIGURE 14.8 Anterior displacement of the disc without reduction. MR images obtained in oblique sagittal plane using a T1-weighted, spin echo pulse sequence. This kinematic MRI examination shows the posterior band of the disc anteriorly displaced relative to the condylar head in the closed-mouth view (1). The disc remains in front of the condylar head as the mouth incrementally opens and the condyle translates anteriorly (2 to 7).

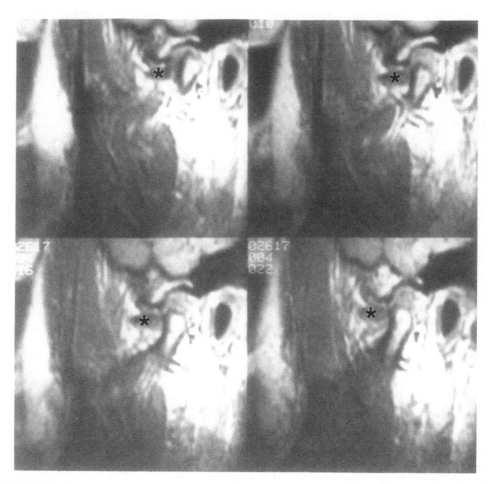

FIGURE 14.9   Severe anterior displacement of the disc without reduction. MR images obtained in oblique sagittal plane using a T1-weighted, spin echo pulse sequence. This kinematic MRI examination shows substantial anterior displacement of the disc relative to the condylar head in the closed-mouth view (asterisk, top left). The disc remains in front of the condylar head as the mouth incrementally opens (top right, bottom left, bottom right). Additionally, the disc is severely deformed.

Asymmetrical motion may be associated with lateral deviation of the mandible as the mouth opens (Figure 14.12) or other more unusual or complex movements. For example, there may be progressive anterior translation of one condyle as the mouth opens, while the other condyle remains in a fixed position or moves in a retrograde manner. To identify and characterize asymmetrical motion, it is necessary to perform kinematic MRI using the simultaneous, bilateral imaging technique.[11,18,19,28,29]

Asymmetrical motion of the TMJ may be caused by muscle spasm, shortened or atrophic muscles, fibrous adhesions, fibrotic contractures, or other mechanisms. A reduced range of motion is often found with this functional abnormality and may occur with or without disc displacement.

E.   TMJ ABNORMALITIES SECONDARY TO WHIPLASH

Hyperextension and hyperflexion of the cervical spine, or "whiplash," typically occurs during rear-end motor vehicle collisions and is the most common cause of injuries related to automobile accidents. During the initial hyperextension phase of whiplash, as the vehicle is accelerated by the rear-end collision, the mandible moves backward at a slower rate than the movement of the head. This results in excessive mouth opening and a downward and forward displacement of the

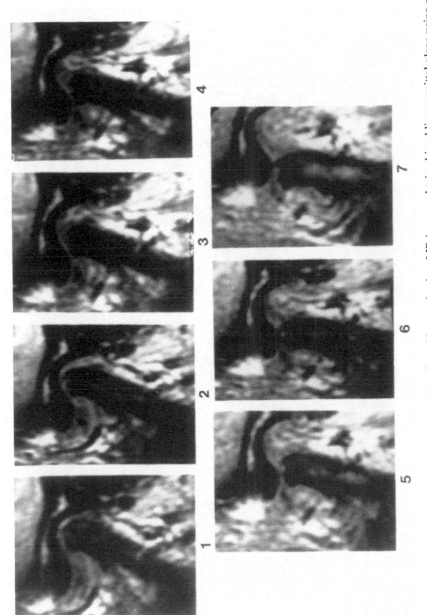

FIGURE 14.10 Severe osteoarthritis and anterior displacement of the disc without reduction. MR images obtained in oblique sagittal plane using a T1-weighted, spin echo pulse sequence. This kinematic MRI examination shows marked anterior displacement of the disc relative to the eroded condylar head in the closed mouth view. The severely deformed disc remains in front of the condylar head as the mouth incrementally opens (2 to 7). Note the low signal intensity of the condyle resulting from marrow fat loss associated with advanced degenerative changes.

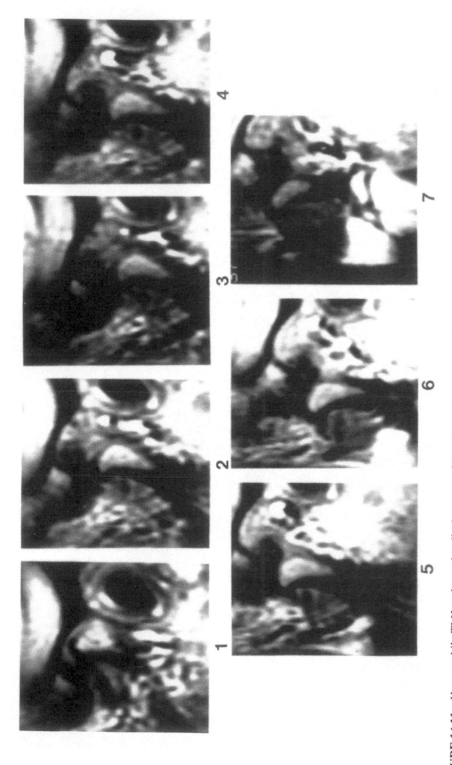

FIGURE 14.11 Hypermobile TMJ and anterior displacement of the disc with reduction. MR images obtained in oblique sagittal plane using a T1-weighted, spin echo pulse sequence. This kinematic MRI examination shows anterior displacement of the disc relative to the condylar head in the closed mouth view (1). The disc is recaptured early (2, the condylar head moves onto the intermediate zone), as the mouth incrementally opens and the condyle translates anteriorly (2 to 7). Notably, the condylar head translates beyond the articular eminence (7, full opened mouth view), indicating a hypermobile TMJ. This condition is a predisposition to internal derangement.

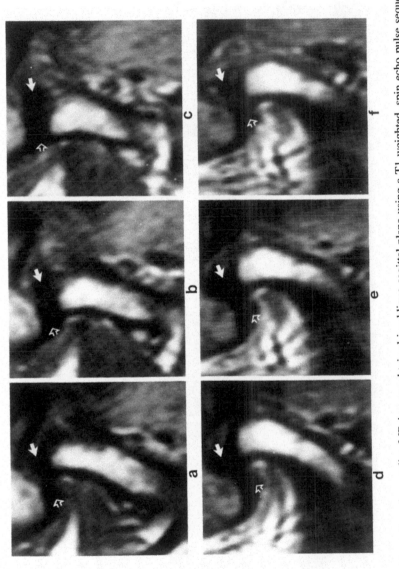

FIGURE 14.12 Asymmetric motion abnormality. MR images obtained in oblique sagittal plane using a T1-weighted, spin echo pulse sequence. This kinematic MRI examination shows selected images obtained during simultaneous, bilateral examination of the TMJ: (a) closed mouth views, right TMJ; (b) partially opened mouth views, right TMJ; (c) fully opened mouth views, right TMJ; (d) left TMJ; (e) left TMJ; (f) left TMJ (posterior band of the disc, bold arrow; anterior band of the disc, open arrow). Note the relative positions of each condylar head relative to the articular eminence. In the closed mouth views, the condyle of the right TMJ (a) is situated more posteriorly than the condyle of the left TMJ (d). In the partially opened mouth views, the right condyle (b) is near the bottom of the articular eminence, while the position of the left TMJ (e) has changed very little. In the fully opened mouth views, the right condylar head is at the bottom of the articular eminence (c), while the left condylar head shows relatively little anterior translation (f). This illustrates asymmetrical motion and is typically associated with lateral deviation of the mandible during mouth opening.

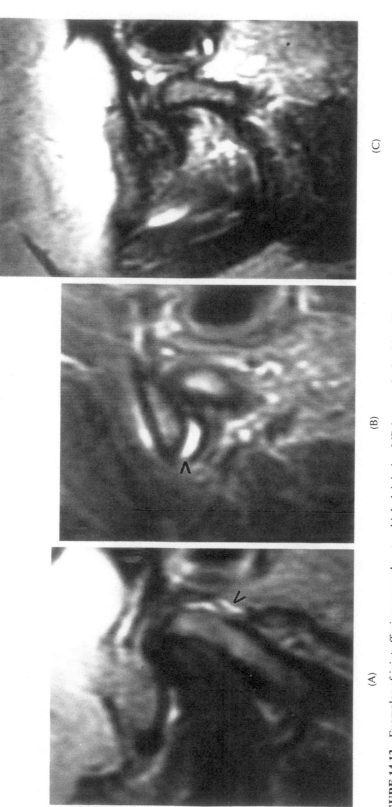

(A)

(B)

(C)

FIGURE 14.13 Examples of joint effusions secondary to whiplash injuries. MR images obtained in oblique sagittal plane using inversion recovery, fast spin echo pulse sequences. (A) Focal effusion secondary to whiplash injury in posterior joint space (arrow head). (B) Focal effusion secondary to whiplash injury in anterior joint space (arrow head). (C) Diffuse effusion secondary to whiplash injury.

disc-condyle complex relative to the cranium.[46-50] Excessive mouth opening, in turn, leads to over-stretching and possible tearing of the posterior attachments of the disc, as well as loosening or tearing of the discal attachments to the medial and lateral condyle.[46-50]

During the hyperflexion phase of whiplash, as the vehicle decelerates either due to braking or striking an object in front, the head is rapidly propelled forward. This causes further abrupt movement of the mandible and also can cause injury to the soft tissues of the TMJ.[46-50] For example, the previously displaced disc and/or the posterior tissues may be crushed between the mandibular condyle and glenoid fossa.

In consideration of the biomechanical aspects of cervical whiplash, it is apparent that the extreme and rapid changes in mandibular position that occur during rear-end collisions are likely to damage the TMJ.[46-50] In cases where there may be a pre-existing, albeit asymptomatic, internal derangement of the TMJ, whiplash can aggravate the condition.

Notably, patients frequently complain of TMJ-related symptoms following cervical whiplash injuries caused by rear-end motor vehicle collisions.[46-49] In a study by Pressman et al.,[51] patients with suspected TMJ abnormalities secondary to cervical whiplash were evaluated using static view and kinematic MRI examinations (Figure 14.13). These patients had no direct trauma to the jaw, mouth, head, or face during the automobile accident and had no prior history of TMJ dysfunction. Findings indicated that the majority of the patients had some form of TMJ abnormality that included displacement of the disc and/or abnormal joint fluid[51] (Figure 14.13).

A more recent study conducted by Garcia and Arrington[52] also used MRI to examine the relationship between whiplash and TMJ injuries. Similar to the study by Pressman et al.,[51] this patient group did not sustain direct trauma to the face, head, or mandible and had no TMJ complaints prior to the motor vehicle accident.[52] Garcia and Arrington reported a high percentage of TMJ abnormalities associated with whiplash.[52]

Thus, MRI-based investigations have demonstrated that patients who experience whiplash have a high frequency of disc displacements as well as abnormal joint fluid.[51,52] In consideration of this research, patients with TMJ symptoms secondary to whiplash injuries should be evaluated routinely using static view and kinematic MRI techniques.

IV. SUMMARY AND CONCLUSIONS

Abnormalities that affect the TMJ are associated primarily with the position of the disc relative to the condyle head. Successful treatment of patients with TMJ dysfunction greatly depends on accurately diagnosing and staging the specific problem. While the use of clinical criteria to document TMJ abnormalities is often problematic, objective diagnostic information pertaining to anatomic and functional disorders that affect the TMJ may be obtained in a thorough, comprehensive manner using static view and kinematic MRI examinations.[18,19,28,29]

REFERENCES

1. Helms, C. A., Richardson, M. L., Moon, K. L., and Ware, W. H., Nuclear magnetic resonance imaging of the temporomandibular joint: preliminary observations, *J. Craniomand. Pract.*, 2, 219, 1984.
2. Harms, S. E., Wilk, R. M., Wolford, L. M., Chiles, D. G., and Milam, S. B., The temporomandibular joint: magnetic resonance imaging using surface coils, *Radiology*, 157, 133, 1985.
3. Harms, S. E. and Wilk, R. M., Magnetic resonance imaging of the temporomandibular joint, *Radio-Graphics*, 7, 521, 1987.
4. Westesson, P. L, Katzberg, R. W., Tallents R. H., Sanchez-Woodworth R. E., Svensson, S. A., and Espeland, M. A., Temporomandibular joint: comparison of MR images with crysectional anatomy, *Radiology*, 164, 59, 1987.
5. Katzberg, R.W., Temporomandibular joint imaging, *Radiology*, 170, 297, 1989.
6. Fulmer, J. M. and Harms, S. E., The temporomandibular joint, *Topics Magn. Reson. Imag.*, 1, 75, 1989.

7. Katzberg, R. W., Westesson, P. L., Tallents, R. H., Anderson, R., Kurita, K., Manzione, J. V., and Totterman, S., Temporomandibular joint: MR assessment of rotational and sideways disc displacements, *Radiology*, 169, 741, 1988.

8. Sanchez-Woodworth, R. E., Tallents, R. H., Katzberg, R. W., and Guay, J. A., Bilateral internal derangements of temporomandibular joint: evaluation by magnetic resonance imaging, *Oral Surg. Oral Med. Oral Pathol.*, 65, 281, 1988.

9. Schellhas, K. P., Wilkes, C. H., Fritts, H. M., Omlie, M. R., Heithoff, K. B., and Jahn, J. A., Temporomandibular joint: MR imaging of internal derangements and postoperative changes, *Am. J. Roentgenol.*, 150, 381, 1988.

10. Schellhas, K. P. and Wilkes, C. H., Temporomandibular joint inflammation: comparison of MR fast scanning with T1- and T2-weighted imaging techniques, *Am. J. Neuroradiol.*, 10, 589, 1989.

11. Shellock, F. G. and Pressman, B. D., Dual-surface-coil imaging of bilateral temporomandibular joints: improvement in the imaging protocol, *Am. J. Neuroradiol.*, 10, 595, 1989.

12. Schellhas, K. P., Wilkes, C. H., Fritts, H. M., Omlie, M. R., and Lagrotteria, L. B., MR of osteochondritis dissecans and avascular necrosis of the mandibular condyle, *Am. J. Roentgenol.*, 152, 551, 1989.

13. Schellhas, K. P., Piper, M. A., and Omlie, M. R., Facial skeletal remodeling due to temporomandibular joint degeneration: an imaging study of 100 patients, *Am. J. Neuroradiol.*, 11, 541, 1990.

14. Drace, J. E., Young, S. W., and Enzmann, D. R., TMJ meniscus and bilaminar zone: MR imaging of the substructure-diagnostic landmarks and pitfalls of interpretation, *Radiology*, 177, 73, 1990.

15. Helms, C. A. and Kaplan, P., Diagnostic imaging of the temporomandibular joint: recommendations for use of the various techniques, *Am. J. Roentgenol.*, 154, 319, 1990.

16. Rao, V. M., Farole, A., and Karasick, D., Temporomandibular joint dysfunction: correlation of MR imaging, arthrography, and arthroscopy, *Radiology*, 174, 663, 1990.

17. Marguelles-Bonnet, R. E., Carpentier, P., Yung, J. P., Defrennes, D., and Pharaboz, C., Clinical diagnosis compared with findings of magnetic resonance imaging in 242 patients with internal derangement of the TMJ, *J. Orofac. Pain*, 9, 244, 1995.

18. Harms, S. E., Temporomandibular joint, in *Magnetic Resonance Imaging,* Vol. II, 3rd edition, Stark, D. D. and Bradley, W. G., Jr., Eds., Mosby, New York, 1999, chap. 33.

19. Stoller, D. A. and Jacobson, R. L., The temporomandibular joint, in *Magnetic Resonance Imaging in Orthopaedics and Sports Medicine,* 2nd edition, Stoller, D. W., Ed., Lippincott-Raven, Philadelphia, 1997, p. 995.

20. Westesson, P. L. and Brooks, S. L., Temporomandibular joint: relationship between MR evidence of effusion and the presence of pain and disc displacement, *Am. J. Roentgenol.*, 159, 559, 1992.

21. Pressman, B. D., Schames, M., Schames, J., and Shellock, F. G., Evaluation of TMJ trauma by MRI, *J. Magn. Reson. Imag.*, 8 (Suppl. 1), 19, 1990.

22. Schellhas, K. P., Temporomandibular joint injuries, *Radiology*, 173, 211, 1989.

23. Rao, V. M., Imaging of the temporomandibular joint, *Semin. Ultrasound CT MR*, 16, 513, 1995.

24. Westesson, P. L., Larheim, T. A., and Tanaka, H., Posterior disc displacement in the temporomandibular joint, *J. Oral Maxillofac. Surg.*, 56, 1266, 1998.

25. Palicious, E., Valvassori, G. E., Shannon. M., and Reed, C. F., *Magnetic Resonance Imaging of the Temporomandibular Joint*, Thieme, New York, 1990.

26. Drace, J. E. and Enzmann, D. R., Defining the normal temporomandibular joint: closed-, partially open-, and open mouth MR imaging of asymptomatic subjects, *Radiology*, 177, 67, 1990.

27. Burnett, K. R., Davis, C. L., and Read, J., Dynamic display of the temporomandibular joint meniscus by using "fast-scan" MR imaging, *Am. J. Roentgenol.*, 149, 959, 1987.

28. Pressman, B. D. and Shellock, F. G., The temporomandibular joint, in *MRI of the Musculoskeletal System: A Teaching File,* Mink, J. H. and Deutsch, A. L., Eds., Raven Press, New York, 1990, p. 521.

29. Shellock, F. G., Kinematic magnetic resonance imaging, in *Magnetic Resonance Imaging in Orthopaedics and Sports Medicine,* 2nd edition, Stoller, D. W., Ed., Lippincott-Raven, Philadelphia, 1997, chap. 13.

30. Bell, K. A., Miller, K. D., and Jones, J. P., Cine magnetic resonance imaging of the temporomandibular joint, *Cranio*, 10, 313, 1992.

31. Conway, W. F., Hayes, C. W., and Campbell, R. L., Dynamic magnetic resonance imaging of the temporomandibular joint using FLASH sequence, *J. Oral Maxillofac. Surg.*, 46, 930, 1988.

32. Ren, Y. F., Westesson, P. L., and Isberg, A., Magnetic resonance imaging of the temporomandibular joint: value of pseudodynamic images, *Oral Surg. Oral Med. Oral Pathol. Oral Radiol. Endodontics.* 81, 110, 1996.
33. Dorsay, T. A. and Youngberg, R. A., Cine MRI of the TMJ: need for initial closed mouth images without the Burnett device, *J. Comput. Assist. Tomogr.,* 19, 163, 1995.
34. Vogl, T. J., Eberhard, D., Bergman, C., and Lissner, J., Incremental hydraulic jaw opener for MR imaging of the temporomandibular joint, *J. Magn. Reson. Imag.,* 2, 479, 1992.
35. Benito, C., Casares, G., and Benito, C., TMJ static disc: correlation between clinical findings and pseudodynamic magnetic resonance images, *Cranio*, 16, 242, 1998.
36. Shellock, F. G., Schatz, C. J., and Hahn, P., MRI evaluation of traumatic TMJ abnormalities: comparison between T2-weighted and STIR pulse sequences, *J. Magn. Reson. Imag. (Suppl.),* S25, 1994.
37. Crabbe, J. P., Brooks, S. L., and Lillie, J. H., Gradient echo MR imaging of the temporomandibular joint: diagnostic pitfall caused by superficial temporal artery, *Am. J. Roentgenol.,* 164, 451, 1995.
38. Rao, V. M., Vinitski, S., Liem, M., and Rapoport, R., Fast spin-echo imaging of the temporomandibular joint, *J. Magn. Reson. Imag.*, 5, 293, 1995.
39. Schwaighofer, B. W., Tanaka, T. T., and Klein, M. V., MR imaging of the temporomandibular joint: a cadaver study of the value of coronal images, *Am. J. Roentgenol.,* 154, 1245, 1990.
40. Pressman, B. D., Shellock, F. G., Schames, J., and Schames, M., Value of coronal plane MR images for the evaluation of TMJ trauma, *J. Magn. Reson. Imag.*, 1, 220, 1991.
41. Fourcart, J. M., Carpentier, P., Pajoni, D., Marguelles-Bonnet, R., and Pharaboz, C., MR of 732 TMJs: anterior, rotational, partial, and sideways disc displacements, *Eur. J. Radiol.*, 28, 86, 1998.
42. Musgrave, M. T., Westesson, P. L., Tallents, R. H., Manzione, J. V., and Katzberg, R. W., Improved magnetic resonance imaging of the temporomandibular joint by oblique scanning planes, *Oral Surg. Oral Med. Oral Pathol.*, 71, 525, 1991.
43. Tasaki, M. M. and Westesson, P. L., Temporomandibular joint: diagnostic accuracy with sagittal and coronal MR imaging, *Radiology*, 186, 723, 1993.
44. Brooks, S. L. and Westesson, P. L., Temporomandibular joint: value of coronal MR images, *Radiology*, 188, 317, 1993.
45. Manzione, J. V., Tallents, R. F., Katzberg, R. W., Oster, C., and Miller, T. L., Arthrographically guided therapy for recapturing the temporomandibular joint meniscus, *Oral Surg. Oral Med. Oral Pathol.*, 57, 235, 1984.
46. Schneider, K., Zernicke, R. F., and Clark, G., Modeling of jaw-head-neck dynamics during whiplash, *J. Dent. Res.*, 68, 1360, 1989.
47. Weinberg, S. and Lapointe, H., Cervical extension-flexion injury (whiplash) and internal derangement of the temporomandibular joint, *J. Oral Maxillofac. Surg.,* 45, 653, 1987.
48. Balla, J. I., The late whiplash syndrome, *Aust. NZ J. Surg.,* 50, 610, 1980.
49. Mannheimer, J., Attanasio, R., Cinotti, W. R., and Pertes, R., Cervical strain and mandibular whiplash: effects upon the craniomandibular apparatus, *Clin. Prev. Dent.,* 11, 29, 1989.
50. Weinberg, L. A., Tempormandibular joint injuries, in *Whiplash Injuries. The Cervical Acceleration/Deceleration Syndrome,* Foreman, S. M. and Croft, A. C., Eds., Williams & Wilkins, Baltimore, 1988, pp. 347–383.
51. Pressman, B. D., Shellock, F. G., Schames, J., and Schames, M., MRI evaluation of TMJ abnormalities associated with cervical hyperextension-hyperflexion (whiplash) injuries, *J. Magn. Reson. Imag.,* 2, 569, 1992.
52. Garcia, R., Jr. and Arrington, J. A., The relationship between cervical whiplash and temporomandibular joint injuries: an MRI study, *Cranio*, 14, 233, 1996.

Part VII

Wrist

15 The Wrist: Functional Anatomy and Kinesiology

Elizabeth F. Souza

CONTENTS

I. INTRODUCTION

The wrist is one of the most complex joints in the human body. It provides final positioning for the hand so that it can grasp and manipulate objects. Composed of eight irregularly shaped bones, the articulations that constitute the wrist must provide a stable base for the hand to achieve the mobility, dexterity, and strength required for this joint to function effectively.

Discussions regarding the interrelationships of the carpal bones with regard to normal and pathological movement are controversial. There are two main theoretical constructs regarding carpal structure and function. The "classical" construct views the carpal bones as lying in two distinct rows (proximal and distal) and describes the movement between the carpals of each row. The "carpal link" construct views the wrist as a series of longitudinal rays composed of the carpal bones and metacarpals. This chapter draws upon both approaches in describing the normal and abnormal functional anatomy and pathokinesiology of the wrist.

0-8493-0807-0/01/$0.00+$.50
© 2001 by Frank G. Shellock

II. FUNCTIONAL ANATOMY

A. OSSEOUS STRUCTURE

The osseous structure of the wrist is composed of the distal ends of the radius and ulna, eight carpal bones, and the bases of the metacarpals. The "true" wrist joint is the articulation between the articular surface of the radius with the scaphoid and lunate and the articular surface of the ulna with the triangular fibrocartilage complex. The triangular fibrocartilage complex then articulates with the lunate and triquetrum. The articular surface of the distal end of the radius is oriented with 10 to 25 degrees of volar tilt and 15 to 25 degrees of angulation towards the ulna.[1] It has two articular facets for the scaphoid and lunate, forming the radiocarpal articulations.

The distal end of the ulna does not directly articulate with any of the carpal bones but, instead, articulates with the triangular fibrocartilage which is located in the space between the distal end of the ulna and the triquetrum. This fibrocartilage acts as an articular disc and inserts into the base and tip of the ulnar styloid process.[2] The triangular fibrocartilage assists in transmission of compressive loads from the distal ulna to the lunate and triquetrum.

The carpal bones form a proximal and distal carpal row. The proximal row consists of the scaphoid, lunate, triquetrum, and pisiform while the trapezium, trapezoid, capitate, and hamate form the distal carpal row. Together, the carpals are arranged such that each carpal bone has several articulations with surrounding bones. This arrangement results in a total of 19 intercarpal articulations (Figure 15.1).

Although not considered part of the wrist joint, the distal radioulnar joint has functional importance. The movements of forearm pronation and supination occur through the combined motion of the proximal and distal radioulnar joints and are required to place the hand in either a palm-up or palm-down posture. During pronation, the distal end of the ulna translates distally and

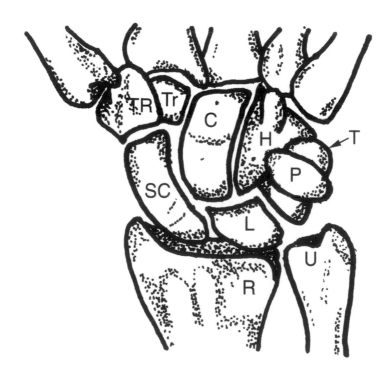

FIGURE 15.1   The carpal bones (left palmar view). Proximal carpal row: scaphoid (SC), lunate (L), triquetrum (T), pisiform (P). Distal carpal row: trapezium (TR), trapezoid (Tr), capitate (C), hamate (H), ulna (U), radius (R).

dorsally. These translations can become significant when evaluating joint space and load transmission through the ulnar aspect of the wrist.

B. Ligamentous Structures

The stability of the wrist complex is essential for precise positioning of the hand for fine motor skills, as well as grip strength. Stability is provided by osseous geometry and ligamentous structures. With the exception of the flexor carpi ulnaris muscle inserting onto the pisiform, there are no direct muscular attachments onto the carpal bones.

The volar ligaments are thicker and stronger than the dorsal ligaments. The volar ligaments stabilize the joint against hyperextension, while the dorsal ligaments prevent volar instability.[3] The ligaments of the wrist can be categorized as either intrinsic or extrinsic. Volarly, the extrinsic radioscaphocapitate, radioscapholunate, radiolunate, ulnolunate, and radiocollateral ligaments traverse the radius to the carpals and metacarpals (Figure 15.2A). On the dorsal surface, there are the radioscaphoid, radiolunate, radiocapitate, and radiotriquetral ligaments which reinforce the capsule dorsally (Figure 15.2B).

The intrinsic ligaments originate and insert on the carpals themselves.[4] The intrinsic ligaments, by the nature of their attachments, act to stabilize intracarpal motion. Taleisnik[3] described the V-shaped deltoid ligament, which originates from the volar aspect of the capitate with a segment branching to both the scaphoid and the triquetrum. The deltoid ligament is also known as the volar intercarpal ligament or the arcuate ligament.

The interosseus ligaments of the proximal row, the scapholunate and lunotriquetral ligaments, bind the scaphoid to the lunate and lunate to the triquetrum, respectively (Figure 15.3). There are three short intrinsic ligaments, the trapeziotrapezoid, trapeziocapitate, and capitohamate ligaments, which connect the bones in the distal carpal row into a single functional unit[3] (Figure 15.3).

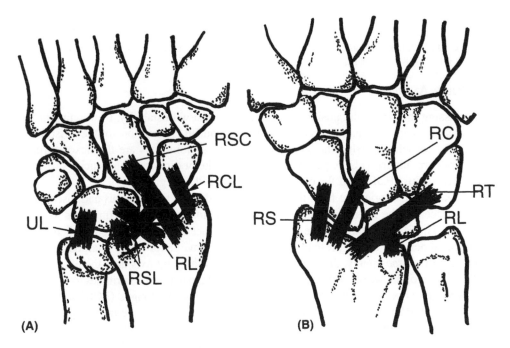

FIGURE 15.2 (A) The extrinsic wrist ligaments (volar surface of the right hand): radioscaphocapitate (RSC), radioscapholunate (RSL), radiolunate (RL), ulnolunate (UL), and radiocollateral (RCL) ligaments. (B) The extrinsic wrist ligaments (dorsal surface of the right hand): radioscaphoid (RS), radiocapitate (RC), radiotriquetral (RT), and radiolunate (RL) ligaments.

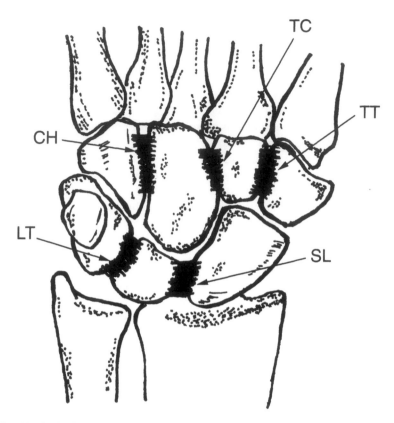

FIGURE 15.3   The intrinsic wrist ligaments (volar surface of the right hand): scapholunate (SL), lunotri-quetral (LT), trapeziotrapezoid (TT), trapeziocapitate (TC), and capitohamate (CH) ligaments. (From Ruby, L K. et al., Relative motion of selected carpal bones: a kinematic analysis of the normal wrist, *J. Hand Surg. Am.*, 13(1), 1988. With permission.)

C. MUSCULAR ANATOMY

Muscles crossing the wrist joint position the hand and assist with stability. Positioning of the wrist in the frontal and sagittal planes is accomplished by balanced contractions of the wrist flexors and extensors. The muscles crossing the wrist joint volar to its joint axis are the flexor carpi radialis (FCR), flexor carpi ulnaris (FCU), palmaris longis (PL), flexor digitorum superficialis (FDS), flexor digitorum profundus (FDP), and flexor pollicis longus (FPL) (Figure 15.4).

The FCR and FCU originate from the medial epicondyle of the humerus and insert distally on the volar surfaces of the metacarpal bases. The palmaris longus primarily functions to tighten the palmar fascia. The FDS and the FDP are finger flexors and act as wrist flexors only when dysfunction (e.g., peripheral nerve injury) is present. The FPL is the prime flexor of the interphalangeal joint of the thumb. As the names imply, the FCR crosses radial to the joint axis and, therefore, contributes to radial deviation of the wrist, while the FCU is positioned ulnarly and contributes to ulnar deviation.

The prime movers for wrist extension, extensor carpi radialis longus (ECRL), extensor carpi radialis brevis (ECRB), and extensor carpi ulnaris (ECU), originate at the lateral epicondyle of the elbow and insert distally on the dorsal surfaces of the metacarpals (Figure 15.5). The ECRL and ECRB are oriented radial to the joint axis and contribute to radial deviation while the ECU contributes to ulnar deviation due to its joint axis orientation. Also crossing the wrist on the dorsal surface are the extensor digitorum communis (EDC), extensor pollicis longus (EPL), extensor pollicis brevis, and the abductor pollicis longus (APL). The EDC's primary role is extension of the digits at the metacarpalphalangeal joints.

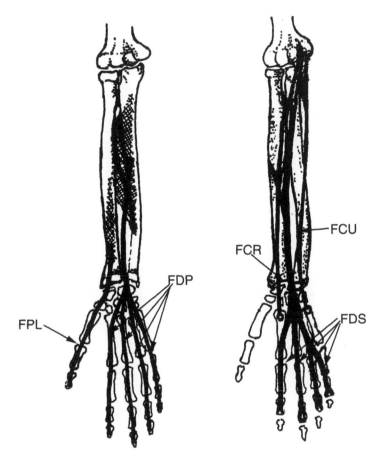

FIGURE 15.4   Muscles that produce flexion of the wrist joint (volar surface, right hand). The prime movers are flexor carpi radialis (FCR) and flexor carpi ulnaris (FCU). Additional muscles that may assist with wrist flexion: flexor digitorum superficialis (FDS), flexor digitorum profundus (FDP), and flexor pollicis longus (FPL).

III. NORMAL JOINT KINESIOLOGY

A. GLOBAL WRIST MOTIONS

Movement of the wrist/hand complex with respect to the distal end of the radius is considered global wrist motion. The global wrist movements of flexion, extension, radial deviation, and ulnar deviation are not the result of pure angular carpal displacements. Rather, for these motions to occur, the carpal bones must move simultaneously along three joint axes.

Although not considered global movements of the wrist, the individual carpal bones pronate and supinate. Pronation and supination occur in the horizontal plane with an axis of motion that lies along the shaft of the radius (Figure 15.6). The axis of motion for the sagittal plane motions of wrist flexion and extension lies parallel with the transverse axis of the forearm when the radial and ulnar styloid processess are in alignment from a lateral view. The sagittal axis of rotation is perpendicular to that of pronation and supination (Figure 15.7).

Wrist radial and ulnar deviation occur in the coronal plane with an axis of motion that is perpendicular to both of the above axes. The axes of rotation of all three motions pass through the head of the capitate, although each axis is slightly offset from the others[5,6] (Figure 15.8).

As with all physiologic movements, wrist movement patterns are coupled. Unrestrained wrist flexion is coupled with ulnar deviation, while wrist extension and radial deviation are coupled.

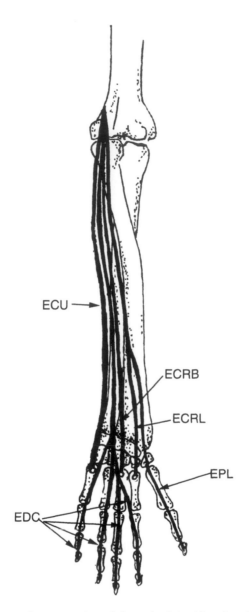

FIGURE 15.5   Muscles that produce extension of the wrist joint (dorsal surface, right hand). The prime movers are extensor carpi radialis longus (ECRL), extensor carpi radialis brevis (ECRB), and extensor carpi ulnaris (ECU). The extensor digitorum communis (EDC) and extensor pollicis longus (EPL) also have the ability to assist with wrist extension.

Active muscle contraction of antagonist muscles is required for motion to occur purely within a given plane.

B. Carpal Movement

Global wrist motion is the result of radiocarpal, intercarpal, and intracarpal motion. Radiocarpal motion refers to movement between the proximal row of carpals and the distal end of the radius. Movement between the proximal and distal carpal rows is referred to as intercarpal motion. Movement between carpals located in the same row is defined as intracarpal motion.

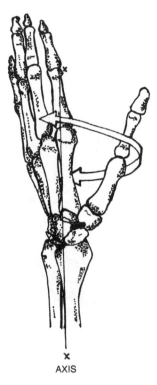

FIGURE 15.6 The axis of rotation for horizontal plane movements (wrist pronation and supination) lies along the shaft of the radius and travels through the head of the capitate (x-axis). (From An, K. N., Berger, R. A., and Cooney, W. P., Eds., *Biomechanics of the Wrist Joint*, Springer-Verlag, New York, 1996, 12. With permission.)

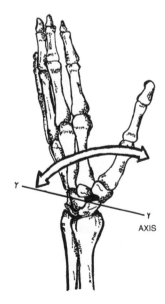

FIGURE 15.7 The axis of rotation for sagittal plane movements (wrist flexion and extension) lies parallel to the transverse axis of the forearm when the radial and ulnar styloid processes are in alignment from a lateral view (y-axis). This axis is oriented at a 90 degree angle to the x-axis. (From An, K. N., Berger, R. A., and Cooney, W. P., Eds., *Biomechanics of the Wrist Joint*, Springer-Verlag, New York, 1996, 12. With permission.)

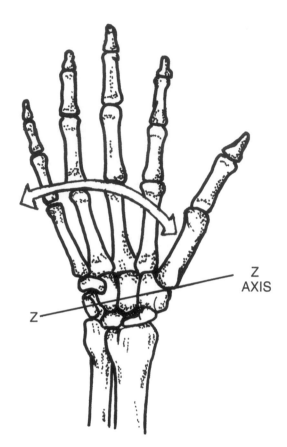

FIGURE 15.8   The axis of rotation for coronal plane movements (wrist radial and ulnar deviation) travels through the head of the capitate (z-axis) and is perpendicular to both the x and y axes. (From An, K. N., Berger, R. A., and Cooney, W. P., Eds., *Biomechanics of the Wrist Joint*, Springer-Verlag, New York, 1996, 12. With permission.)

Very little intracarpal motion occurs between the carpal bones of the distal row. Therefore, the distal row can be thought of as a fixed unit.[6,7] The proximal carpal row can be considered an intercalated segment between the relatively fixed distal row and the distal radial-ulnar complex.[8]

The carpal-link construct views the wrist as a series of longitudinally oriented articular chains.[3] Each chain contains a carpal bone from the proximal carpal row which can be viewed as an intercalated segment. The radial chain consists of the scaphoid interposed between the radius proximally, and the distal trapezium and trapezoid bones distally (Figure 15.9). The ulnar chain consists of the triquetrum interposed between the ulna and triangular fibrocartilage complex complex proximally and the hamate distally (Figure 15.9). In the central chain, the lunate acts as the intercalated segment; it lies between the radius proximally and the capitate distally (Figure 15.9).

The radiocarpal ligaments, intrinsic ligaments, and the joint surface geometry assist in stability of the proximal carpal row. The carpal-link construct is helpful in understanding how movements at both the radiocarpal and midcarpal levels are interdependent. The proximal carpal bones must constantly adapt and alter their position according to the changing needs of the surrounding structures. Much of the adaptation necessary is due to the specific geometric shapes of the proximal carpal bones.

C. Wrist Flexion/Extension

Flexion of the wrist is initiated by the tendonous pull of the FCR on the palmar bases of metacarpals two and three and by the pull of the FCU on the palmar surface of the pisiform, hamate, and fifth

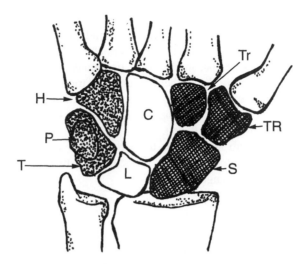

FIGURE 15.9 The carpals can be viewed as lying in longitudinal chains. The medial chain consists of the triquetrum (T), pisiform (P), and hamate (H). The central chain consists of the lunate (L) and capitate (C). The lateral chain consists of the scaphoid (S), trapezium (TR), and trapezoid (Tr).

metacarpal. This motion occurs at the midcarpal joint[9] and results in a palmar rotation of the distal carpal row, along the Y-axis, into a flexed position.[6] The proximal row acts as an intercallated segment between the distal carpal row and the distal end of the radius; it follows the distal row into flexion by rotating palmarly.

Kobayashi et al.[10] studied the intercarpal motion throughout the entire range of motion and noted that, at 60 degrees of flexion, the proximal carpal row rotated into slight ulnar deviation. The relative contributions of the radiocarpal and midcarpal joints to the overall global flexion of the wrist are not equal.

During flexion of the joint, the distal carpal row flexes at a 3-to-2 ratio with the proximal row.[6,11] Thus, the midcarpal joint contributes 60% of the overall flexion while the radiocarpal contribution is 40%.[7,9,12]

Wrist extension is initiated by the pull of the ECRL, ECRB, and ECU on the dorsal bases of the second, third, and fifth metacarpals, respectively.[9] As in flexion, this motion is initiated at the midcarpal joint. Motion at the midcarpal joint accounts for approximately 33% of global wrist extension, while the radiocarpal joint is responsible for 66% of global wrist extension.[9] The proximal carpal row adapts to the distal row motion and rolls into an extended position.[6] The proximal carpal row radially translates as the wrist moves into extension thus coupling wrist extension with radial deviation in the absence of co-contraction.[10]

Intracarpal motion in the distal carpal row during wrist flexion/extension is very limited. Kobayashi et al.[10] reported very similar degrees of sagittal plane rotation for each of the bones in the distal carpal row during both flexion and extension. Kobayashi et al.[10] also found less than 2 degrees of distal carpal row supination relative to the distal end of the radius during wrist flexion/extension. These findings are consistent with others,[5,6] supporting the view that the distal carpal row functions and should be considered as a fixed unit.

The carpal bones of the proximal row do not all exhibit the same degree of sagittal plane motion resulting in an increased amount of intracarpal motion. Of the proximal row carpals, the scaphoid exhibits the greatest amount of rotation about the flexion axis, during global wrist flexion. The lunate flexes the least.[6,10,11,13,14] This discrepancy in motion appears to be important in maintaining the overall range of wrist flexion. Synchronizing the scapholunate movement by carpal transfixion severely decreases the overall flexion range of the wrist.[15]

In the transverse plane, the scaphoid moves in the opposite direction of the lunate and triquetrum during flexion. The scaphoid pronates from neutral to end range flexion while the lunate and triquetrum supinate relative to the distal end of the radius.[10,12]

During wrist extension, intracarpal motion is again limited to the proximal carpal row. The scaphoid extends significantly more than either the lunate or triquetrum, with the lunate extending the least.[9] The magnitude of scaphoid extension relative to the radius is almost equal to that of the distal row. Sarrafian et al.[9] report that the scaphoid functionally belongs to the distal row during extension and the proximal row during flexon.

The scaphoid and triquetrum supinate as the wrist moves into extension while the lunate pronates.[10] This effectively separates the palmar surfaces of the two bones[12] and places tension on the scapholunate ligament at end-range extension.

D. RADIAL AND ULNAR DEVIATION

The coronal plane movements of the wrist, radial and ulnar deviation, are more complex than flexion/extension of the wrist. The magnitudes of distal carpal row rotation about the radial/ulnar deviation axis are much greater than those of the proximal carpal row, indicating greater midcarpal motion than radiocarpal motion.[6,11]

The distal carpal row rotates about the radial/ulnar deviation axis in the direction of hand motion during both movements. This rotation brings the scaphoid and trapezium into approximation with the distal end of the radius during radial deviation, while the triquetrum and hamate approximate the distal end of the ulna during ulnar deviation.

The radial styloid process extends more distally than the styloid process of the ulna, limiting radial deviation to approximately 20 degrees as opposed to the 30 degrees available for ulnar deviation.[16] Youm et al.[5] reported that radial deviation occurs at the midcarpal joint, while there are contributions from both the midcarpal and radiocarpal joints during ulnar deviation.

The amount of out-of-plane motion, by both the proximal and distal carpal rows, during coronal plane movements increases the complexity of these motions. During ulnar deviation, the distal carpal row flexes in relation to the radius. In radial deviation, the distal carpal row extends from the flexed posture of ulnar deviation but does not reach neutral.[11] The proximal carpal row has more motion along the flexion-extension axis in radioulnar deviation than it has motion along the radial/ulnar deviation axis.[6]

Ruby et al.[6] reported that most of the flexion/extension motion occurs between neutral and ulnar deviation, rather than from neutral to radial deviation. Various investigators disagree on the direction of transverse plane motion during radioulnar deviation. Some researchers report that the distal carpal row supinates during radial deviation and pronates during ulnar deviation.[10-12] Others report pronation with radial deviation and supination during ulnar deviation.[13,14,17]

The distal carpal row has a negligible amount of intracarpal motion and again can be viewed as a fixed unit.[6] The carpals in the proximal row do not rotate about the various axis to the same degree resulting in intracarpal movement. The increased flexion of the scaphoid during radial deviation allows for the necessary decrease in radiocarpal length as the scaphoid and trapezium approximate the radius.[18] The interosseous scapholunate ligament forces the lunate and scaphoid into flexion during radial deviation and extension during ulnar deviation. The triquetrum motions mimic those of the lunate[18] but are less in magnitude.[17]

The scaphoid has the greatest magnitude of movement in the transverse plane (pronation/supination) while the lunate rotates the most about the axis of flexion and extension. In comparison to global wrist flexion/extension the amount of intracarpal motion between the scaphoid and lunate is relatively small.[10]

IV. PATHOKINESIOLOGY: CLINICAL RELEVANCE AND IMPLICATIONS

With regard to the functional aspects of the wrist, disruption of the delicate balance of carpal alignment and motion during joint movements results in several different clinical presentations. In the past, diagnosis was difficult and often limited to utilization of the patient's history, subjective complaints, and unreliable clinical tests. The use of kinematic MRI permits direct visualization of carpal movement and relationships. This section provides an overview of the clinical relevance and implications of the pathokinematic conditions that affect the wrist.

A. DISTAL RADIOULNAR JOINT INSTABILITY

Loss of the integrity of the triangularfibrocartilage complex, the ulnotriquetral ligament, or the ulnolunate ligament can disrupt the stability of the distal radioulnar joint. Traumatic disruption of these structures is often associated with fractures to the distal end of the radius and ulna. The result may be increased dorsal translation of the ulna during pronation and increased volar translation during supination.

In distal radioulnar joint instability, the patient often complains of pain with end-range pronation/supination and during gripping activities. The amount of passive glide available between the distal radius and ulna is normally greatest in mid-position. Furthermore, the patient will have increased passive dorsal/volar glide of the ulna with the radius stabilized in a pronated or supinated position, respectively.

B. EXTENSOR CARPI ULNARIS TENDON SUBLUXATION

The patient with extensor carpi ulnaris tendon subluxation will present with ulnar-side wrist pain during activities that require pronation/supination. During pronation, the ECU tendon rests on the medial side of the ulnar head. With supination, the tendon becomes angled and is stabilized from moving laterally over the dorsal surface of the ulnar head by fascial restraints. However, if the fascial restraints become attenuated, the tendon may snap over the ulnar head laterally with supination. Initially, this condition is more annoying than symptomatic but as it continues, tenosynovitis develops and the condition becomes painful.

C. ULNOCARPAL IMPACTION

Alignment of the distal radial ulnar complex affects load transmission through the wrist. Experimental studies evaluating forces acting across the wrist joint have shown that approximately 80 to 90% of the force is transmitted across the radiocarpal joint, while 10 to 20% is transmitted across the radioulnar joint.[2,19]

Generally, the radial styloid process exceeds the length of the articular end of the ulna by 9 to 12 mm. However, at the site of articulation with the lunate, the articular surfaces of the radius and ulna are on the same level. This is termed neutral ulnar variance. Occasionally, the ulna projects more proximally (negative ulnar variance) or more distally (positive ulnar variance).[1] Fractures of the distal radius with a loss of radial length can result in a positive ulnar variance.

A positive ulnar variance results in increased load transmission through the triangular fibrocartilage complex, lunate, and the ulnar side of the wrist. The long-term sequelae of this increased load can include thinning or tears of the articular disk; chondromalacia of the lunate, triquetrum, and ulnar head; and ulnocarpal arthritis. Patients with this condition demonstrate increased symptoms during power grip secondary to the compressive pull of the finger flexors and wrist extensors which translates the radius proximally, effectively increasing ulnar variance (1 to 2 mm)[20,21] and load transmission. Clinically, power grip may be decreased in pronation compared to a neutral or supinated position. The distal glide of the ulna during pronation[22] may provide the biomechanical rationale for this.

D. KEINBOCK'S DISEASE

Avascular necrosis of the lunate, or Keinbock's disease, can be caused by trauma or dislocation of the lunate impairing its blood supply. The development of Keinbock's disease may not be solely attributable to extrinsic trauma as this condition has also been correlated with negative ulnar variance.[18] Patients with negative ulnar variance may be predisposed to developing Keinbock's disease as a result of compression of the lunate against the irregular articular surface created by the discrepancy in radial and ulnar lengths.[1] These patients generally complain of dorsal wrist pain and painful and weakened grip and have tenderness to palpation directly over the lunate without any evidence of a fracture. Wrist extension is usually the most painful motion for these patients.

E. CARPAL INSTABILITY

As mentioned previously, the volar carpal ligaments, dorsal carpal ligaments, and intrinsic interosseous ligaments serve to stabilize the carpal bones. When carpal ligament integrity is lost, the carpals tend to collapse into characteristic predetermined patterns with resulting degenerative changes.[23] The resulting consequences are pain and decreased grip strength.

Carpal instabilities can be classified as predynamic, dynamic, and static. Predynamic carpal instabilities are conditions in which a disruption of the normal stabilizing structures has occurred without a change in the overall movement patterns of the carpals. Diagnosis of such instabilities is made based on history and clinical findings. Dynamic instabilities are conditions where disruption of the stabilizers has altered the movement characteristics of the carpal bones. These can be seen with cinemaradiography and kinematic MRI but cannot be detected on plain films. Static instabilities are defined as disruption in normal carpal alignment that can be detected on static plain films.

Approximately 95% of all degenerative arthritis of the wrist is associated with conditions that affect the scaphoid.[24] The normal orientation of the scaphoid with respect to the axis of rotation for the proximal and distal carpal rows provides a linkage that ensures synchronous motion of the two carpal rows during wrist flexion and extension. Alteration of the scaphoid or lunate orientation as a result of tears in the scapholunate or lunotriquetral ligament disrupts this synchronous motion and decreases the stability of the midcarpal joint.[25] Scapholunate disassociation, dorsal intercalated segmental instability (DISI), and volar intercalated segmental instability (VISI) are the most common instability patterns.

1. Scapholunate Disassociation

Scapholunate disassociation is the most common pattern of carpal instability. Scapholunate disassociation is often the result of a fall on an outstretched (extended) and ulnarly deviated wrist. The radioscapholunate and scapholunate ligaments that support the proximal pole of the scaphoid are torn, allowing it to flex palmarly. The lunate may rotate into extension creating a DISI alignment.

2. Dorsal Intercalated Segmental Instability (DISI)

The scaphoid is the most commonly fractured carpal bone and the scapholunate ligament is the most commonly injured ligament in the wrist. Both structures are often injured during a fall on the outstretched hand (full wrist extension). Fracture of the scaphoid, resulting in a loss of osseous integrity, or dysfunction of the scapholunate ligament results in a predictable pattern of abnormal carpal kinematics. A complete disruption of the scapholunate ligament results in the lunate assuming an extended or dorsally tilted position in neutral wrist position with the scaphoid frequently assuming a palmar-flexed position[26] (Figure 15.10B). This altered alignment is referred to as dorsal intercalated segmental instability or DISI.

The patient with DISI may complain of wrist pain (especially with extension), snapping or clicking with movement, and decreased grip strength. This local abnormality in many cases progresses to generalized arthritis in a predictable fashion, called scapholunate advanced collapse (SLAC) wrist.[24,27]

3. SLAC Wrist

Loss of scaphoid stability from fracture or ligamentous trauma results in an alteration of the contact areas between the radius and scaphoid. Normally, the radius makes contact with the entire articular facet on the radius. With decreased scaphoid stability, the scaphoid rotates and its articular surface

A.NORMAL

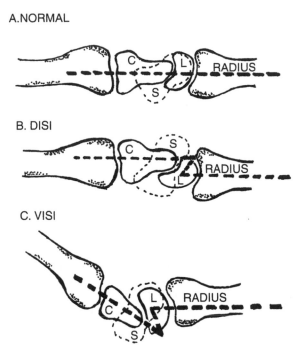

B. DISI

C. VISI

FIGURE 15.10 (A) Normal alignment of the distal radius with the scaphoid (S), lunate (L), and capitate (C). (B) In dorsal intercalated segmental instability (DISI), the lunate rotates dorsally and the scaphoid rotates palmarly. (C) In volar intercalated segmental instability (VISI), the lunate rotates volarly and the scaphoid rotates dorsally.

is no longer congruous with the radial articular facet. The contact area is limited to the lateral margins of the radius.[24] The result is increased stress and corresponding degenerative changes in the radial portion of the radioscaphoid joint. This, in turn, is followed by degenerative changes in the rest of the radioscaphoid joint and then the capitolunate joint.[24,27]

4. Volar Intercalated Segmental Instability (VISI)

Volar intercalated segmental instability (VISI) refers to either a volar tilt of the lunate with the wrist in neutral or a failure of the lunate to tilt dorsally with ulnar deviation[28] (Figure 15.10C). Isolated tears of the lunotriquetral ligament[1,28] or tears in conjunction with the ulnar half of the volar arcuate ligament[28] will cause the lunate to tilt volarly. Dorsal tilt of the capitate in neutral can be seen in conjunction with VISI.[1] Patients with VISI most often complain of nonspecific wrist pain and decreased grip strength. This type of instability pattern is less common than the DISI pattern.

V. SUMMARY AND CONCLUSIONS

The complex anatomy and arthrokinematics of the wrist allow for stability and load transmission throughout a large range of motion. From a basic understanding of the arthrokinematics of the wrist it is not difficult to see why the normal function of the wrist can be easily disrupted leading to significant dysfunction and degenerative changes. Visualization of carpal movement through kinematic MRI can enhance both diagnostic accuracy and rehabilitation efficiency.

REFERENCES

1. Greenspan, A., *Orthopedic Radiology,* 2nd ed., Raven Press, New York, 1992.
2. Berger, R. A., The anatomy and basic biomechanics of the wrist joint, *J. Hand Ther.,* 9, 84, 1996.
3. Taleisnik, J., The ligaments of the wrist, *J. Hand Surg.,* 1, 110, 1976.
4. Stuchin, S. A., Wrist anatomy, *Hand Clin.,* 8, 603, 1992.
5. Youm, Y. et al., Kinematics of the wrist. I. An experimental study of radial-ulnar deviation and flexion-extension, *J. Bone Joint Surg. Am.,* 60, 423, 1978.
6. Ruby, L. K. et al., Relative motion of selected carpal bones: a kinematic analysis of the normal wrist, *J. Hand Surg. Am.,* 13(1), 1, 1988.
7. Patterson, R. M. et al., High-speed, three-dimensional kinematic analysis of the normal wrist, *J. Hand Surg. Am.,* 23(3), 446, 1998.
8. Kauer, J. M. G. and deLange, A., The carpal joint. Anatomy and function, *Hand Clin.,* 3, 23, 1987.
9. Sarrafian, S. K., Melamed, J. L., and Goshgarian, G. M., Study of wrist motion in flexion and extension, *Clin. Orthop.,* 126, 153, 1977.
10. Kobayashi, M. et al., Normal kinematics of carpal bones: a three-dimensional analysis of carpal bone motion relative to the radius, *J. Biomech.,* 30, 787, 1997.
11. Kobayashi, M. et al., Intercarpal kinematics during wrist motion, *Hand Clin.,* 13, 143, 1997.
12. Berger, R. A., Crowninshield, R. D., and Flatt, A. E., The three-dimensional rotational behaviors of the carpal bones, *Clin. Orthop.,* 167, 303, 1982.
13. Kauer, J. M. G., The interdependence of carpal articulating chains, *Acta Anat.,* 88, 481, 1974.
14. DeLange, A., Dauer, J. M. G., and Huiskes, R., Kinematic behavior of the human wrist joint: a roentgen-stereophotogrammetric analysis, *J. Orthop. Res.,* 3, 56, 1985.
15. Seradge, H., Owens, W., and Seradge, E., The effect of intercarpal joint motion on wrist motion: are there key joints? An in vitro study, *Orthopedics,* 8, 727, 1995.
16. Norkin, C. C. and White, D. J., *Measurement of Joint Motion: A Guide to Goniometry,* F.A. Davis, Philadelphia, 1986, p. 138.
17. Feipel, V. et al., Bi- and three-dimensional CT study of carpal bone motion occurring in lateral deviation, *Surg. Radiol. Anat.,* 14, 341, 1993.
18. Reicher, M. A. and Kellerhouse, L. E., Normal wrist anatomy, biomechanics, basic imaging protocol, and normal multiplanar MRI of the wrist, in *MRI of the Wrist and Hand,* Reicher, M. A. and Kellerhouse, L. E., Eds., Raven Press, New York, 1990, chap. 3.
19. Schuind, F. et al., Force and pressure transmission through the normal wrist. A theoretical two-dimensional study in the posteroanterior plane, *J. Biomech.,* 28, 587, 1995.
20. Friedman, S. L. et al., The change in ulnar variance with grip, *J. Hand Surg. Am.,* 18, 713, 1993.
21. Schuind, F. A. et al., Changes in wrist and forearm configuration with grasp and isometric contraction of elbow flexors, *J. Hand Surg.,* 10A, 698, 1992.
22. Epner R. A. et al., Ulnar variance: the effect of wrist positioning and roentgen filming technique, *J. Hand Surg.,* 7A, 298, 1982.
23. Watson, H. and Black, D. M., Instabilities of the wrist, in *Hand Clinics: Management of Wrist Problems,* Vol. 3, Taleisnik, J., Ed., W.B. Saunders, Philadelphia, 1987, 103.
24. Watson, H. K. and Ryu, J., Degenerative disorders of the carpus, *Orthop. Clin. North Am.,* 15, 337, 1984.
25. Linscheid, R. L. et al., Traumatic instability of the wrist: diagnosis, classification, and pathomechanics, *J. Bone Joint Surg.,*, 54A, 1612, 1972.
26. Wright, T. W. and Michlovitz, S. L., Management of carpal instabilities, *J. Hand Ther.,* 6, 148, 1996.
27. Watson, H. K., Weinzweig, J., and Zeppieri, J., The natural progression of scaphoid instability, *Hand Clin.,* 13, 39, 1997.
28. Trumble, T. et al., Kinematics of the ulnar carpus related to the volar intercalated segment instability pattern, *J. Hand Surg.,* 15A, 384, 1990.

16 Kinematic MRI of the Wrist

John D. Reeder

CONTENTS

I. INTRODUCTION

Symptomatic musculoskeletal instability tends to occur in response to specific positional and/or loading force demands placed upon a joint. Although multiplanar magnetic resonance imaging (MRI) performed with static views has contributed greatly to the evaluation of musculoskeletal injuries, kinematic MRI examinations provide a means to better study the dynamic or functional nature of articular relationships, especially with regard to position-dependent pathology or abnormalities.[1]

The complex articular anatomy of the wrist permits coordinated movement in multiple planes, including flexion and extension, pronation and supination, and radial and ulnar deviation. Disruption of the critical synergy of bone, muscle, tendon, and ligament results in biomechanical instability and consequent accelerated chondromalacia and osteoarthritis, as well as irreversible functional impairment.[2-5] Early detection of pathologic carpal relationships is essential in preventing the development of chronic disabling sequelae. Notably, MRI plays an integral part in the assessment of the patient who presents with physical signs and symptoms of wrist pathology.[2]

The combination of static view MRI with a kinematic MRI examination of the wrist offers an extremely effective diagnostic means of evaluating this joint. In this chapter, the technical aspects and clinical applications of kinematic MRI of the wrist are presented.

II. TECHNIQUE

A. POSITIONING DEVICES AND RADIOFREQUENCY COILS

The use of an MR-compatible positioning device is crucial for standardized, repeatable kinematic MRI examinations of the wrist. Fortunately, there are several different types of commercially

0-8493-0807-0/01/$0.00+$.50
© 2001 by Frank G. Shellock

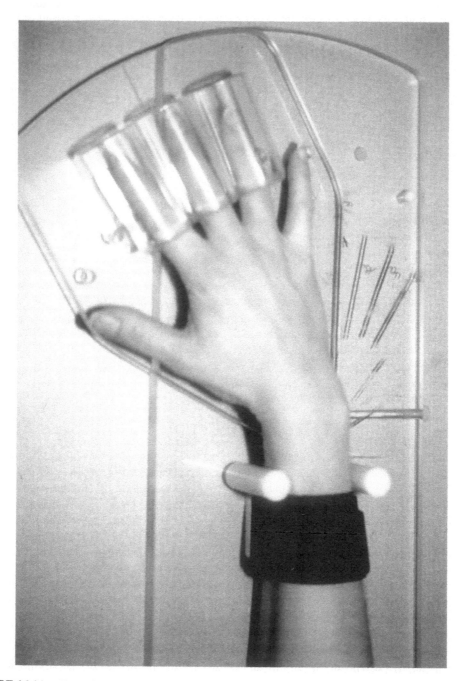

FIGURE 16.1A   Example of a positioning device used for kinematic MRI of the wrist. Plastic positioning device consisting of interchangeable components that permit movements of the wrist from radial to ulnar deviation as well as flexion and extension. This device uses two 3-in. or 5-in. circular coils placed on upper and lower sides of the wrist for the kinematic MRI procedure.

available positioning devices that have been developed for this kinematic MRI application (Figures 16.1A, B, and C). The positioning device essentially supports and stabilizes the extremity, permitting movement of the joint in precise, reproducible increments. With some designs, the positioning device also may impose a load or stress that can improve sensitivity in detecting joint instabilities or abnormal motion patterns.

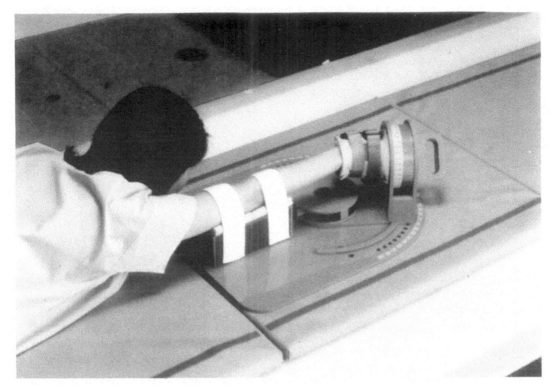

FIGURE 16.1B   Positioning device designed for incremental positions of the wrist (General Electric Medical Systems, Milwaukee, WI). This device supports and stabilizes the upper extremity and permits progressive movements of the wrist through single or multiple ranges of motions. A circumferential receive-only surface coil is typically used with this positioning device.

The small size of the wrist makes it necessary to use a radiofrequency (RF) coil to obtain adequate signal-to-noise for the small field of view and high resolution images necessary for the kinematic MRI examination. Possible RF coils used for kinematic MRI studies include single or dual 3- or 5-in. receive-only, circular surface coils; flexible, wrap-around coils; or transmit/receive extremity coils.[2] Obviously, the RF coil configuration must be of adequate size and shape to be acceptable for use with a particular positioning device. Furthermore, it is advantageous to employ the same coil equipment to obtain high-resolution MR images, thus combining static view and kinematic MRI examinations for a comprehensive evaluation of the wrist.

B. THE MAGNETIC RESONANCE SYSTEM

The first kinematic MRI applications for the wrist were developed for use on high-field-strength MR systems.[2] However, the increased availability of dedicated positioning devices and the improved image quality achieved with the current generation, low-field-strength "open" MR systems have contributed significantly to the development of clinically relevant kinematic MRI procedures for the wrist. Additionally, performing kinematic MRI with an open MR system provides more efficient and convenient access to the positioning device during the examination and permits evaluation of a greater range of joint motion than possible with most high-field-strength MR systems.

C. IMAGING PARAMETERS AND PROTOCOL

Since it is currently not possible to rapidly obtain MR images using imaging parameters that provide the high signal-to-noise required to assess the wrist dynamically, an incremental passive positioning

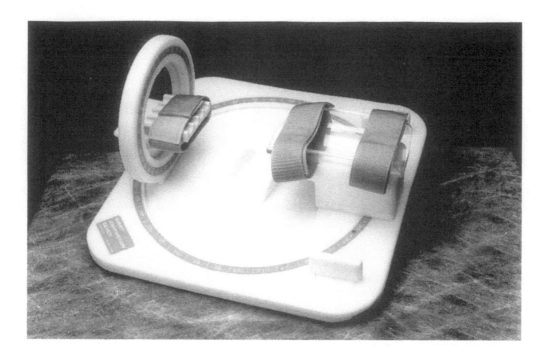

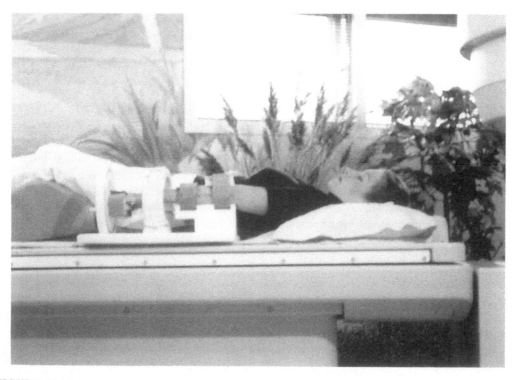

FIGURE 16.1C Positioning device designed for incremental positions of the wrist (top, CHAMCO, Inc., Cocoa, FL). This device supports and stabilizes the upper extremity and permits progressive movements of the wrist through single or multiple ranges of motion. Several different types of surface coils may be utilized with this positioning device. (bottom) A subject prepared for kinematic MRI of the wrist using an open MR system.

kinematic MRI technique is typically used to examine this joint.[2] Using this technique, the wrist is incrementally moved using the positioning device at 5 to 10 degree intervals through a specified range of motion in a specific plane of interest.

A variety of pulse sequences is acceptable for the incremental, passive positioning kinematic MRI technique, including conventional T1-weighted or T2-weighted spin echo, T1-weighted or T2-weighted fast spin echo, gradient echo, or fast gradient echo pulse sequences. Obviously, the selection of the specific imaging parameters used to evaluate the wrist is highly dependent on the suspected or known pathology or abnormality that is present. A small section thickness (e.g., 2 to 4 mm) and small field of view (e.g., 8 to 10 cm) are also requirements for this procedure.

With regard to the plane of imaging, adjustments need to be made based on the anatomy and abnormality that is being assessed. For example, to evaluate distal radioulnar joint instability, axial plane images of the distal radioulnar joint are acquired with the wrist incrementally placed into pronation and supination. To examine carpal instability or impingement syndromes, coronal plane images (i.e., selected from a view showing the carpal bones) are acquired with the wrist progressively moved in radial and ulnar deviation. Additionally, sagittal plane images may be obtained with the wrist placed in flexion and extension and in radial and ulnar deviation to identify instability patterns.

Similar to other types of kinematic MRI studies, the images that are acquired for examination of the wrist may be viewed individually or in a cine-loop format.[2] Notably, the cine-loop display is best for demonstrating subtle instability patterns or transient subluxations of the carpal bones.

III. CLINICAL APPLICATIONS

A. DISTAL RADIOULNAR JOINT INSTABILITY

The distal ulna represents the fixed reference point for rotation of the distal radioulnar joint. In a fully pronated position, slight volar translation of the distal radius relative to the distal ulna may occur. While in a fully supinated position, slight dorsal translation of the distal radius relative to the distal ulna may be observed.[5] However, during pronation of the normal wrist, less than 25% of the distal ulna should be identified dorsal to the dorsal aspect of the radius at the level of the distal radioulnar joint (Figure 16.2).

A tear of the volar distal radioulnar ligament, typically a result of hyperpronation, results in dorsal dislocation of the ulna relative to the distal radius. A tear involving the dorsal distal radioulnar ligament, secondary to hypersupination injury, permits volar dislocation of the distal ulna relative to the distal radius. However, severe hyperpronation or hypersupination injuries may be sufficient to tear both dorsal and volar ligaments, permitting multidirectional instability of the distal radioulnar joint.[5]

The identification of subluxation or dislocation of the distal radioulnar joint using conventional radiography, computed tomography (CT), or conventional MRI is dependent upon the relative position of the wrist during the examination. Dorsal subluxation of the distal ulna is elicited during pronation and reduction occurs during supination (Figure 16.3). With volar subluxation of the distal ulna, reduction of the articular incongruence occurs with pronation.

To evaluate distal radioulnar relationships using kinematic MRI, axial plane images are obtained during progressive rotation of the wrist at 5 to 10 degree intervals from pronation to supination. Borderline laxity of the distal radioulnar joint may be observed in some subjects, as evidenced by a 25% dorsal translation of the ulna relative to the radius. Physiologic laxity is typically observed bilaterally.[5] Therefore, if there is doubt about the significance of apparent ulnar subluxation, comparison is needed with the kinematic pattern of the patient's asymptomatic wrist.

Distal radioulnar joint injuries also may involve the extensor carpi ulnaris tendon, located within the dorsal groove of the distal ulna. Although static MRI views may adequately allow detection

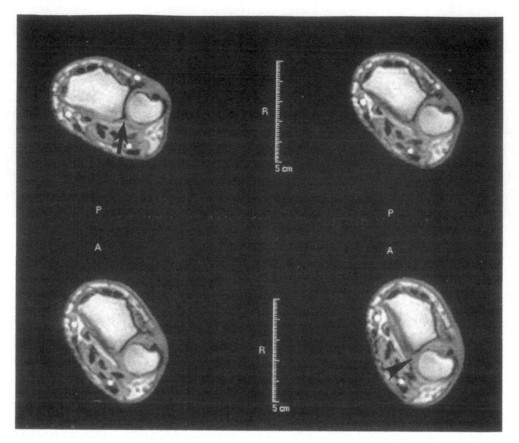

FIGURE 16.2   Kinematic MRI of the wrist performed using axial plane imaging (gradient echo) with passive, incremental movements. This example shows a normal distal radioulnar joint. Normal alignment of the distal radioulnar joint (upper left image, arrow) is observed with the wrist in pronation. As the wrist is progressively moved towards supination (upper right, lower left, and lower right images) note the slight dorsal translation of the radius relative to the ulna (arrowhead).

and characterization of tears and tenosynovitis of the extensor carpi ulnaris tendon, the kinematic MRI examination improves the sensitivity of identifying tendon subluxation. This finding is frequently dependent upon the rotational position of the wrist (Figure 16.3).

B. CARPAL INSTABILITY

Carpal instability patterns have been classified as either static or dynamic.[6-8] Static instabilities are recognizable on conventional radiographs because of fixed carpal malalignment.[7,8] Dynamic instabilities require a particular stress or movement to produce symptoms associated with abnormal carpal orientation. Kinematic MRI techniques can be applied to the evaluation of both static and dynamic carpal instabilities, with imaging performed during the relevant wrist motion.[1,2]

Ventral intercalated segmental instability (VISI) represents a type of static carpal instability in which abnormal volar angulation of the distal lunate bone is observed.[6] The capitolunate angle is increased (greater than 30 degrees) and the scapholunate angle measures less than that normally observed (less than 30 degrees). Acquiring MR images in the sagittal plane through the lunate axis with the wrist in radial and ulnar deviation and in flexion and extension permits differentiation between normal and pathologic carpal motion.[6-8]

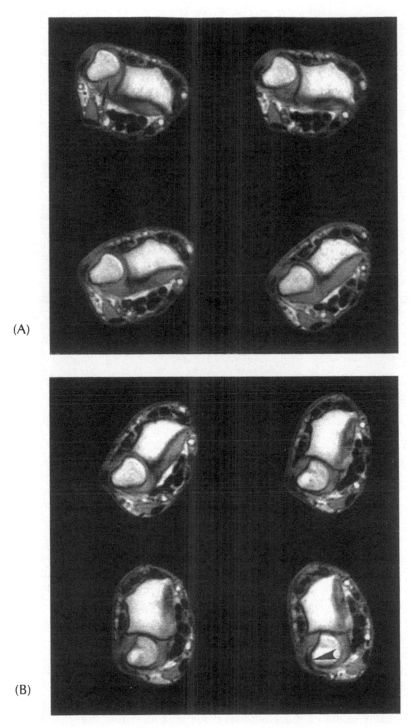

(A)

(B)

FIGURE 16.3 Kinematic MRI of the wrist performed using axial plane imaging (gradient echo) with passive, incremental movements. This example shows an abnormal distal radioulnar joint. In pronation, dorsal subluxation of the ulna (A, upper left image, arrow) relative to the radius is identified. As the wrist supinates, reduction of the distal radioulnar joint incongruence is observed but progressive subluxation of the extensor carpi ulnaris tendon occurs (B, lower right, arrowhead).

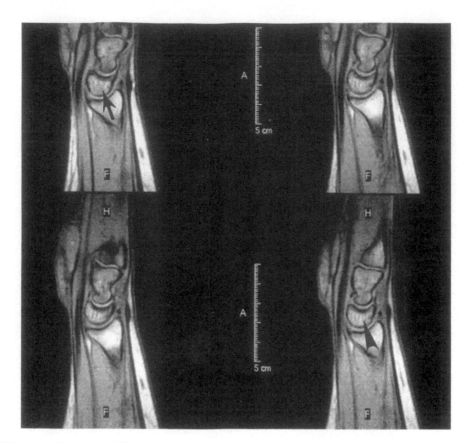

FIGURE 16.4 Kinematic MRI of the wrist performed using sagittal plane imaging (gradient echo) with passive, incremental movements. This example shows a normal capitolunate angle. Note that the capitolunate angle remains normal as the wrist is sequentially moved from ulnar deviation to radial deviation. In addition, with the wrist in ulnar deviation (upper left image, arrow), the lunate normally exhibits a greater dorsal tilt with respect to the distal radius than it does with the wrist in radial deviation (lower right image, arrowhead).

The capitolunate relationship and angle are assessed at different phases of positional stress. Normally, the lunate exhibits a greater dorsal tilt in ulnar deviation relative to neutral positioning or radial deviation (Figure 16.4). During flexion and extension, the capitate should flex and extend relative to the lunate and the lunate should flex and extend relative to the distal radius. Similar to the diagnostic imaging evaluation of the distal radioulnar joint, performing a kinematic MRI procedure on a patient's asymptomatic wrist may prove helpful in demonstrating pathologic asymmetry of dynamic intercarpal relationships.

Dorsal intercalated segmental instability (DISI) represents a pattern of static instability, more frequently encountered than the VISI configuration, in which abnormal dorsal tilt of the distal lunate is identified.[6-8] The scapholunate angle is increased (greater than 80 degrees) and the capitolunate angle also may appear abnormal, measuring greater than 30 degrees. Because the lunate axis normally exhibits a relative dorsal tilt in ulnar deviation, comparison with kinematic MRI of the asymptomatic wrist may prove necessary to confirm the presence of excessive capitolunate angulation in equivocal cases.[6]

With MR imaging of flexion and extension in the sagittal plane, the capitate should normally flex and extend with respect to the lunate axis and the lunate should flex and extend relative to the axis of the distal radius. As discussed in the evaluation of the VISI pattern, documentation of these sagittal relationships is important in the assessment of any suspected instability of the wrist (Figure 16.5).

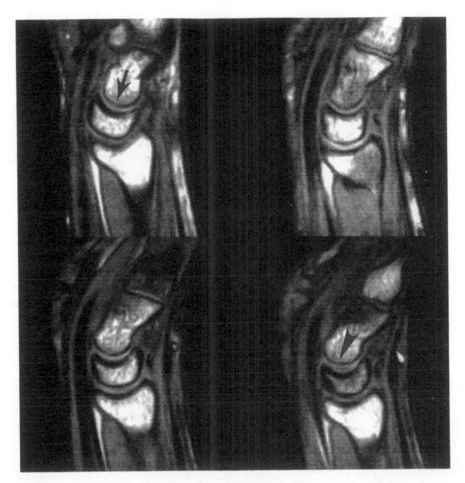

FIGURE 16.5 Kinematic MRI of the wrist performed using sagittal plane imaging (gradient echo) with passive, incremental movements. This example shows carpal instability. In this patient with a clinical presentation of wrist pain and carpal instability, the capitolunate angle appears normal with the wrist in an ulnar deviation position (upper left image, arrow) but becomes abnormal (greater than 30 degrees) as the wrist progressively moves into a radial deviation position (lower right image, arrowhead).

Scapholunate dissociation, another relatively common form of carpal instability, is often encountered in association with DISI. Ligamentous injury involving the stabilizers of the proximal pole of the scaphoid can result in either static or dynamic instability.

Clinical findings include a positive Watson scaphoid shift test. That is, with the forearm in a pronated position, as the wrist is passively positioned from ulnar deviation towards radial deviation, a palpable dorsal subluxation of the proximal pole of the scaphoid can be detected.[7] This maneuver typically reproduces the patient's pain.

If the scapholunate dissociation remains static, an anteroposterior radiograph of the wrist reveals increased scapholunate diastasis and foreshortening of the scaphoid. On the lateral radiograph, the scapholunate angle is increased, usually measuring greater than 80 degrees, and a DISI configuration is often observed.

Suspected dynamic scapholunate subluxation represents an indication for a kinematic MRI procedure, as a positional and/or loading stress is required to elicit abnormal carpal alignment and resultant symptoms. Sagittal imaging through the plane of the scaphoid is performed as the wrist is positioned from ulnar to radial deviation. With radial deviation, the scaphoid abruptly shifts into a plane almost perpendicular to the long axis of the wrist and is associated with dorsal subluxation of the proximal pole of the scaphoid. Clenching of the fist may occasionally be required to produce a loading force necessary to reproduce this dynamic carpal instability pattern.

C. SCAPHOLUNATE AND LUNOTRIQUETRAL LIGAMENT TEARS

A tear of the scapholunate ligament is frequently associated with both static and dynamic carpal instability. In the absence of a fixed rotatory subluxation of the scaphoid, conventional radiographs remain normal. High resolution, small field-of-view, MR imaging techniques have improved the detection of scapholunate ligament tears, but kinematic MRI improves sensitivity by imaging during the application of a tensile stress applied to the ligament.[9,10]

Coronal plane kinematic MRI is performed at the level of the scapholunate joint while moving from progressive radial to ulnar deviation. Normally, the scaphoid and lunate bones move in concert with the intercarpal distance remaining constant (Figures 16.6 and 16.7). In the presence of a scapholunate ligament tear or pathologic ligamentous laxity, a dynamic scapholunate diastasis develops as tensile stress increases during ulnar deviation (Figure 16.8). Radial deviation of the wrist applies tensile stress to the lunotriquetral ligament, thereby improving the probability of detecting lunotriquetral ligament tears and laxity with kinematic MRI.[5]

Close attention to intercarpal spacing on coronal plane images with the wrist positioned from radial to ulnar deviation also may provide evidence of an abnormality.[1,2] Spacing should be evenly distributed between the carpal bones, without any significant or uneven intercarpal widening, proximal or distal movement, or anterior or posterior displacement of the carpal bones.[1,2,8] The

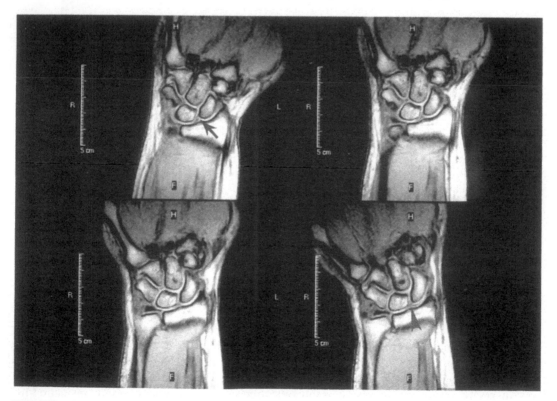

FIGURE 16.6 Kinematic MRI of the wrist performed using coronal plane imaging (gradient echo) with passive, incremental movements. This example shows a normal scapholunate joint. The scapholunate distance remains constant as the wrist moves from radial deviation (upper left image, arrow) to ulnar deviation (lower right image, arrowhead).

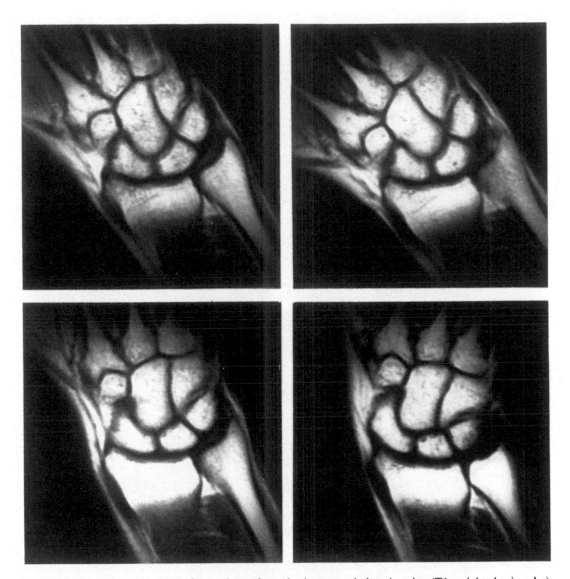

FIGURE 16.7 Kinematic MRI of the wrist performed using coronal plane imaging (T1-weighted spin echo) with passive, incremental movements. This example shows a normal kinematic MRI of the wrist with the joint positioned in radial deviation (upper left image) and progressively moved to ulnar deviation (lower right image). Note that the carpal bones move in a smooth arc formed and bordered by the radius and ulna. There is no abnormal widening of any of the intercarpal spaces and there is no distal or proximal displacement of the carpal bones with the wrist in these positions. Additionally, there is no evidence of positive or negative ulnar variance.

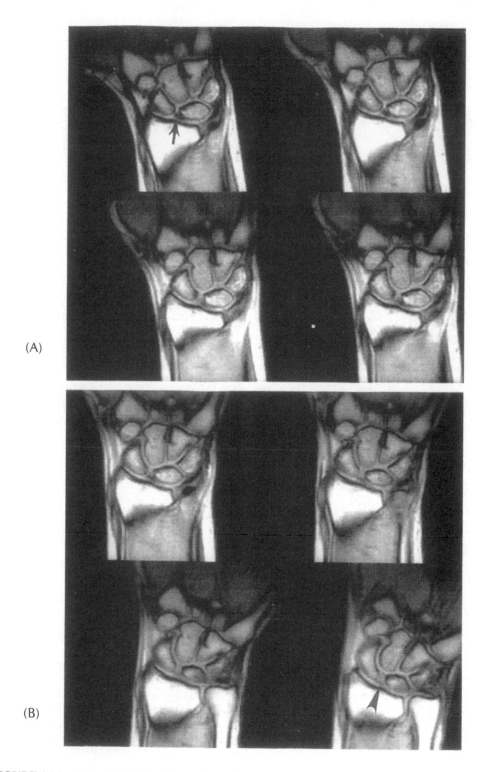

(A)

(B)

FIGURE 16.8   Kinematic MRI of the wrist performed using coronal plane imaging (gradient echo) with passive, incremental movements. This example shows a scapholunate ligament tear. With the wrist in radial deviation, the scapholunate distance appears normal (A, upper left image, arrow). As the wrist moves towards ulnar deviation, the scapholunate joint widens (B, lower right image, arrowhead), indicating a tear of the scapholunate ligament and resultant scapholunate instability.

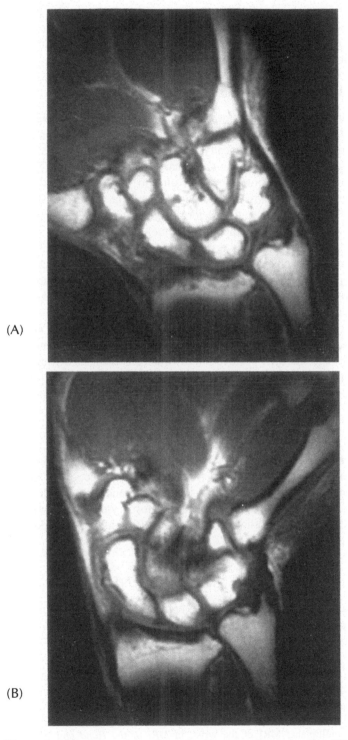

(A)

(B)

FIGURE 16.9   Kinematic MRI of the wrist performed using coronal plane imaging (T1-weighted spin echo) with passive, incremental movements. This example shows the wrist positioned in radial deviation (A) and ulnar deviation (B). This kinematic MRI examination shows cystic degeneration of the triquetrum. Additionally, positive ulnar variance is noted. Impaction between the distal ulna and triquetrum occurs during ulnar deviation (B). (From Shellock F. G., Kinematic MRI of the joints, in *Magnetic Resonance Imaging in Orthopaedics and Rheumatology,* 2nd edition, Stoller, D. W., Ed., Lippincott-Raven, Philadelphia, 1996. With permission.)

normal intercarpal space is approximately 1 to 2 mm wide. Increased joint space is suggestive of an abnormal ligament, increased joint fluid, synovial hypertrophy, or other form of pathokinematics.[1,8] Notably, decreased joint space may be caused by loss of ligament integrity, loss of cartilage, carpal coalition, or dislocated or subluxated carpal bones.[1,8]

D. ULNOLUNATE IMPACTION SYNDROME

Coronal plane images obtained using kinematic MRI techniques during examination of radial and ulnar deviation of the wrist also contribute to the evaluation of ulnolunate impaction syndrome.[1,2,13] Ulnolunate impaction syndrome is typically associated with positive ulnar variance and patients present with a history of pain involving the ulnar aspect of the wrist (Figure 16.9). Abnormal compressive forces transmitted from the distal ulna to the lunate and triquetrum result in the development of secondary osteoarthritis and chondromalacia. Chronic findings, demonstrable on static MRI views, include intraosseous cyst formation, marrow edema, and reactive fibrovascular proliferation involving the osseous components of the ulnar aspect of the wrist.[2,12,13]

Coronal plane kinematic MR images acquired during radial and ulnar deviation permit detection of abnormal ulno-carpal abutment prior to the development of the irreversible structural findings that are evident on static MRI views. Documenting the resolution of an abnormal dynamic ulno-carpal relationship following ulnar-shortening osteotomy or ulnar head resection is an additional application for kinematic MRI of the wrist.

The presence of ulnar variance, whether positive or negative, should always be noted on the kinematic MRI study of the wrist because it may provide an indication of the mechanism responsible for the abnormality. For example, positive ulnar variance is associated with tears of the triangular fibrocartilage complex and articular erosions of the lunate and triquetrum.[1] Alternatively, negative ulnar variance is often seen with Keinbock's disease or avascular necrosis of the lunate.[1]

IV. SUMMARY AND CONCLUSIONS

Kinematic MRI has been applied in a variety of manners to examine the function of the wrist.[1,2,13] To date, this experience has been reported to be useful for detection of subtle abnormalities of carpal motion, instability patterns, transitory subluxation, and other conditions that are not seen using routine static MRI views. To improve the diagnostic yield of the MRI examination of the wrist, a kinematic MRI procedure should be used to assist in identifying additional conditions that affect this joint.

ACKNOWLEDGMENTS

The author gratefully recognizes the invaluable contribution of Donna Mushinshy, R.T., (R)(MR) to this project in protocol development and in the performance of clinical and research-oriented kinematic MRI studies.

REFERENCES

1. Reicher, M. A. and Kellerhouse, L. E., Normal wrist anatomy, biomechanics, basic imaging protocol, and normal multiplanar MRI of the wrist, in *MRI of the Hand and Wrist*, Reicher, M. A. and Kellerhouse, L. E., Eds., Raven Press, New York, 1990.
2. Shellock, F. G., Kinematic MRI of the joints, *Semin. Musculoskeletal Radiol.*, 1, 143, 1997.
3. Linscheid, R. L., Dobyns, H., Beabout, J. W., and Bryan, R. S., Traumatic instability of the wrist, *J. Bone Joint Surg. [Am.]*, 54, 1612, 1972.
4. Culver, J. E., Instabilities of the wrist, *Clin. Sports Med.*, 5, 725, 1986.

5. Bruckner, J. D., Alexander, A. H., and Lichtman D. M., Acute dislocation of the distal radio-ulnar joint, *J. Bone Joint Surg.,* 77A, 958, 1995.
6. Zanetti, M., Hodler, J., and Gilula, L. A., Assessment of dorsal or ventral intercalated segmental instability configurations of the wrist: reliability of sagittal MR images, *Radiology,* 206, 339, 1998.
7. Truong, N. P. et al., Wrist instability series: increased yield with clinical-radiologic screening criteria, *Radiology,* 192, 481, 1994.
8. Gilula, L. A., Carpal injuries: analytic approach and case exercises, *Am. J. Roentgenol.,* 133, 503, 1977.
9. Totterman, S. M. S. and Miller, R. J., Scapholunate ligament: normal MR appearance on three-dimensional gradient-recalled-echo images, *Radiology,* 200, 237, 1996.
10. Tjin, A., Ton, E. R. et al., Interosseous ligament: device for applying stress in wrist MR imaging, *Radiology,* 196, 863, 1995.
11. Lichtman, D. M., Noble, W. H., and Alexander, C. E., Dynamic triquetrolunate instability, *J. Hand Surg. [Am.],* 9, 185, 1984.
12. Imaeda, T. et al., Ulnar impaction syndrome: MR imaging findings, *Radiology,* 201, 495, 1996.
13. Shellock, F. G., Kinematic MRI of the joints, in *Magnetic Resonance Imaging in Orthopaedics and Rheumatology,* 2nd edition, Stoller, D. W., Ed., Lippincott-Raven, Philadelphia, 1996.

Part VIII

Special Procedures

17 Kinematic MRI of the Knee: Preliminary Experience Using the Upright, Weight-Bearing Technique

Wadi M. W. Gedroyc and Andrew Williams

CONTENTS

I. INTRODUCTION

The conventional use of magnetic resonance imaging (MRI) has profoundly changed musculo-skeletal diagnostic imaging, to the extent that MRI is now the primary investigational tool in this field. An immense amount of information may be gathered using high resolution MRI in standard MR systems with the joints in static positions. However, the drawback of this MR system configuration is that the image provides only a "snapshot" or single view of the joint at rest, without visualization of the effects of the application and influence of muscular stress or body weight to that joint. Additionally, the typical "closed-tunnel" shape of standard MR systems prevents substantial movements in the magnet bore. If movements do take place, it is difficult to maintain the anatomic area within the imaging plane because of the lack of a technical means of accomplishing this.

Clearly, many symptomatic patients do not have obvious findings on static view MR images. However, it is possible that such patients may have abnormalities that are evident only in a loaded and/or a dynamic condition, particularly when the torsional forces of activity are imposed.[1,2] Notably, if these types of stress could be applied to the joint, many abnormalities that are evident only under such conditions could be assessed.

Recently, several different types of "open" MR systems have become available with a variety of static magnetic field strengths. These MR systems permit motion of the large joints for MR imaging, thus allowing acquisition of information during dynamic joint movements. Unfortunately, the typical configuration of an open MR system with its limited vertical access does not allow significant weight bearing or application of force to a joint. Thus, the degree of information that is obtained is somewhat limited.

0-8493-0807-0/01/$0.00+$.50
© 2001 by Frank G. Shellock

Currently, it is not possible to examine the stresses of weight bearing and antigravity muscular activity using the typical open-configured MR system. While it is possible to obtain kinematic MR images using this approach,[1,2] the results from such work in joints that normally function under axial loading (e.g., the knee, hip, and ankle) must be viewed with caution until they can be supplemented by upright, weight-bearing kinematic MRI examinations. This chapter describes preliminary work performed on the knee with regard to MRI conducted in an upright, weight-bearing position. This was accomplished using a unique MR system with a large vertical opening and specialized imaging techniques.[3-7]

II. TECHNIQUE

Recently, investigations have been conducted using a vertically opened MR system (Signa SP, General Electric Medical Systems, Milwaukee, WI) that has both vertical and horizontal space around the patient (Figure 17.1). This MR system was specifically designed for MR-guided interventional and intraoperative applications.[3,6,7] It has a 56 cm vertical gap between two vertically placed ring magnet components and operates using a superconducting magnet at a static magnetic field strength of 0.5 Tesla.[3,6]

Using this specialized MR system, patients may be imaged either vertically or horizontally or anywhere in between, as long as the area of interest corresponds to the area between the magnet components. While this MR system was intended for MR-guided procedures, serendipitously it was noted that it provides sufficient patient access to allow upright, weight-bearing MRI examinations to be conducted (Figure 17.2).

This particular MR system design has two different methods of image acquisition that allow images to be obtained continuously, directly from the area of interest. For example, a joint may be

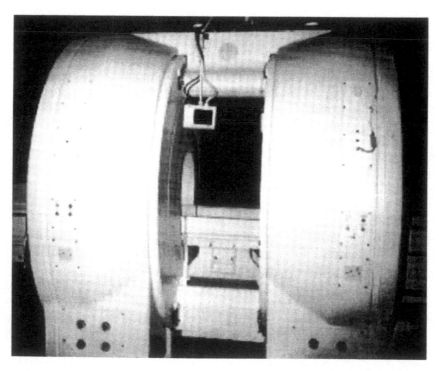

FIGURE 17.1 Vertically opened MR system (General Electric Medical Systems, Milwaukee, WI) with vertical and horizontal access to position the patient between two magnet components for the upright, weight-bearing kinematic MRI examination. Note the presence of the in-bore monitors that facilitate the MRI procedure.

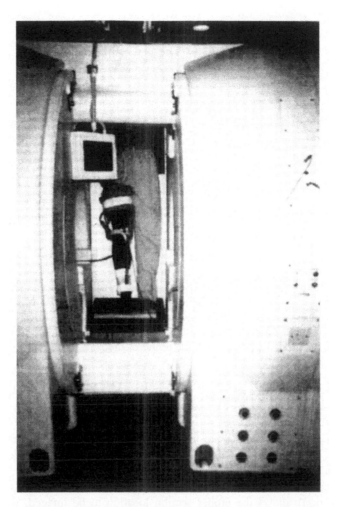

FIGURE 17.2 Open MR system with the patient in the upright position for imaging of the weight-bearing knee. Note that the table has been removed and the patient is leaning against a backboard (see Figure 17.3) to provide support in the near-vertical position. A flexible transmit-receive coil is applied to the knee and the Flashpoint Tracking device is positioned over the anterior tibia for image registration during the MRI procedure.

assessed during movement despite substantial motion between individual MR images (i.e., the plane of imaging) in the field of view. Again, while these image acquisition techniques were initially designed to facilitate MR-guided procedures, they worked equally well for kinematic MRI examinations.[4,5]

The first technique of image acquisition is called Flashpoint Tracking.[6] This technique uses light emitting diodes (LEDs) placed within a plastic rod of known dimensions. There are infrared sensitive video cameras in the roof of the magnet that visualize and track the LEDs. This information is conveyed to a workstation that, by a triangulation process, calculates exactly where the LEDs are within the MR imaging volume.

If the Flashpoint Tracking device is attached to a particular body part (e.g., the middle section of the knee) (Figure 17.3), the magnet will always scan towards that selected position as long as the video cameras can communicate with the LEDs and the Flashpoint Tracking device maintains its relationship to the selected slice location.

The second method of acquiring MR images is called MR Tracking.[7] This technique uses small active coils incorporated into a plastic plate or catheter in a triangular configuration. The small coils produce a relatively small MR signal that is localized using a Fourier analysis and provides a positional coordinate to direct the plane of imaging.

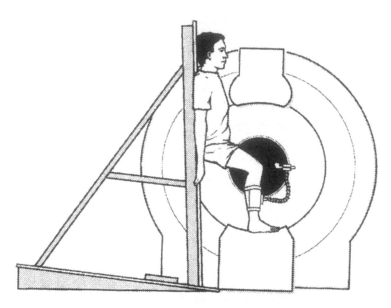

FIGURE 17.3   Side view schematic of the patient placed upright in the MR system leaning against a supporting back board. With the patient within the MR system, the Flashpoint Tracking device is used to show how the area of interest is placed within the center of the bore of the magnet, at the maximum site of optimal image quality.

If three active coils are used such that x, y, and z axis information is obtained, MR imaging can be performed in imaging planes that are orthogonal, oblique, and compound oblique angles. Compound obliquity is particularly useful when performing MR imaging of complex joint structures. For example, the anterior cruciate ligament has an alignment that does not conform to a simple orthogonal plane. Thus, the use of this image localization technique greatly facilitates imaging of this anatomic structure.

The MR Tracking device (which can be incorporated into a rod or a plate attached to the patient in the desired position) allows the proper section location to be imaged, while overcoming the problems of motion artifacts that may be present in the imaging field. This particular method has two further advantages. First, visual contact with the coils is not required as it is with the Flashpoint Tracking device. Therefore, the system can be used in positions where the upper body is between the LEDs and the video cameras. Second, the software used with the MR Tracking device allows a series of section locations to be obtained through the area of interest, rather than just a single selected slice, as is the case when the Flashpoint Tracking device is used.

With respect to the actual MRI method, fast gradient echo pulse sequences are typically used to permit rapid acquisition of images. For musculoskeletal applications, either fast-spoiled gradient recalled echo in the steady state (GRASS) or inversion recovery (IR) prepared gradient echo images are usually used. These pulse sequences provide T1-weighted images at the rate of approximately one image every two seconds. There are many instances where it would be useful to have more T2-weighted, gradient echo sequences applied at a rapid rate, but this currently is difficult to obtain using the vertically opened MR system.

Combining the above techniques allows MR imaging during upright, weight bearing of the knee to be performed easily. While there is not enough space to permit the patient to stand fully upright or erect in this MR system, slight backward angulation of the trunk (i.e., 5 to 10 degrees) allows near-weight-bearing images to be obtained (Figures 17.2 and 17.3). Notably, this positioning scheme may be accomplished without the patient's requiring support from the upper extremities.

For the upright, weight-bearing kinematic MRI examination, the patient is placed in a near-vertical position to provide axial loading of the knee. A flexible transmit and receive radiofrequency

(RF) coil is suspended around the joint (Figure 17.2). MR images are then obtained in the desired imaging plane by the MR system operator, placing one of the image acquisition devices in the proper place and fixing it into the exact position on the patient. Subsequent MR images are continuously obtained using the above-mentioned pulse sequences through a series of movements involving small incremental changes between each subsequent position. This procedure is repeated in an incremental manner until the desired range of motion is evaluated.

From a biomechanical consideration, the implications of this near-vertical positioning scheme compared with full upright loading of the knee have yet to be determined. Admittedly, the "normal" biomechanical aspects for the knee may not be accomplished using near-vertical positioning. Nevertheless, certain aspects of upright, weight-bearing forces are imposed on the knee in consideration of the constraints of the available MR technology. For the knee, the positions from full extension to approximately 90° of flexion in a single sagittal or oblique plane of imaging can be acquired in approximately 3 min. The MR images obtained during this examination may be viewed individually as single section locations or put in a paging format and visualized as a cine-loop display of the incremental positions.

With the unique ability to image the knee in an upright, loaded position, our group initiated studies to assess pathological conditions that may be revealed using this procedure that could otherwise not be identified using conventional, static view MR imaging.[8,9] However, before this issue can be reliably addressed, the normal findings associated with this positioning scheme need to be defined for the soft tissues and bones under the upright, weight-bearing conditions. Thus, the remainder of this chapter describes two projects that illustrate how osseous and soft tissues move under upright loading. We believe that this is only the beginning of more detailed biomechanical studies that will expand the understanding of how joints actually function in health and disease.

III. UPRIGHT, WEIGHT-BEARING KINEMATIC MRI OF THE KNEE

A. MENISCAL MOVEMENTS

Previous studies of knee kinematics have been of limited value due to a number of factors. For example, most of the previous work has been unrepresentative of knee kinematics because of the use of cadaveric specimens or, for *in vivo* studies, knees examined using x-ray techniques that provided only a two-dimensional representation of a three-dimensional reality.[10-18] Obviously, the use of conventional MRI to assess the knee in non-weight-bearing also has known limitations, as discussed above. Notably, investigations conducted to define meniscal movements associated with flexion in the cadavaric knee, unloaded knee, or inappropriately loaded knee have yielded confusing and contradictory results.[13-18]

To examine the important aspects of knee kinematics, our first study involved the measurement of meniscal motion during knee flexion.[8] The meniscus is an important multifunctional component of the knee. It has an important role in load transmission, shock absorption, proprioception, maintaining joint stability, and lubrication.[13-18]

The menisci effectively distribute contact forces over the articular surfaces by increasing the surface area of the knee joint. Load distribution over an incongruent joint surface is facilitated by the mensicus conforming to the joint surface and its ability to move as the femur and tibia move, thereby maintaining maximum congruency.[13-18] Movements of the menisci during knee flexion ensures maximum congruency with the articulating surfaces while avoiding injury to these crucial anatomic structures. This capacity to move protects this structure from injury between articulating surfaces. Understandably, the loss of a portion of, or the entire, meniscus results in an increased risk of joint degeneration.

To perform the aforementioned functions efficiently and effectively, the menisci must behave in a dynamic manner. This action is dependent on a variety of factors, including the longitudinal orientation of the meniscal fibers, the attachments of the anterior and posterior horns, and the intermeniscal connections producing a circular construct. The intermeniscal connections produce a circumferential tension as a vertical load is applied during weight bearing.[8,14,17,18]

Using MRI, Thompson et al.[10] were the first to evaluate meniscal movements through a range of motion from extension to flexion in the intact cadaver knee. While earlier cadaveric studies used direct visualization to study meniscal kinematics, this method required considerable dissection that inevitably produced substantial joint instability and altered biomechanics.

With regard to the evaluation of the knee using the unique upright, weight-bearing technique described herein, Vedi et al.[8] examined elite soccer players without known knee pathology. The subjects stood against the specially constructed support frame and the knee was imaged from full-extension to flexion during weight bearing. In addition, using a hinge support positioned behind the knee, the subjects' knees were scanned from flexion to extension during passive positioning while the subjects were seated.

MR images were obtained at 10 degree increments between 0 and 90 degrees of flexion. Initially with the knee extended, sagittal plane MR images were acquired at the level of the mid-medial and mid-lateral compartments to determine the maximal meniscal size. These planes of imaging were then maintained using the Flashpoint Tracker device as the knee was moved. Additionally, coronal plane MR images were obtained from the point of maximal meniscal thickness, again using the Flashpoint Tracker device to maintain the proper section location.

The movements of both menisci were observed in the sagittal plane in the line of their maximal diameter. The perpendicular distance from the outer inferior edge of the meniscus to the outermost edge of the articular cartilage of the tibial plateau for both the anterior and posterior horn was measured (Figure 17.4). Similarly on the coronal plane images, the distance from the outer inferior edge of the meniscus to the edge of the tibial plateau was measured to investigate the extent of radial displacement. The height of the anterior and posterior horn of each meniscus was also measured. The maximum movement of the meniscus through the extension-flexion arc was calculated from the measurements that were obtained (Figures 17.5 and 17.6).

Based on this analysis, in the upright, weight-bearing position, the anterior horn of the medial meniscus moved 7.1 mm, while the posterior horn of the meniscus moved 3.9 mm, with 3.6 mm of mediolateral radial displacement.[8] The height of the anterior horn of the meniscus increased 2.6 mm, and the height of the posterior horn increased 2.0 mm.[8]

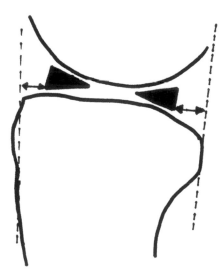

FIGURE 17.4 Schematic showing how meniscal motion is measured using horizontal distances with a vertical line continued along the borders of the tibia.

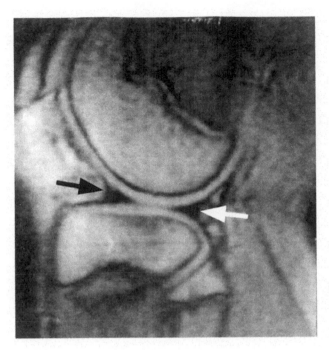

FIGURE 17.5   Upright, weight-bearing MR image (gradient echo pulse sequence) of the lateral knee compartment indicating the degree of posterior motion of the lateral meniscal complex relative to the tibial plateau (black arrow, anterior mensicus; white arrow, posterior meniscus; see Figure 17.6 for additional details).

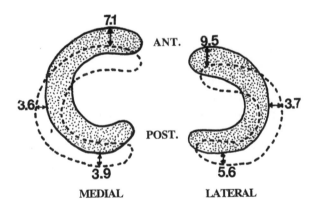

FIGURE 17.6   Schematic showing the mean movement (in mm) that occurs for the medial and lateral meniscal complexes between the fully extended position and the 90° flexed upright, weight-bearing position. Note the greater movement of the lateral meniscus in comparison to the medial meniscus. Additionally, the posterior horn of the medial meniscus is the least mobile portion of the entire complex. These findings suggest why this anatomic site is injured frequently in association with activity. That is, this anatomic site has limited motion capabilities and, therefore, it is trapped easily at the time of trauma. (ANT, anterior; POST, posterior)

The anterior horn of the lateral meniscus moved 9.5 mm, the posterior horn moved 5.6 mm, with 3.7 mm of radial displacement. The anterior horn height increased by 4.0 mm, while the height of the posterior horn increased 2.4 mm. Thus, given these results, the lateral meniscus has a greater excursion with knee movement in comparison with the medial meniscus.[8] Additionally, the posterior horn of the medial meniscus is the least mobile portion of the whole complex (Figure 17.7). These findings suggest that this may be the reason why this anatomic site is injured frequently in

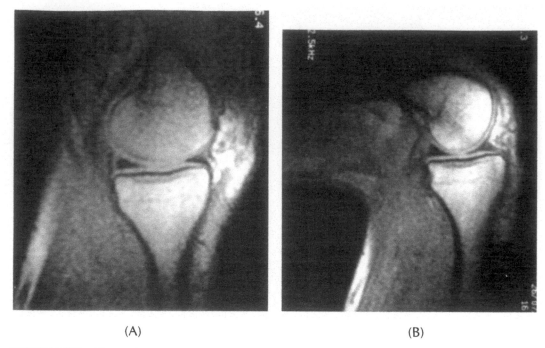

(A)   (B)

FIGURE 17.7 Kinematic MRI of the knee with the subject in an upright, weight-bearing position. MR images were obtained using a gradient echo pulse sequence. (A) The medial compartment of the knee during upright, weight-bearing at full extension. Note the position of the femoral condyle with respect to the tibial plateau. (B) Upright, weight-bearing image in the 75° flexed position of the medial compartment. Note the slight anterior movement of the femoral condyle relative to the tibia without posterior displacement.

association with activity. That is, this anatomic site has limited motion capabilities and, therefore, it is trapped easily at the time of trauma.

The reported meniscal motion obtained with the subjects in an upright, weight-bearing position contrasts with those recently published by Kawahara et al.[11] This group used MRI to study meniscal movements and morphologic changes in healthy knees positioned at extension, 45 degrees, and 90 degrees of flexion.[11] Kawahara et al. reported that the medial meniscus in the unloaded, non-weight-bearing knee had greater excursion compared with the lateral meniscus during flexion.[11] Notably, Bylski-Austrow et al.,[12] in their investigation of cadaveric knees with simulated weight bearing, reported results comparable to ours, but with smaller overall excursion values.

In our non-weight-bearing investigation of the knee,[8] the anterior horn of the medial meniscus moved 5.4 mm, the posterior horn moved 3.8 mm, with 3.3 mm of radial displacement. The anterior horn of the lateral meniscus moved 6.3 mm, the posterior horn moved 4.0 mm, with 3.4 mm of radial displacement. Notably, statistically significant differences were found between weight-bearing and non-weight-bearing conditions for the motion and vertical height of the anterior horn of the lateral meniscus.[8]

In a cadaveric study of the knee, Muhle et al.[19] assessed the effect of the transverse ligament on translation of the menisci. The knees were examined to determine the anterior-posterior excursion before and after transection of the transverse ligament at positions of extension, 30 degrees, 60 degrees, and full flexion using MRI.[19]

There were statistically significant differences in the meniscal excursions before compared with after transection of the transverse ligament.[19] This study demonstrated that the transverse ligament plays an important role in restricting and maintaining the anterior-posterior excursion of the anterior horn of the medial meniscus at the lower increments of knee flexion.

These findings suggest that, unless upright, weight-bearing kinematic MRI is used, the resulting information may be ambiguous in its representation of the normal meniscal motion. Furthermore, evaluating meniscal motion in the unloaded joint may underestimate how much movement there is in a loaded joint.

B. Tibio-Femoral Relationships

Accordingly, data derived from previous *in vitro* and *in vivo* studies of the knee have also led to contradictory information with regard to tibio-femoral relationships. Results from these studies have contributed to the concept of a "roll-back" or posterior motion of the femur on the tibia during knee flexion, facilitated by the cruciate ligament "four-bar linkage" as being established dogma.[13] Although the contact points between femoral and tibial articular surfaces move posteriorly during knee flexion, it is assumed that this equates to a posterior motion of the femur on the tibia during flexion. Notably, this concept is commonly incorporated into the great majority of knee prosthesis designs.

Thus, having established the normal meniscal movement pattern for the upright, weight-bearing knee using kinematic MRI, the motion of the femur relative to the tibia was considered next.[9] Once again, subjects were evaluated in the vertical and horizontal access, open MR system.

Each knee was imaged in the sagittal plane through the mid-medial and mid-lateral compartments of the tibio-femoral joint. Initially, the subjects were placed in a seated position and MR images were obtained with the knee positioned from extension to 90 degrees of flexion in predetermined increments. In addition, with the knee held at 90 degrees of flexion, MR images were obtained with the tibia passively rotated internally and externally.

The movement of the femur relative to the tibia was measured by comparing the positions of fixed points on images of these bones between successive MR images. A fixed point on the tibia was easy to establish. The fixed point on the femur was designated using the method described by Kawahara et al.,[11] whereby circles of best-fit were applied to the sagittal femoral profiles, providing a reproducible center as a reference point on each femoral condyle.

For the non-weight-bearing knees, there was negligible antero-posterior motion of the medial femur on the tibia during flexion, with most of the motion being pure sliding at the joint surface. In contrast, the lateral femoral condyle was seen to move posteriorly 15 to 20 mm. This difference in medial and lateral motion equated to 20 degrees of external femoral rotation as the knee flexed. In terminal knee extension, the most anterior joint surface of the tibia and femur was observed to compress (especially medially) and the posterior femoral condyles exhibited a "lift-off" movement.

The kinematic MRI procedure performed in the upright, weight-bearing knee revealed that the lateral compartment basically moved as already stated for the non-weight-bearing situation. However, the medial femoral condyle actually moved *anteriorly* during joint flexion (Figure 17.8). Again, the relative medial and lateral motion equates to external femoral rotation.

In the non-weight-bearing knee at 90 degrees, the maximum passive internal and external tibial rotation was found to produce an arc of rotation greater than the axial rotation measured during weight-bearing knee flexion. The upright, weight-bearing position with internal tibial rotation (i.e., foot placed inward) simply augmented slightly the tibio-femoral axial rotation. However, full external tibial rotation (i.e., foot placed outward) abolished axial rotation, with the knee flexing like a hinge.

Thus, the axial rotation of the femur on the tibia, which was measured during knee flexion with the tibia in a "comfortable," neutral rotation, is not obligatory and can be abolished by planting the foot in a way that produces external tibial rotation. Therefore, the extent of axial rotation of the femur on the tibia will depend on the rotational position of the tibia as the foot is planted. Therefore, this information demonstrates that the degrees of internal and external rotation must be specified and known when interpreting this type of information as it pertains to the knee.

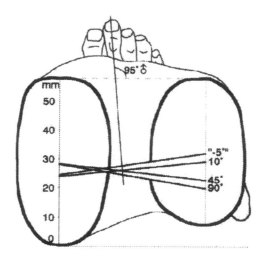

FIGURE 17.8   Diagram depicting the posterior motion of the femoral condyle relative to the tibia in neutral and flexed over the range from hyperextension to 90° in the upright, weight bearing position.

Of interest is that the inherent shapes of the articulating tibial and femoral surfaces fit well with the observed kinematics. Medially, the femoral condyle is effectively a ball "captive" in a socket. Motion between the articulating surfaces is largely by sliding. Laterally, there is minimal constraint between the joint surfaces, which are convex on both sides, and substantial relative motion between femur and tibia occurs with rolling as well as sliding.

These observed kinematics call into question the concepts of the "roll-back" produced by the cruciate ligament "four bar linkage" and "polycentric" motion, which has been described previously.[13] Data obtained from kinematic MRI have obvious implications for understanding cruciate ligament injuries and reconstruction, as well as prosthesis design and performance. Also we hypothesize that the repetitive cyclic compressive loading of the anterior joint surfaces of the medial compartment of the knee during late extension may explain the site (antero-medial) of the early lesion in osteoarthritis in the knee with an intact anterior cruciate ligament.

IV. SUMMARY AND CONCLUSIONS

This chapter provides preliminary findings obtained using upright, weight-bearing kinematic MRI of the knee. This powerful new imaging technique has the potential to provide new detail and insights into the function of this joint because of the ability to study the "loaded condition." The data obtained from future studies will ultimately allow an improved understanding of normal joint kinematics and how pathological processes occur and impact the joint. It is hoped that this new information will allow us to understand how to better treat altered joint function and ideally demonstrate how to restore normal joint kinematics.

REFERENCES

1. Shellock, F. G., Kinematic MRI of the joints, *Semin. Musculoskeletal Radiol.*, 1, 143, 1997.
2. Shellock, F. G., Kinematic MRI of the joints, in *Magnetic Resonance Imaging in Orthopaedics and Rheumatology*, 2nd edition, Stoller, D. W., Ed., Lippincott-Raven, Philadelphia, 1996, p. 1023.
3. Schenck, J. F., Jolesz, F. A., Roemer, P. B. et al., Superconducting open-configuration MR imaging system for image-guided therapy, *Radiology*, 195, 805, 1995.

4. Beaulieu, C. F., Hodge, D. K., Bergman, A. G. et al., Glenohumeral relationships during physiologic shoulder motion and stress testing: initial experience with open MR imaging and active imaging-plane registration, *Radiology,* 212, 699, 1999.

5. Pearle, A. D., Daniel, B. L., Bergman A. G. et al., Joint motion in an open MR unit using MR tracking, *J. Magn. Reson. Imag.,* 10, 8, 1999.

6. Silverman, S. G., Collick, B. D., Figuera, M. R., Khorasani, R., Adams, D. F., Newman, R. W., Topoulos, G. P., and Jolesz, F. A., Interactive MR guided biopsy in an open configuration MR imaging system, *Radiology,* 197, 175, 1995.

7. Dumoulin, C. L., Souza, S. P., and Darrow, R. D., The real-time position monitoring of invasive devices using magnetic resonance, *Magn. Reson. Med.,* 29, 411, 1993.

8. Vedi, V., Williams, A. M., Tennant, S. J., Spouse, E., Hunt, D., and Gedroyc, W. M. W., Meniscal movement. An in vivo study using dynamic MRI, *J. Bone Joint Surg. [Br.],* 81-B, 37, 1991.

9. Hill, P., Vedi, V., Iwaki, H., Pinskerova, V., Freeman, M. A. R., and Williams, A. M., The relative movements of the femur and tibia at the knee: a study of the loaded and unloaded living knee using MRI, *J. Bone Joint Surg. [Br.],* (in press).

10. Thompson, W. O., Leland, W., Thaete, F., Fu., F. H., and Dye, S. H., Tibial meniscal dynamics using three-dimensional reconstruction of magnetic resonance image, *Am. J. Sports Med.,* 19, 210, 1991.

11. Kawahara, Y., Uetani, M., Fuchi, K., Eguchi, H., and Hayashi, K., MR assessment of movement and morphologic change in the menisci during knee flexion, *Acta Radiol.,* 40, 610, 1999.

12. Bylski-Austrow, D., Ciarelli, M., Kayner, D., Mathews, L., and Goldstein, S., Displacements of the menisci under joint load: an *in vitro* study in human knees, *J. Biomech.,* 27, 421, 1994.

13. Nordin, M. and Frankel, V. H., *Basic Biomechanics of the Musculoskeletal System,* 2nd edition, Lea & Febiger, Philadelphia, 1989.

14. Henning, C. E. and Lynch, M. A., Current concepts of meniscal function and pathology, *Clin. Sports Med.,* 4, 259, 1985.

15. Noble, J. and Turner, P. G., The function, pathology, and surgery of the meniscus, *Clin. Orthop.,* 339, 163, 1997.

16. Bessette, G. C., The meniscus, *Orthopedics,* 15, 35, 1992.

17. McBride, I. D. and Reid, J. G., Biomechanical considerations of the menisci, *Can. J. Sports Sci.,* 13, 175, 1988.

18. Walker, P. S. and Erkman, M. J., The role of the menisci in force transmission across the knee, *Clin. Orthop.,* 109, 184, 1975.

19. Muhle, C., Thompson, W. O., Sciulli, R., Pedowitz, R., Ahn, J. M., Yeh, L., Clopton, P., Haghighi, P., Trudell, D. J., and Resnick, D., Transverse ligament and its effect on meniscal motion. Correlation of kinematic MR imaging and anatomic sections, *Invest. Radiol.,* 34, 558, 1999.

18 The Extremity MR System: Kinematic MRI of the Patellofemoral Joint

Frank G. Shellock

CONTENTS

I. INTRODUCTION

Magnetic resonance imaging (MRI) is typically performed using "whole-body" MR systems that permit procedures to be performed on virtually any body part. The development of new metal alloys has permitted the construction of smaller permanent magnets which, in turn, has allowed development of MR systems designed to be physically smaller than conventional, whole-body MR systems.[1] These specialized devices are referred to as "niche," "dedicated," or "extremity" MR systems. The use of an extremity MR system represents a substantial departure from conventional whole-body MR scanning.[1] Importantly, performing MRI procedures with this type of MR system offers distinct advantages that include reduced overall costs, more convenient installation and siting, and greater patient comfort and safety.[1-20]

The first extremity MR system became available on a commercial basis in 1993 (Artoscan®, Esaote, Genoa, Italy and General Electric Medical Systems/Lunar Corporation, Madison, WI). This unique device uses a low-field-strength magnet to image feet, ankles, knees, hands, wrists, and elbows. MRI procedures performed using this MR system have been reported to provide sensitive, accurate, and reliable evaluations of various forms of musculoskeletal pathology.[1-20]

0-8493-0807-0/01/$0.00+$.50
© 2001 by Frank G. Shellock

Recently, a technique was developed to perform kinematic MRI of the patellofemoral joint to assess and characterize patellar tracking abnormalities using the extremity MR system,[12,13] thus expanding the usefulness of this scanner. This chapter describes the unique features of the extremity MR system, presents the technique for kinematic MRI of the patellofemoral joint, and discusses the use of this examination in the clinical setting.

II. TECHNIQUE

A. THE EXTREMITY MAGNETIC RESONANCE SYSTEM

1. Technical and Physical Features

The extremity MR system has several unique design features that are responsible for making it a relatively inexpensive device, especially with regard to siting, installation, and operating costs. The static magnetic field is produced by a 0.2 Tesla, small-bore, permanent magnet that has an ultra-compact fringe field (Figures 18.1 and 18.2). The entire extremity MR system weighs approximately 800 kg. Thus, there is typically no need for structural modifications to site this device. Another major advantage is that it can be sited in a relatively small space (approximately 100 square feet) without the need for a special power source (110 VAC, 60 Hz, 16-amp power is used).

The gradient magnetic fields operate at 12 mT/m, allowing sufficiently small section thickness and fields of view to be obtained for optimal imaging of the musculoskeletal system. The extremity MR system has internal radiofrequency (RF) shielding, which eliminates the need for a Faraday cage or a costly RF screened room. Solenoid RF coils are provided in various sizes to accommodate different body parts and different patient sizes.

A full array of pulse sequences specifically tailored for musculoskeletal examinations is included with the extremity MR system. These sequences include spin echo, fast spin echo, gradient echo, fast gradient echo, three-dimensional gradient echo, magnetization transfer contrast, and fast-pin echo-inversion recovery pulse sequences. In general, using the appropriate imaging parameters and protocols, the image quality and diagnostic performance of the extremity MR system is comparable to mid- and high-field-strength whole-body MR systems.[2-20]

2. Patient Management Considerations

With the expanded clinical use of "niche" or extremity MR systems, Peterfy et al.[1] suggested that these new devices would ultimately offer several important patient-related advantages over MR systems with conventional designs. For example, because the magnetic field and eddy currents generated by the extremity MR system are substantially less than conventional whole-body scanners, risks to patients with ferromagnetic implants are markedly reduced.[1,21,22] Additionally, the ergonomic design of the extremity MR system provides substantially improved patient comfort[1] (Figure 18.1).

To empirically assess these contentions, investigations have been performed to evaluate the relative safety of performing MRI procedures using the extremity MR system in patients with ferromagnetic aneurysm clips, cardiac pacemakers, and implantable cardioverter defibrillators (ICDs).[23,24] Additionally, because only the patient's limb is inserted into the MR system for the MRI procedure (Figure 18.1), sensations of claustrophobia and anxiety often associated with examinations performed using whole-body MR systems may be minimized or eliminated.[1,21,25] A study was conducted by Shellock et al.[25] to assess subjective perceptions associated with MRI examinations performed using the extremity MR system.

a. Aneurysm clips

Aneurysm clips are typically used for the surgical management of intracranial aneurysms and arteriovenous malformations. It is well known that ferromagnetic aneurysm clips are strictly con-

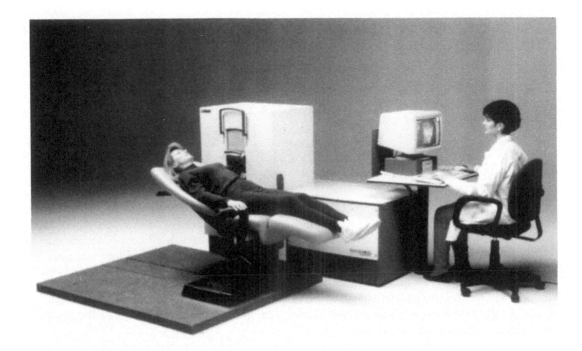

(A)

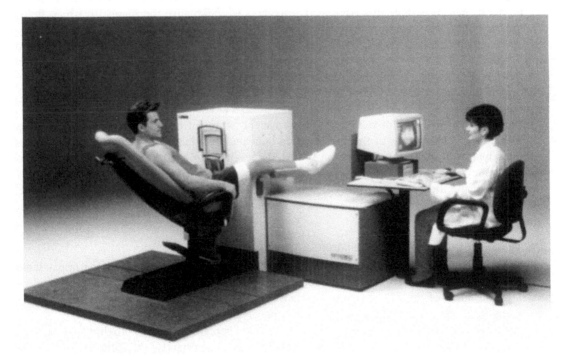

(B)

FIGURE 18.1   The 0.2 Tesla, extremity MR system (Artoscan®, Esaote, Genoa, Italy and General Electric Medical Systems/Lunar Corporation, Madison, WI). These photographs show MRI examinations being performed on the wrist (A) and knee (B). Note that only the body part that requires imaging is placed inside of this specialized MR system.

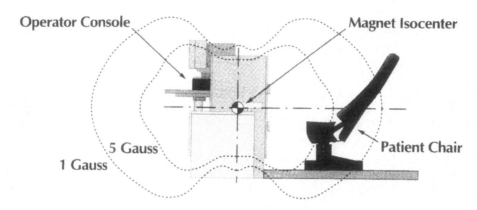

FIGURE 18.2   Fringe fields for the 0.2 Tesla extremity MR system (Artoscan) showing the 1 and 5 Gauss levels. The distribution and contour of these fringe fields are not substantially affected by various external influences (i.e., proximity to large masses of metal, support beams, etc.), like magnets for whole-body MR systems. The 5 Gauss fringe field is well contained with respect to proximity to the extremity MR system.

traindicated for patients and individuals in the MRI environment.[21-23,26] Strong magnetic forces and torque associated with conventional MR systems can move or displace these metallic implants, resulting in serious injury or death.[21-23,26]

It should be noted that the distribution of the magnetic fringe fields, especially for the 1 and 5 Gauss levels (Figure 18.2), is relatively close to the magnet bore of the extremity MR system. By comparison, fringe fields associated with conventional MR systems may be 10 times these values at comparable distances to the magnets.[1,21,22] Because the magnetic fringe fields for the extremity MR system are "contained" in close proximity to the magnet bore (Figure 18.2), the same magnet-related hazards associated with conventional MR systems are not present with this system.[1,21,22]

To demonstrate this, a study was conducted to assess 22 different aneurysm clips for magnetic field interactions associated with the extremity MR system.[23] Aneurysm clips selected for evaluation included older types (e.g., Heifetz and Yasargil, Model FD aneurysm clips), as well as versions currently used in patients for temporary or permanent treatment of aneurysms or arteriovenous malformations.[23] The results of this investigation indicated that there would be no risk to patients or individuals with respect to movement or dislodgment for the aneurysm clips that were tested for magnetic interactions. Therefore, in consideration of how patients are positioned for MRI procedures using the extremity MR system (i.e., the head does not enter the magnet bore), it was deemed safe to perform MRI examinations in patients with the specific aneurysm clips that had undergone evaluation.

b. Pacemakers and implantable cardioverter defibrillators

In general, patients with permanent cardiac pacemakers (i.e., pulse generators) or implantable cardioverter defibrillators (ICDs) are restricted from entering the MRI environment.[21,22] The electromagnetic fields of the MR systems may cause these devices to malfunction, creating serious problems for patients or resulting in lethal consequences.[21,22,24]

As previously mentioned, the magnetic fringe field is contained in close proximity to the low-field-strength magnet of the extremity MR system. More importantly, this MR system has an integrated Faraday cage that prevents RF interference of body parts that are not exposed to the MRI procedure. Importantly, it is not possible for the gradient or RF electromagnetic fields associated with the extremity MR to induce currents in a pacemaker or ICD because the patient's thorax (where the pacemaker or ICD is typically implanted) remains outside the MR system during the MRI examination.

In consideration of the factors and because of the need and desire to use MRI in patients with cardiac pacemakers or ICDs, an investigation was conducted using *ex vivo* testing techniques to determine if the extremity MR system could be used to safely image patients with these devices.[24] Cardiac pacemakers and ICDs were selected for testing because they represent older and newer devices.[24] Magnetic field interactions and various functional aspects of the pacemakers and ICDs were evaluated.

The findings indicated that the pacemakers paced normally before, during, and after MRI.[24] There was no alteration of the programmed parameters or inhibition of the pacing outputs and there were no electromagnetic interference signals identified. Likewise, the ICDs did not display any inappropriate events nor were there electrical resets of the programmed parameters. Furthermore, there were no MR imaging artifacts produced as a result of the operation of cardiac pacemakers and ICDs. Therefore, it would appear to be safe to perform MRI in patients with the specific pacemakers and ICDs tested.[24]

c. Claustrophobia and anxiety

Dysphoric psychological reactions may be encountered by up to 65% of the patients examined by MRI.[21] Of the various forms of psychological distress experienced by these patients, claustrophobia, anxiety, or panic attacks tend to be the most debilitating. As a result, as many as 20% of the patients attempting to undergo an MRI procedure cannot complete it secondary to claustrophobia or other similar psychological sensation.[21] Admittedly, this 20% figure reported in the literature mostly pertains to patient experiences with "tunnel-shaped" conventional MR systems.

Sensations of claustrophobia or anxiety have been reported to originate from one or more factors involved in the MRI examination performed using a conventional MR system. These problems may be related to the confining dimensions of the magnet bore, restriction of movement required during the procedure, the gradient magnetic field-induced acoustic noise, and environmental conditions (e.g., temperature and humidity).[21] Additionally, the "tunnel shape" of the MR system may produce a feeling of sensory deprivation, also known to be a precursor of severe anxiety states.

The architecture of the extremity MR system has no confining features or other aspects that would create patient-related problems as described above (see Figure 18.1). A study conducted by Shellock et al.[25] evaluated the subjective perceptions of patients undergoing MRI procedures using this MR system. Using the extremity MR system, all of the examinations were completed without interruptions or cancellations. In fact, none of the patients reported feeling anxious, nervous, or claustrophobic. Notably, this study represents one of the largest prospective investigations of patients' subjective perceptions of MRI and is the first to evaluate experiences associated with an extremity MR system.[25] Thus, it is useful to know that, for a patient requiring an evaluation of the extremity, there is the option of having the procedure conducted using an MR system that is unlikely to create sensations of claustrophobia or anxiety.

B. THE POSITIONING DEVICE AND RADIOFREQUENCY COIL

With the extremity MR system, kinematic MRI of the patellofemoral joint is performed using the *incremental, passive positioning* technique.[12,13,27-34] While it would be preferable to use the *active movement* or *active movement, against resistance* method,[27,30,35] achievement of the temporal resolution and spatial resolution necessary to perform an "active" kinematic MRI examination is currently not possible with the extremity MR system. Nevertheless, the diagnostic information obtained using an incremental, passive positioning technique for identification of patellar tracking abnormalities exceeds that afforded by other standard radiological methods (e.g., compared with "skyline" or Merchant views).[27,29,30-33]

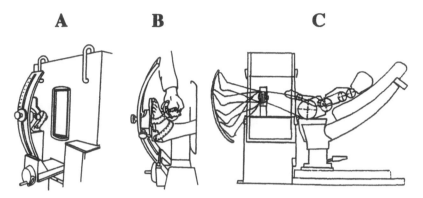

FIGURE 18.3 The leg locking/movement device used to perform the incremental, passive positioning, kinematic MRI examination of the patellofemoral joint. Schematic shows (A) the leg locking/movement device and front of the extremity MR system, (B) the technique for securing the patient's foot in the device in preparation for kinematic MRI, and (C) positioning the patellofemoral joint from extension to approximately 36 degrees of flexion.

The leg locking/movement device, which is a standard accessory provided with the extremity MR system, is used for kinematic MRI (Figure 18.3). This device is normally used to maintain the position of the patient's leg for routine MRI examinations of the knee. Notably, no modifications are required to permit this device to be used for the kinematic MRI procedure.

The patient is seated on the chair of the extremity MR system in a semi-reclined position, with his or her leg placed through a medium or large solenoid RF coil into the foot holder of the leg locking/movement device (Figure 18.3). The leg locking/movement device is then used to maintain the extremity in extension and various evenly spaced positions of flexion (Figure 18.3).

C. Imaging Parameters and Protocol

MR images for the kinematic MRI examination are obtained using the following parameters: T1-weighted, spin echo pulse sequence; axial plane; repetition time (TR), 70–120 msec; echo time (TE), 12–20 msec; section thickness, 10 mm; field of view, 18 cm; matrix size, 192 × 128; number of excitations, 2; number of section locations imaged, 4.[12,13]

The basic protocol involves imaging four contiguous section locations through the anatomy of interest (i.e., in relation to the position of the patella) with the patellofemoral joint extended. These section locations are then imaged as the joint is progressively flexed into three equal increments up to approximately 36 degrees of flexion.[12,13] Thus, four different patellofemoral joint positions are imaged at 12 degree increments (total number of images, 16). The entire kinematic MRI procedure can be accomplished in 15 min or less.[12,13]

MR images obtained from the kinematic MRI examination may be viewed individually or in a cine-loop format.[27,30] The cine-loop is created using the software provided on the extremity MR system to "page" images obtained at the same section locations forwards and backwards. Similar to other kinematic MRI examinations, use of the cine-loop is preferable to examining individual MR images because it allows multiple images to be viewed at different section locations in a timely manner. Additionally, subtle patellar tracking abnormalities may be better appreciated on the cine-loop display of the MR images.[27,29,30,34]

D. Interpretation of the Kinematic MRI Examination

Because of the limitations of using quantification techniques (see Chapter 9, Kinematic MRI of the Patellofemoral Joint), the kinematic MRI examination of the patellofemoral joint performed using the extremity MR system is typically interpreted using qualitative criteria.[27-36] Briefly, the following qualitative classifications of patellofemoral relationships are used.

Normal patellar alignment and tracking: The central ridge of the patella is positioned in the center of the femoral trochlear groove. This patellofemoral relationship is maintained throughout the increasing increments of joint flexion.

Lateral displacement of the patella: The central ridge of the patella is laterally displaced relative to the femoral trochlear groove or the centermost part of the femoral trochlea. The lateral facet of the patella overlaps the lateral aspect of the femoral trochlea.

Lateral patellar tilt or excessive lateral pressure syndrome: The patella is tilted, usually towards the dominant lateral facet. Notably, a space is seen between the central ridge of the patella and the femoral trochlear groove or centermost part of the femoral trochlea. A small amount of lateral displacement of the patella may or may not be present during joint flexion.

Medial displacement of the patella: The central ridge of the patella is medially displaced relative to the femoral trochlear groove or the centermost part of the femoral trochlea.

Lateral-to-medial subluxation of the patella: In the initial increments of joint flexion (i.e., 5 to 10 degrees), the central ridge of the patella is laterally displaced relative to the femoral trochlear groove or the centermost part of the femoral trochlea. As the increments of flexion increase, the patella moves into and across the femoral trochlear groove or femoral trochlea, and becomes medially displaced during the highest increments of flexion.

III. CLINICAL APPLICATIONS

Patellofemoral joint abnormalities are a predominant cause of anterior knee pain. Discordant patellofemoral relationships are the primary reason for painful symptoms and joint dysfunction.[37,38] As previously described in Chapter 9 of this textbook, kinematic MRI of the patellofemoral joint provides a useful and objective means of evaluating and characterizing patellar alignment and tracking. Similar to kinematic MRI methods designed for use on whole-body MR systems,[28-36] kinematic MRI of the patellofemoral joint using the extremity MR system may be employed to determine the presence and severity of abnormal patellofemoral relationships.[12,13]

A. ABNORMAL PATELLOFEMORAL RELATIONSHIPS

Various types of abnormal patellofemoral relationships may be identified using extremity MR system to perform kinematic MRI,[12] including: lateral subluxation of the patella (Figure 18.4), lateral patellar tilt, medial subluxation of the patella, and lateral-to-medial subluxation of the patella.[12] As a result of the ability to image the patellofemoral joint during the initial increments of flexion when alignment and tracking abnormalities are the most apparent, this imaging procedure has been demonstrated to exceed the diagnostic capabilities of conventional plain film radiography for evaluation of patients with suspected patellofemoral joint abnormalities.[12,13,27-38] Figure 18.4 shows an example of such a case.

B. EVALUATION OF TREATMENTS

As discussed in Chapter 9, various conservative and surgical treatment protocols have been applied to manage patients with patellofemoral joint pain.[37,38] Importantly, a thorough evaluation of the patient with patellofemoral syndrome, which includes use of kinematic MRI, facilitates the selection of a proper treatment regimen.[13,31,32-36]

In an investigation conducted by Shellock et al.,[13] the extremity MR system was used to assess the effect of a patellar brace to treat patients with abnormal patellofemoral relationships. The

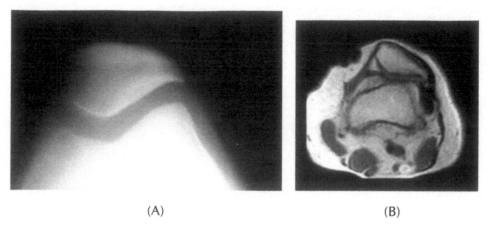

(A)   (B)

FIGURE 18.4   (A) Plain film radiograph showing Merchant view (45° flexion) obtained in a patient with patellofemoral joint symptoms. Note that the position of the patella relative to the femoral trochlear groove is within normal limits. (B) MR image selected from the series of images obtained from the kinematic MRI examination showing patellofemoral joint at approximately 12° of flexion (axial plane; TR/TE, 90/20 msec; 10 mm section thickness). There is marked lateral subluxation of the patella. In addition, the patella is positioned above the femoral groove, indicating the presence of patella alta. This example illustrates the inherent limitations of conventional plain film radiography and the importance of imaging the patellofemoral joint at the earliest increments of joint flexion to identify abnormal patellofemoral relationships.

findings of this study revealed that application of the brace produced centralization or improvement in the position of the patella in the majority of patients.[13] Thus, information provided by kinematic MRI of the patellofemoral joint was used to determine if the selected treatment produced the desired result (e.g., improvement in the position of the patella relative to the femoral trochlear groove). In addition, similar to other kinematic MRI examinations performed using whole-body MR systems, imaging the patellofemoral joint with the extremity MR system was considered helpful for evaluating patients after realignment surgeries or other interventions to assess the effectiveness of the procedures or to determine the reason for persistent symptoms. Further details pertaining to clinical applications for kinematic MRI of the patellofemoral joint that are applicable to the extremity MR system are presented in Chapter 9.

IV. SUMMARY AND CONCLUSIONS

A kinematic MRI of the patellofemoral joint technique has been developed for the extremity MR system and used in the clinical setting.[12,13] Similar to kinematic MRI methods designed for whole-body MR systems, this procedure may be used to determine the presence and severity of patellar malalignment and abnormal tracking patterns. Because there is a high incidence of combined abnormalities of the knee and the patellofemoral joint,[37,38] it may be diagnostically useful to perform both routine MRI examinations of the knee and kinematic MRI procedures using the extremity MR system. This may be particularly helpful for assessment of patients who have confusing or complicated clinical presentations.

A major advantage of the extremity MR system is that it can be sited without radiofrequency shielding or a special power source, in a relatively small space. This permits the device to be installed in a physician's office so that it is readily available for patient use. Accessibility of the extremity MR system permits timely diagnosis and treatment of musculoskeletal disorders. With office-based extremity MR systems, orthopedic surgeons or other clinicians typically have relationships with MRI-trained radiologists to interpret the MRI examinations with the use of teleradiology techniques, facilitating the temporal delivery of healthcare.

REFERENCES

1. Peterfy, C. G., Roberts, T., and Genant, H. K., Dedicated extremity MR imaging: an emerging technology, *Radiol. Clin. North Am.,* 35, 1, 1997.
2. Franklin, P. D., Lemon, R. A., and Barden, H. S., Accuracy of imaging the menisci on an in-office, dedicated, magnetic resonance imaging extremity system, *Am. J. Sports Med.,* 25, 382, 1998.
3. Ahn, J. M., Sartoris, D. J., Kank, H. S. et al., Gamekeeper thumb: comparison of MR arthrography with conventional arthrography and MR imaging in cadavers, *Radiology,* 206, 737, 1998.
4. Masciocchi, C., Barile, A., Navarra, F., Mastantuono, M., DeBac, S., Satragno, L., Lupattelli, L., and Passariello, R., Clinical experience of osteoarticular MRI using a dedicated system, *MAGMA,* 2, 545, 1994.
5. Barile, A., Masiocchi, C., Mastantuono, M., Passariello, R., and Satragno, L., The use of a "dedicated" MRI system in the evaluation of knee joint diseases, *Clinical MRI,* 5, 79, 1995.
6. Maschicchi, C., Mastantuono, M., DeBac, S., Barile, A., Satragno, L., Lupattelli, L., and Passariello, R., Technologic advances in magnetic resonance imaging: permanent low-field magnets dedicated to the study of the joints. Clinical results, *Radiol. Med.,* 89, 593, 1995.
7. Riel, K. A., Kersting-Sommerhoff, B., Reinisch, M., Ottl, G., Golder, W., Lenz, M., Hof, N., Gerhardt, P., and Hipp, E., Prospective comparison of Artoscan-MRI and arthroscopy in knee injuries, *Z. Orthop. Ihre. Grenzgeb,* 134, 430, 1996.
8. Kersting-Sommerhoff, B., Hof, N., Lenz, M., and Gerhardt, P., MRI of peripheral joints with a low-field dedicated system: a reliable and cost-effective alternative to high-field units?, *Eur. Radiol.,* 6, 561, 1996.
9. Maschicchi, C., Dedicated MR system and acute trauma of the musculo-skeletal system, *Eur. J. Radiol.,* 22, 7, 1996.
10. Shellock, F. G., Stone, K., and Crues, J. V., Evaluation of the knee using an extremity MRI system: diagnostic findings compared to arthroscopy, *Med. Sci. Sports Exercise,* 30, S123, 1998.
11. Shellock, F. G., Walgenbach, A., Stone, K., and Crues, J. V., Determination of chondral lesions using a 0.2 Tesla extremity MR system: diagnostic findings compared to arthroscopy, *Radiology,* 214, P07H, 2000.
12. Shellock, F. G., Stone, K., and Crues, J. V., Development and clinical applications of kinematic MRI of the patellofemoral joint using an extremity MR system, *Med. Sci. Sport Exercise,* 31, 788, 1999.
13. Shellock, F. G., Mullen, M., Stone, K., Coleman, M., and Crues, J. V., Kinematic MRI evaluation of the effect of bracing on patellar positions: qualitative assessment using an extremity MR system, *J. Athletic Training,* 35, 44, 2000.
14. Herber, S., Kreitner, K. F., Kalden, P., Low, R., Berger, S., and Thelen, M., Low-field MRI of the ankle joint: initial experience in children and adolescents using an open 0.2 T MR-system, *Rofo Fortschr. Geb. Rontgenstr. Neuen Bildgeb Verfahr,* 172, 267, 2000.
15. Steinborn, M., Heuck, A., Jessel, C., Bonel, H., and Reiser, M., Magnetic resonance imaging of lateral epicondylitis of the elbow with a 0.2-T dedicated system, *Eur. Radiol.,* 9, 1376, 1999.
16. Merhemic, Z., Breitenseher, M., Trattnig, S., Happel, B., Kukla, C., Rand, T., and Imhof, H., MRI of the ankle joint. Comparison of the 1.0-T and the 0.2-T units, *Radiologe,* 39, 41, 1999.
17. Hollister, M. C., Dedicated extremity MR imaging of the knee: how low can you go?, *Magn. Reson. Imag. Clin. North Am.,* 8, 225, 2000.
18. Hottya, G. A., Peterfy, C. G., Uffmann, M., Hackl, F. O., LeHir, P., Redei, J., Gindele, A. U., Dion, E., and Genant, H. K., Dedicated extremity MR imaging of the foot and ankle, *Eur. Radiol.,* 10, 467, 2000.
19. Bretlau, T., Christensen, O. M., Edstrom, P., Thomsen, H. S., and Lausten, G. S., Diagnosis of scaphoid fracture and dedicated extremity MRI, *Acta Orthop. Scand.,* 70, 504, 1999.
20. Bonel, H., Messer, G., Seemann, M., Walchner, M., Rocken, M., and Reiser, M., MRI of fingers in systemic scleroderma. Initial results with contrast-enhanced studies using a dedicated MRI system, *Radiologe,* 37, 794, 1997.
21. Shellock, F. G. and Kanal, E., *Magnetic Resonance: Bioeffects, Safety, and Patient Management,* Lippincott-Raven, New York, 1996.
22. Shellock, F. G., *Pocket Guide to MR Procedures and Metallic Objects: Update 2000,* Lippincott Williams & Wilkins, Philadelphia, 2000.
23. Shellock, F. G. and Crues, J. V., Aneurysm clips: assessment of magnetic field interaction associated with a 0.2-T extremity MR system, *Radiology,* 208, 407, 1998.

24. Shellock, F. G., O'Neil, M., Ivans, V., Kelly, D., O'Connor, M., Toay, L., and Crues, J. V., Cardiac pacemakers and implantable cardiac defibrillators are unaffected by operation of an extremity MR system, *Am. J. Roentgenol.,* 172, 165, 1999.
25. Shellock, F. G., Stone, K. R., Resnick, D., Peterfy, C. G., and Crues, J. V., Subjective perceptions of MRI examinations performed using an extremity MR system, *Signals,* 32(1), 16–21, 2000.
26. American Society for Testing and Materials, Standard specification for the requirements and disclosure of self-closing aneurysm clips, in *Annual Book of ASTM Standards,* American Society for Testing and Materials, 1994.
27. Shellock, F. G., Kinematic MRI of the joints, *Semin. Musculoskeletal Radiol.,* 1, 143, 1997.
28. Shellock, F. G., Mink, J. H., and Fox, J. M., Patellofemoral joint: kinematic MR imaging to assess tracking abnormalities, *Radiology,* 168, 551, 1988.
29. Shellock, F. G., Mink, J. H., Deutsch, A., and Fox, J. M., Patellar tracking abnormalities: clinical experience with kinematic MR imaging in 130 patients, *Radiology,* 172, 799, 1989.
30. Shellock, F. G., Kinematic MRI of the joints, in *Magnetic Resonance Imaging in Orthopaedics and Rheumatology,* 2nd edition, Stoller, D. W., Ed., Lippincott-Raven, Philadelphia, 1996.
31. Shellock, F. G., Mink, J. H., Deutsch, A., Fox, J. M., and Ferkel, R. D., Evaluation of patients with persistent symptoms following lateral retinacular release by kinematic MRI of the patellofemoral joint, *Arthroscopy,* 6, 226, 1990.
32. Koskinen, S. K., Hurme, M., Kujala, U. M., and Kormoano, M., Effect of lateral release on patellar motion in chondromalacia, *Acta Orthop. Scand.,* 61, 311, 1990.
33. Kujala, U. M., Osterman, K., Kormano, M., Komu, M., and Schlenzka, D., Patellar motion analyzed by magnetic resonance imaging, *Acta Orthop. Scand.,* 60, 13, 1989.
34. Brown, S. M. and Bradley, W. G., Kinematic magnetic resonance imaging of the knee, *MRI Clin. North Am.,* 2, 441, 1994.
35. Shellock, F. G., Mink, J. H., Deutsch, A. L., Foo, T. K. F., and Sullenberger, P., Patellofemoral joint: identification of abnormalities using active movement, "unloaded" vs "loaded" kinematic MR imaging techniques, *Radiology,* 188, 575, 1993.
36. Shellock, F. G., Mink, J. H., Deutsch, A. L., Fox, J., Molnar, T., Kvitne, R., and Ferkel, R., Effect of a patellar realignment brace on patellofemoral relationships: evaluation with kinematic MR imaging, *J. Magn. Reson. Imag.,* 4, 590, 1994.
37. Fulkerson, J. P. and Hungerford, D. S., *Disorders of the Patellofemoral Joint,* 2nd edition, Williams & Wilkins, Baltimore, 1990.
38. Fox, J. M. and Del Pizzo, W., *The Patellofemoral Joint,* McGraw-Hill, New York, 1993.

Glossary

Abduction Movement away from the midline of the body.

Adduction Movement towards the midline of the body.

Anterior The direction towards the front of the body in an anatomical coordinate system.

Anteversion A pathologic increase in the angle of torsion of the femur.

Arthrokinematics The movement of one joint surface relative to another.

Articular cartilage A thin, highly hydrated hyaline connective tissue, lining the end of the bone within a diarthrodial joint.

Articulation The joining of two bones (i.e., a joint).

Artifact An appearance or feature seen on an MR image that is not present in the imaged object.

Axial plane Transverse plane defined by the right-left, anterior-posterior body dimensions; the imaging plane that bisects the body into top and bottom parts.

Biomechanics The branch of mechanics applied to biological systems.

Center of rotation A point around which circular motion is described.

Closed-chain Descriptive term referring to when the foot is on the ground (i.e., the tibia is "fixed" during weight-bearing activity).

Compression A loading mode in which equal and opposite loads are applied toward the surface of a structure, resulting in shortening and widening.

Contact area The area of load support or direct surface-to-surface contact.

Contrast The difference in signal intensity between two discrete areas of an image.

Contrast agent Any drug or material that is introduced to change the contrast between two tissues. MR contrast agents shorten the T1 and/or T2 relaxation times of tissue, thus improving the contrast-to-noise ratio of abnormal tissue.

Coronal plane The imaging plane that bisects the body into front and back parts.

Coupled movement The association of one motion (i.e., translation or rotation about an axis of rotation) with another motion about a second axis of rotation.

Cross-sectional area The area of a material on a plane perpendicular to its longitudinal axis.

Diarthrodial joints The freely moving joints of the body. The ends of bony components are free to move in relation to one another because no cartilaginous tissue directly connects adjacent osseous surfaces.

Distraction The movement of two surfaces away from each other.

Dorsiflexion Movement of the foot towards the anterior surface of the tibia while bending the ankle.

Dynamics The study of forces acting on a body in motion.

Echo planar imaging (EPI) A specialized MRI imaging technique or pulse sequence that is capable of producing images at rapid rates.

Echo time (TE) The time between the center of the 90 degree pulse and the center of the spin-echo.

Extension A straightening of a limb in which the bones making up the joint move to a more nearly parallel position.

Fast spin echo (FSE) A multiple echo spin-echo sequence that records different regions of k-space with different echos. Typically, a long repetition time (TR) multispin-echo pulse sequence where each echo is separately phase encoded.

Field of view (FOV) The distance across an image, typically indicated in centimeters or millimeters; the size of the anatomical region that is imaged. The field of view in the frequency and phase encoding directions for an MR image may be different (the dimensions may be square or rectangular).

Flexion The bending of a joint (i.e., the distal segment rotates toward the proximal segment).

Frontal plane The plane passing longitudinally through the body from side to side.

Functional MRI MRI technique used to evaluate or monitor physiological, anatomical, or metabolic processes.

Functional spinal units (FSU) Two neighboring vertebrae and the interconnecting soft tissue, devoid of musculature.

Gadolinium A lanthanide metal that has seven unpaired electrons. This paramagnetic metal is often used in MR contrast agents.

Gradient echo A form of magnetic resonance signal produced by the refocusing of transverse magnetization caused by the application of a specific magnetic field gradient.

Gradient recalled echo sequence; gradient recalled echo in the steady state (GRASS) An MRI pulse sequence that produces signals called gradient echoes as a result of the application of a refocusing echo. This type of pulse sequence is typically used to improve temporal resolution.

Inferior The direction towards the feet in an anatomical coordinate system.

Instantaneous center of rotation The immovable point existing at an instant in time created by one segment (link) of a body rotating about an adjacent segment (i.e., the rotation of all points along a segment about an immovable point).

Inversion time (TI) The time between the inversion pulse and the sampling pulse(s) in an inversion recovery or STIR sequence.

Joint reaction force The internal reaction force acting at the contact surfaces when a joint in the body is subjected to external loads.

Kinematic MRI Any magnetic resonance imaging (MRI) technique used to assess joint function, including imaging the joint through a specific range of motion, during stress, or under loading condition.

Kinematics The branch of mechanics that deals with the motion of a body without reference to force or mass.

Kinesiology The study of normal human movement.

Longitudinal plane *See* Frontal plane.

Magnetic resonance A phenomenon that results in the absorption or emission of electromagnetic energy by nuclei or electrons in the presence of a magnetic field after excitation by a resonance frequency pulse.

Magnetic resonance imaging (MRI) The use of the magnetic resonance phenomenon to produce images of hydrogen or other protons.

Misregistration The incorrect spatial mapping of an acquired MR signal. This artifact may be secondary to motion, chemical shift, or wrap-around.

Number of excitations (NEX) The number of signal averages used during the acquisition of an MR image.

Oblique plane A plane of imaging not perpendicular to the xyz coordinate system.

Open-chain A descriptive term referring to when the foot is off the ground (i.e., the tibia is "free" during non-weight-bearing activity).

Osteokinematics The movement of bones rather than the movement of articular surfaces.

Pathokinematics Abnormal or pathological motion.

Pathokinesiology The study of pathological human movement.

Plantarflexion Movement of the foot away from the anterior surface of the tibia (i.e., straightening of the ankle joint).

Posterior The direction toward the back in an anatomical coordinate system.

Pulse sequence A series of radiofrequency (RF) pulses and magnetic field gradients, and time intervals between pulses applied to a spin system to produce a signal representative of some property of the spin system. For example, a T1-weighted pulse sequence is indicated with the designation of repetition time (msec)/echo time (msec) as TR/TE, 300/20.

Radiofrequency (RF) A frequency band in the electromagnetic spectrum with frequencies in the millions of cycles per second; frequencies of electromagnetic radiation often used in radio and television transmissions. For MRI, the RF used for imaging is dependent on the field strength of the MR system and typically ranges from 0.8 to 85 MHz.

Radiofrequency (RF) coil A device used for transmission or transmission and reception of magnetic resonance signals. RF coils are used to increase signal-to-noise and resolution.

Repetition time (TR) The time between the beginning of one pulse sequence and the beginning of the succeeding pulse sequence at a specified tissue location.

Sagittal plane A tomographic imaging plane bisecting the body into left and right parts.

Screw-home mechanism The combination of knee extension and external rotation of the tibia.

Section thickness; slice thickness The thickness of a slice of an MR image, usually indicated in millimeters.

Spin echo imaging In MR imaging, a spin echo is formed by the sequence of RF pulses and gradient reversals; an MRI sequence whose signal is an echo that results from the refocusing of magnetization after the application of 90 degree and 180 degree RF pulses.

Spoiled gradient echo; spoiled GRASS Heavily T1-weighted gradient echo MR imaging technique, typically used for kinematic MRI examinations that require good temporal resolution.

Static magnetic field The constant magnetic field of an MR system, usually indicated in Tesla.

Statics The study of forces acting on a body in equilibrium.

STIR (short tau inversion recovery, short inversion-time recovery, short T1 inversion recovery) Inversion recovery MR imaging technique in which the T1- and T2-dependent contrasts are additive. This imaging technique is typically used to suppress signal from short T1 tissues (e.g., fat), thus reducing ghost artifacts and improving conspicuity of tissue that has increased fluid content.

Stress Load per unit area that is produced on a plane surface within a structure in response to an externally applied load.

Subluxation Abnormal joint motion, typically the result of joint laxity or other disruptive condition.

Superior The direction towards the head in an anatomical coordinate system.

Surface coil A receive-only RF imaging coil that typically fits against the surface of the object being imaged. The use of receive-only RF coils facilitates imaging by improving signal-to-noise and resolution.

Synovial fluid The fluid in a synovial joint.

T1-weighted image An MR image obtained using a short repetition time and short echo time (short TR/TE) where the contrast is predominantly dependent on the T1 relaxation time of the tissue. Thus, this pulse sequence is commonly used to distinguish between tissues with differing T1 relation times.

T2-weighted image An MR image obtained using a long repetition time and long echo time (long TR/TE) where the contrast is predominantly dependent on the T2 relaxation time of the tissue.

T2* (T-two-star) The spin-spin relaxation time composed of contributions from molecular interactions and inhomogeneities in the magnetic field. Contrast in gradient echo MR imaging depends on the T2* value.

TE *See* Echo time (TE).

TR *See* Repetition time (TR).

Tesla (T) The SI unit of magnetic flux density. One Tesla equals 10,000 gauss (gauss is a cgs unit).

Torsion A loading mode whereby the load is applied to a structure in a manner that causes it to twist about an axis, subjecting it to a combination of tensile, shear, and compressive forces.

Transverse plane The imaging plane that bisects the body into top and bottom portions.

Index